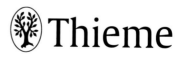

Chinese Medicine in Fertility Disorders

Edited by

Andreas A. Noll
Overseas Visiting Professor
(Chengdu University of TCM/China)
Practice for Chinese Medicine and Naturopathy
Munich, Germany

Sabine Wilms, PhD
Sinologist, Translator, and Lecturer
Ranchos de Taos
New Mexico, USA

With contributions by

Simon Becker, Young-Ju Becker, Stefan Englert,
Kerstin Friol, Walter Geiger, Christian Gnoth,
Dagmar Hemm, Annette Jonas, Andrea Kaffka,
Karin Kielwein, Barbara Kirschbaum, Gudrun Kotte,
Andreas A. Noll, Jacqueline Peineke, Karin Rudzki,
Ruthild Schulze, Hans-Joachim Stelting,
Fransiscus Sulistyo-Winarto, Beatrice Trebuth,
Sabine Wilms, Yuning Wu

Translated by Sabine Wilms, PhD

40 illustrations

Thieme
Stuttgart · New York

Library of Congress Cataloging-in-Publication Data
Chinesische Medizin bei Fertilitätsstörungen. English
   Chinese medicine in fertility disorders / edited
   by Andreas A. Noll, Sabine Wilms ;
with contributions by Simon Becker . . . [et al.] ;
translated by Sabine Wilms.
      p. ; cm.
   Includes bibliographical references and index.
   ISBN 978-3-13-148991-3 (alk. paper)
1. Infertility–Alternative treatment. 2. Medicine,
Chinese. I. Noll, Andreas. II. Wilms, Sabine. III. Title.
   [DNLM: 1. Infertility–therapy. 2. Medicine,
Chinese Traditional–methods. WP 570
C539c 2010a]
   RC889.C4513 2010
   616.6'92–dc22
                              2009035836

This book is an authorized and revised translation of
the German edition published and copyrighted 2008
by Hippokrates Verlag in MVS Medizinverlage, Stuttgart, Germany.
Title of the German edition: Chinesische Medizin bei
Fertilitätsstörungen: Erfolgreiche Behandlung bei unerfülltem Kinderwunsch.

Illustrator: Helmut Holtermann,
Dannenberg, Germany

Important note: Medicine is an ever-changing science undergoing continual development. Research and clinical experience are continually expanding our knowledge, in particular our knowledge of proper treatment and drug therapy. Insofar as this book mentions any dosage or application, readers may rest assured that the authors, editors, and publishers have made every effort to ensure that such references are in accordance with **the state of knowledge at the time of production of the book.**

Nevertheless, this does not involve, imply, or express any guarantee or responsibility on the part of the publishers in respect to any dosage instructions and forms of applications stated in the book. **Every user is requested to examine carefully** the manufacturers' leaflets accompanying each drug and to check, if necessary in consultation with a physician or specialist, whether the dosage schedules mentioned therein or the contraindications stated by the manufacturers differ from the statements made in the present book. Such examination is particularly important with drugs that are either rarely used or have been newly released on the market. Every dosage schedule or every form of application used is entirely at the user's own risk and responsibility. The authors and publishers request every user to report to the publishers any discrepancies or inaccuracies noticed. If errors in this work are found after publication, errata will be posted at www.thieme.com on the product description page.

© 2010 Georg Thieme Verlag,
Rüdigerstrasse 14, 70469 Stuttgart, Germany
http://www.thieme.de
Thieme New York, 333 Seventh Avenue,
New York, NY 10001, USA
http://www.thieme.com

Cover design: Thieme Publishing Group
Typesetting by Druckhaus Götz GmbH,
   Ludwigsburg, Germany
Printed in India by Replika Press PVT LTD

ISBN 978-3-13-148991-3   1 2 3 4 5 6

Contributors

Simon Becker, Dipl Ac and CH
(SBO-TCM, NCCAOM)
President
Swiss Professional Organization for TCM
Waedenswil, Switzerland

Young-Ju Becker, Dipl Ac and CH
(SBO-TCM, NCCAOM)
Private Practice for TCM
Waedenswil, Switzerland

Stefan Englert, MD
Professor
Private Practice
Ravensburg, Germany

Kerstin Friol, MD
Private Clinic
Grevenbroich, Germany

Walter Geiger, MSc (TCM/USA)
Private Practice
Hamburg, Germany

Christian Gnoth, MD
Private Clinic
Grevenbroich, Germany

Dagmar Hemm, PhD, Heilpraktiker /
TCM Practitioner
Private Practice
Munich, Germany

Annette Jonas, Heilpraktiker / TCM Practitioner
Private Practice
Hamburg, Germany

Andrea Kaffka, PhD (Hangzhou University, China)
Private Practice
Munich, Germany

Karin Kielwein, MD
University Clinic Bonn
Bonn, Germany

Barbara Kirschbaum, BAc, FRCHM UK
Private Practice
Hamburg, Germany

Gudrun Kotte, PhD
Sinologist
Berlin, Germany

Andreas A. Noll
Overseas Visiting Professor
(Chengdu University of TCM/China)
Practice for Chinese Medicine and Naturopathy
Munich, Germany

Jacqueline Peineke, Heilpraktiker /
TCM Practitioner
Private Practice
Berlin, Germany

Karin Rudzki, MD
Private Practice
Hamburg, Germany

Ruthild Schulze, Heilpraktiker / TCM Practitioner
Berlin, Germany

Hans-Joachim Stelting, Heilpraktiker /
TCM Practitioner
Private Practice
Hamburg, Germany

Fransiscus X. Sulistyo-Winarto, MD
Private Practice
Dormagen, Germany

Beatrice Trebuth, Heilpraktiker /
TCM Practitioner
Private Practice
Lübeck, Germany

Sabine Wilms, PhD
Sinologist, Translator and Lecturer
Ranchos de Taos
New Mexico, USA

Yuning Wu, MD
Beijing Hospital of TCM
Beijing, China

Foreword

I have great pleasure in writing the foreword for *Chinese Medicine in Fertility Disorders*; my congratulations to these authors on their valuable contribution to this field of Traditional Chinese Medicine (TCM).

In 2002 acupuncture research published in a Western medical fertility journal attracted attention from both medical professionals and the general public. This interest has continued with further research published in reputable journals raising awareness amongst medical personnel about the benefits of working with acupuncturists, and website information stimulating interest from couples undergoing fertility treatment.

This has raised challenges for practitioners working in this area of TCM. While research has raised the profile of acupuncture, the dilemma for many practitioners has been that of successfully integrating the true potential of TCM within a medical system that would prefer to focus on acupuncture point protocols as a method of treatment.

What this book does so well is to offer practitioners a pathway for integration. It does this in two very different but equally important ways: firstly, integration with the Western medicine treatment our patients seek out, assisting practitioners to understand and bridge this medical approach. Secondly, within TCM itself; exploring the richness of our past, the relevance of this literature to modern clinical practice, and an approach throughout that emphasizes the value of using TCM as a whole system—rather than focusing solely on the use of acupuncture. It is very exciting to see such a comprehensive range of work within one text, with scholars of historical texts and experienced practitioners within the field of fertility medicine working together to offer such a wide spectrum of therapeutic approaches.

A quick glance at the contents page illustrates the scope of practice that this book covers and the experience of the contributing authors, reflecting the diversity and potential of Traditional Chinese Medicine as it is being used in practice today.

Chinese Medicine in Fertility Disorders offers practitioners the information to work confidently within a Western medical environment—with extensive chapters covering the physiology and pathology of fertility and reproduction from both a Western and traditional Chinese medical perspective. It also explores the issues of fertility within a traditional social and cultural context, as well as discussing the present day ethical dilemmas faced by practitioners working in this challenging area of medicine.

The depth of knowledge, diversity, and rich experience of the authors shines through their chapters. By allowing each author to explore their subject in such depth this text is unique, with individual chapters that not only examine in detail acupuncture and herbal treatments but also *qi gong*, *tui na*, moxibustion, and Chinese dietetics.

It bodes well for the development of TCM as a profession to have chapters on historical texts, *shen*, and sexuality alongside chapters on treatment for menstrual disorders, the issues surrounding couples undergoing the procedures technology has to offer, including guidelines on assisting couples undergoing the latest assisted reproductive medicine procedures. This comprehensive approach continues through to chapters on treating stress and supporting couples in successful and failed fertility treatment.

As a profession it will be up to those practicing TCM to use the publicity generated from acupuncture research treatment protocols to promote the full potential of our medicine. To shift public perception and medical interest from assisting conception to assisting couples to achieve maximum reproductive health. To shift the focus from becoming pregnant to one that also promotes optimal health during a pregnancy. TCM has the additional benefit of helping couples to cope when their desire for children is not achieved. This timely text offers practitioners the knowledge, whatever their background and preferred mode of practice, to meet this challenge.

With this diverse and informative approach *Chinese Medicine in Fertility Disorders* stands out as a leading text in this field, providing value for both students and experienced practitioners. Having read this book, I have no hesitation in recommending it as an essential text for any practitioner working in the area of fertility and reproductive medicine.

Debra Betts
Wellington, New Zealand

Preface

Ding Tian Li Di (頂天立地—to achieve the extraordinary)

Touching heaven with the head while standing on earth

This Chinese figure of speech vividly illustrates the purpose of this book. The modern methods of reproductive medicine have found human—and therefore earthly—ways of solving a problem that had previously been entrusted to heaven: the passage of time, the *dao*, gods, and saints had the power to make the wish for a child come true. At all times and in all places, medicine was left with the task of preparing as fertile a ground as possible for the seed, which then finally fell out of the sky. And now it seems possible to intervene even here, in the area of new life, in the one aspect—with the exception of death—that had previously been impossible to influence.

The extremely creative field of reproductive medicine is developing new methods at breakneck speed, methods whose refinement appears to vouch irresistibly for their safety and justifiable hopes. Nevertheless, modern biomedicine is at risk of defining the reproductive process exclusively in its biological and technical dimension. Therapists and patients believe in these new possibilities and capabilities, cherish enormous hopes, and then experience corresponding bitter disappointment.

Traditional Chinese Medicine (TCM) holds within it the traditions of a medical system that has integrated different concepts of health and illness from the past 3000 years. It utilizes methods for cultivating health or life (*yang sheng* 養生), that is, for preserving health, and for treating the human body as a "holistic system" in a variety of ways, in order to restore harmony, not only within the individual but also between the individual and the external environment. Harmony, the unimpeded flow of *qi* through its conduits and its absorption and production in the internal organs (*zang* viscera and *fu* bowels) is hence also the most important prerequisite for creating new life —and thereby new *qi*. Different from Western medicine, Chinese medicine—which as a whole includes much more than just modern TCM—considers functioning relationships within and outside the individual to be an essential factor for life and health in and of itself. In contrast to Western medicine, though, and due at least partly to its traditional, vastly different way of looking at the body, on the other hand, it falls short in certain aspects of both diagnostics and therapy that are related to the concrete anatomical structures.

Both medical systems have their advantages— and for the benefit of potential future parents and their child, we should and can make use of both of them; at different stages and with different priorities, but in both cases with a common goal: to fulfill the wish for a child. This book is meant to assist the therapist in the evaluation of those priorities and in choosing the best tools from both medical systems for this purpose.

This book is concrete proof of the progress that has been made in the integration of Chinese medicine with biomedicine and of the powerful rewards that all therapists, whether they come from a traditional Chinese or biomedical background, can reap when they open their eyes and are willing to explore options outside their original field of expertise. The fact that this book is a collection of essays by a large variety of practitioners and scholars furthermore indicates the level of sophistication that the topic of fertility treatment has reached, making it too large an area to be covered exhaustively by any single individual.

In each chapter, we invite you to look at this fascinating topic from a different angle, shaped by the specific academic and clinical experiences of each contributor. The selection of topics covered in this book has been conscious and purposive. Chapters range from historical and anthropological research on the cultural dimensions of Chinese medical notions about fertility to cutting-edge biomedical knowledge and clinical research on TCM treatments as applied in Chinese clinics today. Not ignored either are the particular ethical concerns that modern fertility treatment in all its capabilities and shortcomings brings to the table in our modern society. It is our hope that the inclusiveness and breadth with which we have chosen to approach the complex topic of fertility treatment in the first part of the book will indeed allow therapists to "touch heaven," while the concrete clinical information and advice presented in the second half will enable them to remain "standing on earth," all for the benefit of the patient.

We would like to express our deep gratitude to the authors who have here shared their knowledge and often decades of experience in fertility treatment with the professional public. By doing so, we have succeeded in building a bridge between two medical systems—knowing full well that this is the only way to ensure the best patient care possible. In addition, we would like to thank Thieme Publishers, in particular the Editor Angelika Findgott and Editorial Assistant Anne Lamparter, for their unwavering commitment and encouragement in the production of this book. Sabine Wilms would like to thank her father, Dr. Klaus Wilms, for the inspiration to reach for the sky in the seemingly Herculean task of translating Chinese medical literature, and her daughter Momo for insisting on a healthy balance between work and play, thereby keeping her feet firmly planted in the ground. Andreas Noll is deeply grateful to his parents and his by now grown children and grandchildren for the wonderful experience that made the writing of this book possible in the first place. How important it is for life not only to have roots but also later become a root itself!

Andreas A. Noll
Sabine Wilms

Contents

15 Formula *Shao Fu Zhu Yu Tang*—Decoction for Treating Infertility . 162

5 Fertility Disorders and Treatment Concepts 177

16 Menstrual Disorders—*Yue Jing Bing* 178

17 Early Menopause 220

18 Infertility and Sexual Disorders

19 The Treatment of Male Infertility with TCM

20 Endometriosis—*Nei Ji*

occasionally uncomfortable (smoky and pungent!) but generally indispensable tool. **Annette Jonas**, in Chapters 9, 10, and 11, has compiled practical guidance on these subjects.

If you find new ideas on the application of otherwise rarely used acupuncture points in the contribution by **Andreas A. Noll** in Chapter 12, this will certainly be a great enrichment of your therapeutic arsenal. Dietetics also plays an important role in fertility treatment—nutritional and behavioral habits quite frequently exhaust reserves that are essential for reproduction. Ideas for the daily diet are found in Chapter 13 by **Beatrice Trebuth**.

A correct or adequate administration of Chinese medicinals, on the other hand, requires particular care—for the benefit of mother and child. **Dr. Karin Rudzki** and **Walter Geiger** have focused attention in Chapter 14 on the risks and dangers that are inherent in "standard" prescribing. Chapter 15 by **Simon Becker** and **Young-Ju Becker** on their experiences with a particular prescription in fertility treatment, *Shao Fu Zhu Yu Tang* (Lesser Abdomen Stasis-expelling Decoction), serves as the conclusion to this section.

He Qing He Li (合情合理)
Uniting emotions and reason

To treat the whole person as an individual instead of specific diseases—this is the basic concept of TCM that enthralls patients as well as therapists, and allows us to look for alternatives and/or supplements to Western biomedicine, especially in questions of fertility problems. It is nevertheless important to look more closely at individual diseases and corresponding treatment concepts. In particular, they require additional consideration of differential diagnosis—otherwise not always imperative in TCM—that are based on methods of Western medicine and are then translated into TCM patterns.

In Section 5, you can read discussions on fertility disorders commonly seen in clinic and their treatments. **Andrea A. Kaffka** discusses disorders of the menstrual cycle in Chapter 16 in detail,

since regulating the menstrual cycle is a central aspect of any fertility treatment. **Professor Stefan Englert** deals with premature menopause in Chapter 17, **Andreas A. Noll** with frequently concurring sexual disorders in Chapter 18, **Hans-Joachim Stelting** with that half of couples who tend to appear in clinic only secondarily—that is, men—and with the treatment of their infertility, in Chapter 19. Further disharmonies in women are dealt with by **Barbara Kirschbaum** (endometriosis, Chapter 20) and **Jacqueline Peineke** (polycystic ovaries, Chapter 21). **Professor Yuning Wu** concludes this section in Chapter 22 with extensive deliberations on and experiences in supporting IVF with TCM methods, especially medicinal therapy.

Xin Ping Qi He (心平氣和)
With a peaceful heart and harmonious *qi*

For most couples, fulfilling the wish for a child can be a very lengthy and wearing process and therefore requires us to pay special attention to any relevant circumstances that can arise during this time. The ups and downs of hope and bitter disappointment hence also confront treatment with questions like "Why?," "Why not in our case?," and "When?"—and sometimes, in spite of all efforts, when we realize their futility—also the question, "What happens afterwards?"

Any therapist in fertility practice will have experienced how seemingly "hopeless cases" all of a sudden become pregnant, and conversely how even the best preconditions (chemical and hormonal) are unable to achieve a pregnancy. In this context, **Ruthild Schulze** and **Gudrun Kotte** in Section 6, Chapter 23, pursue the question of the "heavenly spark"—*shen*. **Andreas A. Noll** in Chapter 24 introduces a stress treatment concept with a few pre-eminent acupuncture points that was developed on the basis of Confucian thought. And, together with **Gudrun Kotte** in Chapter 25, he has contemplated the time afterwards; on the basis of classical medical texts and practical experiences, their contribution deals with supporting couples in cases of success and failure.

Introduction

1

1 Fertility Treatment—Its Social and Cultural Context

Andreas A. Noll

This introductory chapter is intended to survey the meanings and problematic of the wish for a child in the context of its social and cultural environments. We have found that ethical-moral views colored by social as well as religious paradigms significantly affect reproductive and sexual behavior. Traditional Chinese Medicine (TCM) draws not only on the experiences of a complex treatment system transmitted over 2500 years, but also, a holistic view of the individual that is rooted in notions from our time and context.

TCM can be utilized in fertility consultations as an alternative as well as supplement to other medical methods. In this context, it benefits from the fact that the unusual reception of TCM in the West has integrated aspects of psychological diagnosis and care, in addition to the therapeutic application of acupuncture/moxibustion and Chinese medicinals, into a special treatment concept.

■ Reduced Fertility— Epidemiology—Causes

Involuntary childlessness refers to a state that is characterized by the condition of barrenness (also called infertility or sterility). In 1967, the Scientific Group on the Epidemiology of Infertility of the WHO recognized involuntary infertility (inability to fertilize or conceive) as a disease. According to the WHO definition, infertility/sterility is diagnosed when a couple is unable get pregnant against their explicit wishes after more than 24 months in spite of regular unprotected sexual intercourse (ICD-10 Diagnosis: Female sterility [N97.x], male sterility [N46]).

In Germany, 15% of all couples have problems with fertility.[16] In the United States, a 2002 survey by the National Center for Health Statistics of the Centers for Disease Control (CDC) and Prevention found that about 12% of women of reproductive

age (7.3 million) had difficulty getting pregnant or carrying a baby to term. It is becoming evident that fertility problems will increase further in the coming years because women, those with a higher level of education in particular, are delaying the question of having a child until the time that biomedicine tends to associate with approaching menopause. Meanwhile, in Germany, 40% of all women aged 35–39 and 43% of women aged 40–44 remain childless from choice. In the United States, the figure is 41.6% for all women of childbearing age. (**Table 1.1** shows the proportion of childless women among persons born in 1955 in various EU countries.)

From 1961–1999, the average age of primaparas (first pregnancies) in Germany rose from 24.9 to 28.9, and the figures are similar in many other developed countries. One reason for this development is the fact that people prioritize economic and societal success when planning their personal lives. The limit for this goal keeps getting pushed forward into the years between ages 30 and 40, as a result of which there is hardly any time left in this short span of 10–20 years for the attention that could be focused on producing a child. Another aspect, though, is the notion that the "wish child" is supposed to serve as much as possible the fulfillment of parents' needs for maximum social conformity and the completion of their own life plans, hence requiring it to arrive as "planned." Behind this idea we often find a mechanistic understanding of the extremely complex process that can ultimately lead to the creation of new life; an understanding that is further promoted and propagated by artificial techniques regardless of their minute success rates.

Success rates refer to the so-called "baby take-home" rate. In Germany, this amounts to an average 16% per embryo transfer. According to the German IVF Register 2002, this comprised 17.49% for IVF, 19.79% for ICSI, and 10.28% for the re-implantation of originally cryoconserved ovums in the pronuclear stage. Hence, we see a baby take-home rate of a good 15% per started cycle in IVF (in vitro fertilization) and ICSI (intracytoplasmic sperm injection).[5] In 2006, Canadian clinics achieved a live birth rate of 27% for IVF treatments.*

This illusion of realizability at will reduces the process of fulfilling the wish for a child to a clockwork mechanism that merely has to be set in motion at the crucial time. Nevertheless, many couples are greatly disappointed when they find that their wish for a child does not come true at the intended time.

After sometimes decades of birth control and the strains of work (stress, shift work, etc.) and the environment (toxins, nutrition, etc.), women's hormone production and menstrual cycle and men's sperm production are not like those of a 25-year-old (**Table 1.2**). It is assumed that the release of stress-related hormones (like prolactin or cortisol) can trigger endocrinologic or immunologic mechanisms (such as antibodies in the cervix), which in turn lead to reduced fertility. In addition, the role of social security as the foundation for long-term life planning has been limited considerably by unemployment as well as increasing demands for mobility and flexibility.

These developments have given rise to a variety of different assumptions: from a threatened "ex-

Table 1.1 Proportion of childless women (voluntary and involuntary) among persons born in 1955 in some countries of the EU

Country	Proportion
Germany (all states)	22%
Finland	18%
Netherlands	17%
United Kingdom	17%
Denmark	13%
Ireland	13%
Sweden	13%
Belgium	11%
Spain	11%
Italy	11%
France	8%
Portugal	7%

Source: Eurostat 2001; quoted after Engstler and Menning.[10]

Table 1.2 Indications for IVF/ICSI treatment (multiple indications)

Diagnosis in the Woman	Frequency	Diagnosis in the Man	Frequency
IVF			
Normal[a]	23.4%	Normal[a]	53.2%
Tubal pathology (fallopian tube damage)	40.2%	Reduced spermiogram (reduced sperm quality determined during an examination of sperms)	39.6%
Endometriosis	10%	Urogenital abnormalities (abnormalities of the urinary or reproductive organs)	0.3%
Pathological menstrual cycle (disrupted cycle)	15.6%	Pathological function tests (function tests with pathological changes)	0.3%
Cervical factor (changes in the cervical mucus or the width of the cervix)	0.7%		
Other	9.22%	Other	6.6%
ICSI			
Normal[a]	52.1%	Normal[a]	9.8%
Tubal pathology	13.6%	Reduced spermiogram	82.4%
Endometriosis	6.2%	Urogenital abnormalities	1.5%
Pathological menstrual cycle	16.2%	Pathological function tests	0.3%
Cervical factor	0.6%		
Other	9.7%	Other	

Note: [a]Negative findings.
Source: German IVF Register 2003[12]; data pertaining to the year 2002.

---

* Canadian Press, December 15, 2008.

tinction of the population" and the "social duty" of parenthood, to the insinuation that voluntary childlessness signals egocentrism and antisocial behavior. Parenthood, by contrast, is presumed to signify maturity and a sense of responsibility towards society at large. Involuntarily childless couples may therefore suffer stigmatization and often feel pushed into social isolation because of their problems.

Due to an attitude of high personal hopes, an age-related reduction in fertility, and social expectations, many couples develop an overwhelming desire to have a child, for the sake of which they are prepared to make many personal or financial sacrifices. "Most commonly, this group is composed of couples who are extremely successful in society, highly oriented towards social norms, and with a great need for functionality and self control."[6]

Reproduction and Sexuality

In the West—Christianity, Enlightenment, and the "Pill"

Sexuality is an innate power that gives humans the possibility to gain pleasure. This energy reaches its peak with the onset of sexual maturity. This does not mean, however, that it is not present before or after this time span. A child also gains pleasure, just as older people past their reproductive age can have a fulfilled sex life. In this respect, human sexuality is something that can first be lived out independently from reproduction. In our context, however, it is important that sex— irrespective of autoerotic activities—is per se directed at a partner and in this aspect acquires a social and cultural dimension.

In the recent past, the "sexual revolution" and the contraceptive pill in particular have separated sex from reproduction. "Free love" created the possibility of having sex without begetting a child, while modern biomedicine now promises a child without sex. We must apparently distinguish here between two terms—sexuality and reproduction—which in fact exist separately from each other but are nevertheless intimately interwoven.

The close connection between sexuality and reproduction was formed in our culture under the influence of Christianity. Hinduism likewise postulates "chastity in marriage," as a result of which sexuality was shifted into the realm of extramarital activities like prostitution, a process that was and is certainly also found in the Greco-Roman-Christian cultural complex as a result of sexual asceticism.

The Christian Church proceeded from a black-and-white image of woman as holy mother or evil temptress. However, this development only occurred with the increasing institutionalization of Christianity into a church, while women enjoyed a status of fundamental equality in the early stages of this religion. In this regard, early Christianity was influenced by stoicism, whose basic premises were the absence of passion, the primacy of reason, virtue, and a lifestyle in correspondence with nature. Philon of Alexandria, for example, a Greek Jewish theologian, postulated that sexual intercourse in marriage should only take place for the purpose of producing offspring, not for the sake of pleasure.

Similarly, according to Clement of Alexandria (2nd–3rd century CE), marital sex should only take place for the sake of reproduction, and man and woman should live like brother and sister the rest of the time. Particularly significant for Christian moral theology was Aurelius Augustinus who branded any type of pleasure as sinful and evil (4th–5th century CE). In early Greece of the 6th century CE, Pythagoras, as well as later Xenophon, Plato, Aristotle, and Hippocrates alike, shared the view that excessive sexual intercourse was harmful. Influenced by these Greek traditions, the apostle Paul finally relegated women to the above-mentioned roles. For centuries thereafter, the "evil" prostitute and sexual temptress on the one side, coexisted with the "holy" mother in the service of reproduction on the other.

The notion that the male seed (just like a seed of grain) already contained all life and that women therefore merely served as a fertile field survived into the 17th century. Thomas Aquinas (13th century) imagined the sexual act in paradise without any sensation of pleasure and considered matrimony as the will of God, as long as it serves the begetting of children. Martin Luther also saw sexual pleasure as resulting from the Fall of Man, but tolerated marriage also "for the sake of harlotry," as a medicine against unchastity. This purposive-rational attitude continues to survive in Calvinism and in radical Puritanism (in the United States).

In the course of enlightenment, which demanded in the 17th and 18th centuries, a "free man, absolved from a self-imposed immaturity" (Kant, 1724–1804), sexuality experienced a partial redefinition in the relationship between man and woman, in the sense that it stressed emotional, sensual relationships based on respect and mutuality. This development was continued by the Romanticists in the 18th century.

A very different view, however, was taken by Sigmund Freud (1856–1939). In his work and on the basis of psychoanalytic reasoning, he created new notions about sexuality that have deeply influenced our thinking even to this day. Influenced by mechanistic ideas, terms like "drive," "suppression," "the unconscious," and so on, are deeply anchored in our use of language. Freud "mechanized" and (pathologized) sexuality as a source of neuroses as well as of cultural developments. Many couples in fertility treatment appear to give more priority to these aspects than to a lively sexuality; and sexual intercourse itself as well as fertilization become increasingly mechanized in the course of the various attempts, and are performed with a purposive attitude.

In the East—Confucianism, Buddhism, Daoism, and Modern China

In China as well, issues of reproduction and sexuality have been determined significantly by the culture as a whole, which since the 5th century BCE, was shaped by the two great religious-philosophical currents, namely Confucianism and Daoism, and later, since the 1st century CE, by Buddhism.

Confucianism

Founded by Kongzi in the 5th century BCE, Confucianism is rooted in a worldview that defines the individual as part of society, and not only on a synchronic plane, that is, during the person's lifetime, but also in terms of obligations towards ancestors and descendants. All individual efforts should serve first and foremost the creation and preservation of a good and just society by a system of mutual, carefully graded rights and responsibilities. The personal fulfillment of wishes and claims of the individual was secondary to this, unlike in the West, where the individual was the governing force since Plato. All human efforts, hence also sexuality, had to be subordinated to this overarching benefit to society as a whole. Reproduction assumed a central role until the modern age, especially since neo-Confucianism developed around the 12th century in the Song dynasty. Concepts of sexuality, on the other hand, were primarily developed in Daoism.

Confucianism, which should in fact be considered a philosophical and social concept rather than a religion, moreover incorporated ancestor worship, practiced in China since thousands of years. This tradition is based on a system of mutual obligations within families, far beyond the present existence. The "begetting of sons" (see pp. 18 ff) was therefore an indispensable part of this system. With regard to reproduction, Confucian thought also influenced the other two great religions in China, Daoism and Buddhism.

Daoism

Daoism is designed much more loosely than Confucianism. We can distinguish between several developments since its creation by Laozi and Zhuangzi, most likely contemporaries of Kongzi:
- sociopolitical developments (Laozi)
- philosophical teachings (Zhuangzi)
- a religion with a particular world of deities (assimilated from popular religion, which also included the *fangshi* ["magicians"] widely popular until the Qing period)
- the ability to cultivate life (*yang sheng*)
- religious cult with sometimes sexual practices, and so on

In particular, with regard to the aspect of "cultivating life" (*yang sheng*), which included efforts to achieve longevity and immortality, numerous strategies were developed in the areas of sexuality and reproduction. More details on this topic and on Confucianism can be found in the contributions of Dagmar Hemm (pp. 18 ff).

Buddhism (Mahayana)

For Buddhism, all life is suffering. This suffering has four causes, of which the second cause is desire, or thirst, that is, for the so-called "lusts of the five senses," for existence, for becoming, and for non-existence. The goal of Buddhism is liberation from the eternal cycle of rebirth. This is achieved by practicing the "eight-fold path of right conduct":

- right insight
- right intent
- right speech
- right actions
- right livelihood
- right efforts
- right mindfulness
- right concentration

In this context, Confucian ideas about descendants and ancestors are just as irrelevant as Daoist ideas about longevity and immortality. Hence, Buddhist monks are not allowed to touch women or spend time with a woman in a secret or non-public place, let alone engage in sexual intercourse. In Buddhism, sexuality is not seen as reprehensible per se, but only as part of general badness that must be overcome because it stands in the way of enlightenment.

We also need to mention that Tantric Buddhism, a school of Buddhism, consciously cultivated sexuality in "red" or "left-handed" Tantra and engaged in sexual practices to unite the polarities. But not all forms of Tantrism include real sexual intercourse, such as Buddhist and Hindu Tantrism. During the time of Kublai Khan (1216–94 CE), this school exerted considerable influence, which, however, declined afterwards and partly continued to exist in turn in Daoist communities like the Quanzhen order.

Syncretism

Throughout Chinese history, the combination of these three great philosophical-religious currents in a great variety of ways led to alternating sexually liberal and repressive periods, as happened for different ideological reasons in European history as well.

Modernity

Since the 17th century, that is, with the end of the Confucian-influenced Ming dynasty and the beginning of the Manchu Qing dynasty, the influence of Western thought has grown, especially due to the activities of mostly Protestant missionaries. Nevertheless, their influence has remained marginal until today.

With the foundation of the socialist People's Republic of China in 1949, and most vividly during the Cultural Revolution since the middle of the 1960s, the large family with many children was propagated as a socialist ideal. The subsequent "one-child policy" successfully slowed down population growth, sometimes with abortive methods up until the last months of pregnancy that are quite severe from a Western perspective. The continued existence of the "wish for sons" (see pp. 18 ff), however, has promoted a selective practice of abortions on the one hand, and the intensive implementation of fertility-enhancing methods from Western and Traditional Chinese Medicine, on the other.

Integration: TCM

TCM as practiced here in the West is rooted in a complex medical system with 2500 years of transmitted experience. This system is linked inseparably to Chinese culture and history. The knowledge and ideas that stem from our own cultural background serve as an additional source. The process of familiarizing ourselves with ideas that are initially foreign to us, however, crystallizes the relativity of our own thinking. New horizons can open up when we surmise the dilemma of Western thinking—to mention just a few, the ethics debate over gene technology, abortion, or pre-implantation diagnosis—as a dead-end inherent in the system. Rooted in our time and environment, the initially vague discomfort that we experience towards mechanistic and particularizing ideas gives rise to a longing for a holistic conception of the human being. This desire originated in and becomes more concrete precisely in the acceptance of or at least confrontation with, even if only partial and quite selective, an often exoticized and glamorized paradise of the East; it can thus point to new perspectives. This synthesis of East and West, which might arise in a few branches, can offer new impulses here as there.

Reception—Opportunities

The comments at the beginning of this chapter clearly show that modern biomedicine and complementary medicine, here referring to TCM, can both contribute to our efforts at fertility treatment. Chinese medicine offers us the chance to build bridges between the deconstructed view of the human body in the West and the fragments of ancient Chinese medicine that will have to be at least partially reconstructed. The reason for this is that it was also influenced by Confucianism, Daoism, and Buddhism, even if not always in a way that we find desirable. In this context, the deconstructed view of the human body in the West concerns on the one hand the relationship between man and woman, in the private and public realm alike, which covers innumerable different areas. On the other hand, however, it also concerns desolate notions about the functioning of a body or its individual parts with neither connection to spirit or soul nor to other parts of the organism. In general, the goal of medicine should be to restore health and thereby the unimpeded life of the organism in all aspects, internally and externally. This goal should be our first maxim, especially in a process as sensitive and affected by multilayered aspects as the creation of new life, of a new autonomous being. Interventions into this extremely complicated set of rules may be necessary, but should always be undertaken with the following quote from Goethe's (1797) poem "The Sorcerer's Apprentice" in the back of the mind:

"I have need of Thee!
From the spirits that I called,
Sir, deliver me!
"Back now, broom,
into the closet!
Be though as though
wert before!
Until I, the real master
call thee forth to serve once more." *

---

* Translation copyright Brigitte Dubiel, http://german. about.com/library/blgzauberl.htm, accessed April 24, 2009.

Bibliography

1. Beier KM, Bosinski HAG, Loewit K. *Sexualmedizin.* 2nd ed. Munich: Urban & Fischer; 2005.
2. Brand M von. *Der Chinese in der Öffentlichkeit und der Familie, Wie er Sich Selbst Sieht und Schildert.* Berlin: Reimer; ca. 1910.
3. Deutsches Hygiene-Museum Dresden (editor). *Sex. Vom Wissen und Wünschen.* Ostfildern: Hatje Cantz; 2001.
4. Eberhard W. *Guilt and Sin in Traditional China.* Berkeley: University of California Press; 1967.
5. Felberbaum R. Fortpflanzungsmedizin: Methoden der Assistierten Reproduktion Werden Sicherer. *Deutsches Ärzteblatt.* 2004;101:A-95/B-83/C-82. http://www.aerzteblatt.de/v4/archiv/artikel.asp?id= 40 109 (accessed April 24, 2009).
6. Gebhard U, Hößle C, Johannsen F. *Eingriff in das Vorgeburtliche Menschliche Leben.* Neukirchen-Vlyun: Neukirchener Verlagsgesellschaft; 2005.
7. Goldin PR. *The Culture of Sex in Ancient China.* Hawaii: University of Hawaii Press; 2002.
8. Granet M. *Die Chinesische Zivilisation. Familie, Gesellschaft, Herrschaft. Von den Anfängen bis zur Kaiserzeit.* Frankfurt: Suhrkamp; 1985.
9. Kang C. *Man and Land in Chinese History. An Economic Analysis.* Stanford: Stanford University Press; 1986.
10. Leutner M. *Geburt, Heirat und Tod in Peking.* Berlin: Reimer; 1989.
11. Linck G. *Frau und Familie in China.* Munich: Beck; 1988.
12. Rieder A, Lohff B (editors). *Gender Medizin.* 2nd ed. Vienna: Springer; 2007.
13. Ruan F-F. *Sex in China.* New York: Plenum Press; 1991.
14. Schnitzer C (editor). *Mannes Lust & Weibes Macht.* Dresden: Sandstein; 2005.
15. Strauß B, Beyer K. Ungewollte Kinderlosigkeit. *Gesundheitsberichterstattung des Bundes.* 2004;20.
16. Thöne C, Rabe T. *Wir Wollen ein Kind! Unfruchtbarkeit: Ursachen und Behandlung.* Munich: dtv; 1996.
17. Wile D. *The Chinese Sexual Yoga Classics including Women's Solo Meditations Texts.* New York: State University of New York Press; 1992.

Fertility treatment is closely tied to ethical issues. These extend from therapeutic assistance in itself to IVF (e.g., regarding surplus embryos) and are discussed extensively by society with regard to pre-implantation diagnosis or cloning. Given the almost worldwide "tourism" of numerous help-seeking patients, the practitioner here is also confronted with diverse moral and legal views.

Reproductive medicine has opened up new possibilities in the last few years to bring about the fertilization of ovums with techniques in vivo and in vitro, that is, inside and outside the human body. Previously beyond the reach of intentional human intervention (coincidental), this event has become plannable and thereby been delivered to the responsibility of humans themselves. This responsibility implicates the question of ethical standards to regulate how we deal with "failed attempts" or "surplus."

The qualities of an embryo are now judged according to standards that are not left to science alone. They result from a societal consensus of right and wrong, good and bad.

◼ Human Dignity

Human dignity is closely tied to the exact point in time when a human being is created. This raises the following question: At which moment in the connection of sperm and ovum is it considered that a human life is created? Scientific, religious, and philosophical perspectives diverge greatly from each other in their ideas.

Circumstances of Conception—Criteria

The first question that arises in this context concerns the beginning of human life: from which

moment on are we no longer dealing with lifeless building blocks but with a living being?

"A living human being is endowed with a right to life and human dignity. However, we can only speak of a being's right to life if this being has been granted 'dignity.' Being granted dignity can mean nothing else, as far as the legal realm is concerned, than that the bearer of this dignity is, to use Kant's term, 'Selbstzweck' (an end in itself), or in other words, that any action implemented on him by other people must be justified to him. He has the status of a subject with rights, not of a tool for other people's purposes; and also not of a mere object of care, as is prescribed in laws for the protection of animals."[4]

Determining the beginning of human life thus means that from this point on, he or she can no longer be used for other purposes, that he or she is endowed with comprehensive liberties and rights, regardless of the possibilities to take advantage of them. Unborn life is therefore as much endowed with these rights as someone failing in physical and mental capabilities due to old age. As Thomas Jefferson writes in 1776 in his declaration of independence for the United States:

"All men are created equal ... and are endowed ... with certain unalienable Rights, that among these are Life, Liberty ... and the pursuit of Happiness." (Virginia Bill of Rights, United States 1776)

Criteria for the beginning of life are constructed by:
- the natural sciences
- religions
- philosophies

Scientific Criteria

These arise from the stages of conception, which can certainly serve as the basis for a graduated protection of life: accordingly, law and morality are universally binding even if they are not embedded in the context of a specific view of the world and of humanity. If we follow these secular standards, given the fact that we live in an ideologically pluralistic society, we have to accept the concept of a graduated protection of life for prepersonal human life.[1]

Germany's Embryo Protection Law determines in Article 1 Section 8 that the fertilized viable human ovum from the time of cell union as well as any totipotent cell that has been removed from an embryo must be considered an embryo. Article 4.1 in the American Convention on Human Rights from 1978 states, "Every person has the right to have his life respected. This right shall be protected by law and, in general, from the moment of conception" (**Table 2.1**).

Religious Ideas

These most commonly begin from the infusion of the soul, which happens at different stages in the formation of human life. The origin of the soul is seen in God, in the parents, but also in the seed of the father (**Table 2.2**).

Table 2.1 Developmental stages of the embryo

Point of Time	Event	Significance
Fertilization	Fusion of ovum and sperm cell	Individual potential is created
4th– 5th day	Nidation	Implantation in the uterus, fusion with the mother
13th– 14th day	Embryo can no longer divide	Hereafter, formation of twins is no longer possible Complete individuality
3 weeks	Heartbeat	Cardiac circulation as mechanistic criterion for life
15th– 42nd day	Nervous system	Precondition for psychological facilities
16th week	Movements of the child	Mother can feel the new life
20th week	Extra-uterine viability	Viability independent of the mother's body
Birth	Own digestion, breathing	Extra-uterine life

Table 2.2 Criteria for the beginning of life

Development of the Idea	Term/Source	Formation of Human Life
St. Thomas Aquinas	Creationism	Soul is lowered into the embryo by God: – in men on the 40th day – in women on the 80th day
Catholic Christianity	Simultaneous animation	Only one soul "forma unica" since conception
Protestant Christianity	Image of God	Embryo is an image of God and worthy of protection
Judaism	Halacha	Life only from implantation in the uterus onwards
	Jewish-orthodox philosophy	Divine breath on the 49th day
Islam	Koran, Central Council of Muslims	40 days drop of seed 40 days blood clot 40 days piece of flesh Breathing in the life spirit: either 40 or 120 days until the formation of human life
Buddhism	Ngawang	The process of becoming human begins with conception, from that point on worthy of protection

Different Concepts

Culture, religion, and philosophy therefore have different ideas about the point in time when life begins and must be protected:

- Absolute positions—**integrity from conception** onwards—advocated by the Christian churches and, for example, also by the philosopher R. Spaemann quoted above.
- Graduated ideas deduce the **right to protection from a specific developmental stage**. They differentiate between human dignity (not qualifiable) and right to life (limitations, e. g., in self-defense, are possible). Considerations are also informed, for example, by the individuation of the embryo, brain function (life and death), or birth.
- A **modified protection of the embryo** is advocated, for example by the philosopher J. Habermas, quoted below, who distinguishes between the "dignity of human life" and "human dignity." "Dignity" is shown and awarded like "reverence" and "respect," while "human dignity" is an inalienable right and exists in and of itself, independent of allocation.

■ Instrumentalization— Intervention in Fertility Treatment

The second question that can confront the practitioner is the basic consideration of the extent to which he or she should intervene in the creation of new life at all. Where are the limits of personal responsibility and ethics? Are there limits to therapeutic action?

We can see the relevance of this question in the case of pre-implantation diagnosis (PID)—prohibited in Germany and objected to by many social and religious conservatives in the rest of the world. This procedure means that fertilized egg cells can be selected by their genetic quality. Habermas outlines the potential consequences:

"Let us suppose that parents will some day be able to select genetic designs to pre-natally determine certain traits, dispositions, or abilities for their planned child.

The adolescent who later learns of such programming then might encounter genetically fixed intentions that he does not want to adopt as part of his own identity. The musically gifted person who would rather become a professional athlete can blame his parents for not having provided him with athletic skills."

And further on:

"Nobody can justify decisions that irrevocably affect the social fate of another person. Nobody can predict whether something will turn out to be a curse or blessing in the context of another person's life history— even if it concerns 'basic genetic assets' like memory or intelligence. In some contexts, a mild physical impairment may even yield an advantage for a child. The results cannot be calculated because the allocation of genetic resources affects realms in which another person will some day make use of her ethical liberty to shape her life in her own direction. In cases of conflict, a programmed person would no longer be able to see herself as the complete author of her own life."[1]

These questions regarding the possibilities of intervening in the quality of the future person arise in every IVF procedure. Even limiting the selection criteria to eugenics, which covers genetic disposition to diseases, is questionable at the least, if we consider the immense range of variability for defining "disease":

"To the extent that this development opens up promising chances to treat previously incurable diseases, it probably also offers the questionable options of an improved eugenics. Within the structure of liberal societies, such practices of changing genetic traits would through the market fall into the hands of parents' personal choices. Shopping in the genetic supermarket is a scenario of the future that relevant bioethical discussions in the United States have been addressing for a long time already. If we have any doubts about whether we really want this individualized variety of eugenics, we should pay attention to the contributions of today's practices to this development."[1]

But even if we leave aside for the moment the possibilities of IVF and the availability of surplus embryos resulting from this method, and the drive to research in biomedicine and genetic engineering, other options of medical intervention cause some fundamental problems: what does the naturalness, the God-given origin, the sacredness of life mean for us? Doesn't Chinese medical philosophy also understand the term *ming men*, which is based on a mandate from heaven that humans are supposed to fulfill? Or the *wu wei* of philosophical Daoism, which actually postulates non-intervention? These notions collide with the development of medicine, and the reader of this book can indeed ask about the extent to which they play a role in fertility treatment.

Finally, we should also give some thought to another group of arguments and considerations; reflecting on them illuminates the problem of therapeutic intervention beyond catchphrases. These are the arguments people advance against human interventions from the "principle of randomness in childbirth." There is, for example, "naturalness," "natural healing," "natural birth"—whatever is natural is seen as good. However nature leads the way is well-ordered and "right." This naturalistic ethics is rooted in the notion that the order of nature is the result of divine action and therefore provides the standard for moral judgments. Alteration of this God-given nature is therefore reprehensible and leads to misery.

Arguments that reject the actualization of the possibilities of therapeutic intervention are also often informed by notions of social Darwinism—humans are becoming older and older, which leads to overpopulation and cost explosion in health care. Humans therefore cause their own doom by intervening in "natural evolution." Nevertheless, "human nature," as the totality of our fundamental, original identity as beings belonging to the genus *Homo* is at the same time an important, if barely comprehensible orientation for our actions. We humans continue to see ourselves as the crown of creation. As such, our life is sacrosanct, whether in the Christian notion of the image of God or as a part of nature.

These reflections show that contemporary Western people have developed in flesh and blood, in the deepest layers of our culture-based identity an image of humanity and therefore also an image of life as sacred and worthy of protection that cannot make unconditional claims of general validity. Our Chinese, Korean, and Japanese colleagues view this problem with completely different eyes. When we consider the use of selective abortion, cloning, stem cell experiments, and positive and negative eugenics in the Far East, issues that cause profound moral apprehension about violating human dignity in our cultural context, it becomes obvious how deeply our ideas are rooted in our culture (see p. 8).

Love, Sex, and Reproduction

As described in detail in "Infertility and Sexual Disorders" (Chapter 18), the possibilities of biomedicine, as well as a general social tendency, are increasingly destroying the ideal of a unity of love, sex, and reproduction. As we explain there though, this unity never existed under cultural-religious premises. The Catholic theologian C. Breuer has elaborated on this topic:

"The physical act of procreation necessarily also includes a mental dimension. This mental act of love between man and woman and its expression in the 'language of the body' is tied to the conditions of the body because the body is the 'carrier' of mental acts. This separation of loving union and reproduction, which has taken place especially since the so-called 'sexual' revolution of the 1960s, has caused an instrumentalization of human sexuality (sex without having children). Under opposite auspices, this instrumentalization is now further intensified by the technology of reproductive medicine (having children without sex). Nevertheless, the oneness of loving union and reproduction is a fundamental condition of humanity because it not only facilitates the unity and integration of personal-mental life (in the act of love) and natural life (sexual act), but in addition prevents the creation of human life from becoming an act of 'making' and then 'disposing' of life, in which human life becomes primarily an object."[2]

On the one hand, secularization has caused issues like reproduction that appear to be explainable by technology to indeed be treated as technological problems. They have thereby been freed from the constraints of this complex, with their solution being simply a question of time. In its social-communicative function, sexuality is reduced to sperm production. And love? It appears to continue to remain in the metaphysical realm.

■ Developments

The secularization of morality, the previously mentioned need for personal initiative by the practitioner in areas where religious norms used to provide clear moral guidelines, requires new thinking:

"Up to now, the development of biotechnology has been unfolding a dynamic that continues to overrun the time-consuming processes by which society forms a self-understanding of its moral goals. The shorter the range of time that we are considering, the greater will later be the power of the facts that have then already been created."[1]

We cannot escape from this development, and whatever is doable will be done. Humanity has begun to construct and also to destruct itself. It will not lose the relevant knowledge.

In this book, we introduce the possibilities of Far Eastern medicine for the treatment of infertility—the possibilities of Chinese medicine. On the one hand, this refers to the regulation of the human energetic system. This includes efforts to incorporate physical, mental, and spiritual sensitivities and their changes, for the purpose of regulating the harmony and flow of the life force *qi* to such an extent that new life *qi* can be created. Nevertheless, these efforts are therapeutic interventions in a (natural?) state of non-function as well. The possibilities of Chinese medicine extend, however, also to a supplementary role in IVF, insemination, and other techniques of biomedicine. In the confrontation of Western-mechanistic ideas with Eastern-synthetic concepts that takes place in such cases, we can perhaps discover new paths.

Bibliography
1. Assheuer T, Jessen J. Auf Schiefer Ebene. Vor der Bundestagsdebatte: Ein Gespräch mit Jürgen Habermas über Gefahren der Gentechnik und Neue Menschenbilder. *Zeit.* 2002;5.
2. Breuer C. *Die Moraltheologische Problematik der In-vitro-Fertilisation.* www.kath-theologie.uni-osnabrueck.de/kug/download/breuer.pdf (accessed April 24, 2009).
3. Gebhard U, Hößle C, Johannsen F. *Eingriff in das Vorgeburtliche Menschliche Leben.* Neukirchen-Vlyun: Neukirchener Verlagsgesellschaft; 2005.
4. Spaemann R. Freiheit der Forschung oder Schutz des Embryos? *Zeit.* 2003;48.

3 Guanyin—Goddess of Fertility

Annette Jonas

Introduction

A book about fertility treatment in Chinese medicine would be incomplete if it did not mention Guanyin, the Goddess of Fertility. This would mean that something very important, a part of the whole, were missing. This is because reproduction is not just a technological-functional process, but the mental-spiritual realm also plays an important role. The authors of this book deal with this topic in their individual chapters—the following contribution on the possibilities of involving a Buddhist goddess will contribute substantially to a consideration of this realm.

Even in our own clinical practice, it is not that exceptional that we as practitioners wonder why a therapy—not only in the case of fertility treatment, but in many other disorders as well—fails to prove effective in spite of the best knowledge and polished therapeutic concepts, why the treatment goal is beyond reach and the patients are regarded as "therapy-resistant." In this context, reproduction is one of the most fundamental matters for human beings. The cradle of life already functioned in primeval times, and it is in this area in particular that medicine and technology are not the end of the story. Even if the whole world was created by a big bang, human reproduction always includes a certain "divine spark" in order to create new life. We regard every new human being as a true miracle.

Starting a Family in China

In Chinese culture, starting a family has always been a matter of great significance. People should be married by the age of 30. Beyond this age, they are regarded as unattractive and no longer desirable. It is difficult to accept for older, conservative Chinese when Western visitors past the age of 30 are not yet married. In China, the family still plays a very important role, one that we in the West have lost a long time ago.

During their first social contact, travelers in China always have to answer the standard question about how many children they have. Blank, almost pitying looks follow, if you answer by saying that you are unmarried and have no children. For Chinese people, it used to be almost beyond their imagination to be single. Yin and yang belong together, after all, and a person should not live alone. People should, however, not live in a homosexual relationship since man and woman belong together and you cannot have children otherwise.

After marriage, a Chinese couple should produce offspring after two years at the latest. If the woman has failed to conceive within this time, she is regarded as a so-called "stone woman" (shi nu). This notion is related to the uterus (zi gong). The uterus is closed, solid, and tight like a rock. The cause of infertility is almost always initially sought in the woman.

Many women then begin by enlisting biomedical help. If this approach is unsuccessful, though, and if acupuncture does not help either, they often turn to mostly Buddhist monasteries. If couples in China have not had success with any of the fertility therapies and have exhausted all technological, medicinal treatment strategies, they have one last option left: they can pray to the Goddess of Fertility, Guanyin.

Legend—Who is Guanyin and Where Does She Come From?

Guanyin is also the Goddess of Compassion, of good fortune, and she bestows the blessing of children. Historically, she is the Chinese embodiment of the Bodhisattva Avalokiteshvara who plays an important role in Tibetan Buddhism. There, however, he is venerated as a male Bodhisattva, while in China and Japan, this deity is female. A Bodhisattva is an enlightened being who has learned through meditation and self-absorption how to escape from the endless cycle of death and rebirth. The core of Bodhisattva philosophy (the "great vehicle" of Buddhism) is the ideal not to attain enlightenment for oneself alone but to help all other beings.

The figure of the Bodhisattva Avalokiteshvara stems from a famous Buddhist text, the *Lotus Sutra*. This is one of the key texts of Mahayana Buddhism. Several translations of this *Sutra* into Chinese exist, the earliest from the 3 rd and 4th centuries CE. In that work, the name of the Bodhisattva Avalokiteshvara (literally: "the lord who is observing the world") was translated from Sanskrit into the Chinese name Guanshiyin. After the *Lotus Sutra* was translated, the 25th chapter, devoted to the Bodhisattva of Compassion Avalokiteshvara (Guanyin), became an independent text. Jorinde Ebert[2] writes that the Chinese title of this chapter ("Guan Shi Yin Pu Men Pin") represents both the responsibilities and character of the Bodhisattva. The text states repeatedly that merely calling out the name of the Bodhisattva is enough to be saved: Guanyin will immediately pay attention (*guan*) to the voices (*yin*) in the whole universe (*shi*) and gates (*men*) will open everywhere (*pu*) for the wishes of believers.

There are many legends that tell stories of salvation by Guanyin. Old inscriptions show examples. By calling Guanyin, you can:
- make a thunderstorm disappear in time
- transform a fire pit into a lotus pond
- calm your thoughts and succeed in letting go
- be safe from all harm

- *om*—liberated from suffering in the realm of the gods
- *ma*—liberated from suffering in the realm of the demigods
- *ni*—liberated from suffering in the human realm
- *pad*—liberated from suffering in the animal realm
- *me*—liberated from suffering in the realm of the hungry ghosts
- *hum*—liberated from suffering in the hells

■ Guanyin—A Mother Goddess

When Buddhism, introduced to China in the 1st century CE, combined with Daoism, Avalokiteshvara was equated with a goddess native to China. Thereby, Guanyin was seen as the old mother goddess Nugua, who, together with her brother/husband, is celebrated as the cofounder of Chinese culture, especially of oracles and writing. When the Italian Jesuit fathers arrived in China in the 16th century, the Madonna statues they brought with them were seen as depictions of Guanyin. Subsequently, Chinese artists produced their statues in the image of the Madonnas (**Fig. 3.1**). In Western analytic psychology, Mary is regarded as the mother of God and protectress of humankind, as well as a particularly obvious expression of the mother archetype.

Graphic illustrations of Guanyin often depict her on the shore of the ocean meditating, or holding an infant in her arms. She sits enthroned on a mountain or an island in the Sea of Japan.

■ Goddess of Compassion

In Tibetan Buddhism, Avalokiteshvara is regarded as the embodiment of the compassion of all Buddhas in all ages. The current Dalai Lama is seen as an embodiment of Avalokiteshvara as well. *Om mani padme hum* ("Oh, you jewel in the lotus flower") is a very popular mantra. The jewel stands for all-encompassing compassion; hence, this is the mantra of compassion:

■ Song Zi Niang Niang—The Woman Who Can Bestow Children

While Guanyin is known as a Buddhist goddess, she is venerated also in Daoist monasteries. We can find a beautiful statue of Guanyin in the famous White Cloud Temple in Beijing. This temple is the central temple of Daoism in China. Guanyin

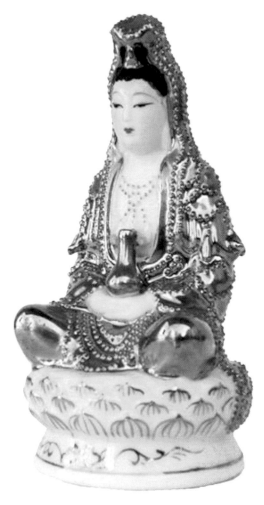

Fig. 3.1 Guanyin

on their inadequacy. But even many men pray here together with their wives. Additionally, people have the option of entering a monastery or taking a statue of Guanyin home to give it a place of honor on the home altar. They are, however, not allowed to buy it, because that would be commerce and hence not proper in this matter. As a rule, Guanyin is borrowed. It is almost as if you have to ask her to come home with you.

Many poor couples, however, do not have the option to acquire a Guanyin because ultimately a statue should be bought at some point. These couples instead go to the temple and pray to her there. A Guanyin statue should be made out of jade or special wood or porcelain. The most expensive version is doubtlessly the jade Guanyin.

■ Times of Prayer

There are specific times for prayers to Guanyin to promote fertility. *Ling,* "magical efficacy," is stronger at the first and 15th days of the Chinese month, during the full moon, and during the new moon. *Shen ling* and *xin ling* (spirit power and heart power) come together and strengthen body and sexuality. The result is *kai guang,* the "opening of light." The Daoists spray water and throw rice grains. These practices are supposed to awaken the spirits and Guanyin. In Buddhist as well as Daoist monasteries, the monk leading the ceremony then blesses the couples. Additionally, Daoist monasteries offer the option to write the birth date of the couple (the Chinese date) on a yellow piece of paper. A monk takes the paper from the couple and prays for them.

It is also possible to rent the entire monastery including the chanting monks for a day. Nevertheless, only wealthy couples can afford this exclusive and costly method. In that case, at least 10 monks pray to bless the couple with children. In Daoist monasteries, this process is repeated up to three times; in Buddhist ones only once. The success rate for couples is supposed to be around 40–50%.

There is another old ritual to promote fertility, called *chen* ("medicinal recipe"). The idea is originally derived from the art of war and relates to a strategic map of the site. In this ritual, the spirits are the enemies of the couple. To influence them,

is known here by a different name, which was given to her "on the street": Song Zi Niang Niang —"the woman who can bestow children."

In Southern China, the name Kuai Zi ("chopsticks") is also often used in Guanyin monasteries. This term incorporates a play on words: *kuai* also means "quickly" and *zi* means "child"—in combination therefore "quickly a child!" The chopsticks are then frequently used as a medium in prayer, and it is said that the soul is already present in them.

This is what worshippers pray for in front of this statue. The prayer is an expression of the plea. Of course, this practice is most commonly performed by women since infertility is blamed individual medicinals are assembled. The executing master in addition requires the following personal information from the couple:

* name
* date of birth
* parents
* siblings
* place of birth

Close attention is paid to the place of residence. Lastly, the location is chosen in which the medicinals, tied together with a red string, are to be buried, such as in the garden or nearby mountains.

Prayers to Guanyin are not limited to fertility. Many people also pray to her after giving birth to a handicapped child. Besides the health of the child, the wish for sons is another common motivation for worshipping Guanyin:

Qi gong master Li Jiacheng told me of a number of cases in which the prayer was said to have been effective. A male acquaintance of his is a realtor and has a lot of money. He paid 300 000 yuan (ca. 44 000 USD) for a prayer ceremony with monks. Subsequently, he had a son. In this case, the sum of money was a great sacrifice. But more important than anything was that the wish for a child came truly from the heart. But the monastery also accepts donations other than money, such as fruit.

It is mostly women who pray, because they are held responsible for 70% of all cases of infertility. But it is also important that the husbands support their wives mentally.

■ Willingness and Openness

In the context of infertility in the West, we often hear: "But a child also has to want to come to you!" Such a statement ascribes a soul to the fetus before it is even conceived. While difficult to accept for some critics, we can at least speak of some sort of potential spiritual energy. But where something is supposed to be received, the door must also be open. From the perspective of Chinese medical philosophy, people who want to conceive a child must be open in the area of the heart, because the heart (xin) is the seat of shen (spirit). If we can follow this line of thinking, we realize that people who are without children or a partner must do something for their heart. They must open their "heart chakra."

The best way to open yourself up is to be relaxed and loose, to feel free, be happy, and able to laugh a lot. The opposite of this is to sit sadly in a corner and take on all the pain of the world, to be very heavy or to doggedly and tensely "want to have" a child or a partner. A child as well as a partner will be more likely to come to a person who is open and radiates happiness than to somebody who has sunk deeply into his or her sadness and depression or lives under extreme tension. We can also express it in this way: the hormones must go haywire, the heart must rejoice, and there must be butterflies in the belly. This is the best precondition for falling in love, opening the heart wide, and becoming pregnant.

Pressure and excessive expectations are extremely detrimental to openness and lightness. Occasionally, a pregnancy occurs at the very moment when a fertility treatment that was associated with a lot of pressure and tension is relinquished. "Letting go" facilitates this openness, as does any distance from everyday life, a change in one's work, or living space, or a vacation with sunshine by the beach. It is better to say, "I can and would like to become pregnant" than "I want to be become pregnant." In this way, life becomes lighter.

A mother can also speak with her wish child: "Yes, I am here, I am open for you, I will take care of you. I invite you to come to me." That would be a very life-affirming attitude.

■ Transmitting Symbolism to the West

In our Western society, religiosity and the feeling of transcendence have been lost or pushed into the private sphere of the home. The widespread aversion to established Christianity and distraction by the tools of our affluent society have caused many people to turn away from traditional religiosity. In retrospect, something is missing, and many people

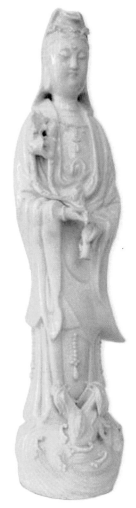

Fig. 3.2 Guanyin statue

are searching for new spiritual meaning. As a result, Buddhism has become quite popular in the West. For many people, identifying with this religion is easier.

Therefore, we can give a picture of Guanyin to female patients who are in treatment for fertility problems. Even if they are not practicing Buddhists, our patients are often quite open-minded, especially since we are most likely in TCM practice to encounter interest and open-mindedness for the different way in which this problem is approached in the homeland of this foreign treatment method.

Small home altars still exist in many Chinese homes. There, we frequently find a statue of Laozi placed right next to one of the Buddha. In practice, it is not that important which religion a person belongs to. It can be a Buddhist deity or a Daoist one, depending on where you are most likely to see your prayers answered. A Buddhist god could easily have been transformed into a Daoist one in the course of many centuries. After all is said and done, we are dealing with a divine presence that is revealing its power and radiance. In prayer, in the simple act of the plea, we are combining our own inherent power with this divine presence. Why shouldn't we in the West also be able to set up a small Guanyin statue (**Fig. 3.2**) and ask to receive a child? In popular religion, Guanyin worship is still alive and well. There were supposedly times when you could find a small porcelain statue of Guanyin in almost every household.

Bibliography

1. Blofeld J. *Das Geheime und Erhabene*. Munich: Goldmann; 1985.
2. Ebert J. Guanyin-Verehrung in China. In: Müller C, Croissant D (editors) *Wege der Götter und Menschen: Religionen im traditionellen China. Begleitbuch zur gleichnamigen Ausstellung*. Berlin: Museum für Völkerkunde; 1989.
3. Scharuk H. *Die Göttin*. Cologne: Taschen; 2001.

4   The Wish for Sons—Woman and Family in Imperial China—*Qiu Zi* (求子)

Dagmar Hemm

■ The Status of Women

Nu jian nan gui (女賤男貴)—"Women are worthless, men are valuable"—a typical statement that was not taken as an insult in ancient China but merely reflected the social position of women. While it is true, as we well know, that half of humanity is female in China, women were apparently quite replaceable in the economic, social, and political realms. This very contrast, between on the one hand being needed for the continuation of society but on the other being redundant in other areas, became a dilemma for women in general but especially so for Chinese women. The only way in which they were able to legitimize their position in the male world was as mothers. And hence, they fell back on the world accessible to them, the one that could not exist without them: the family.

At this point, we already need to correct an image commonly held by Western observers of the Chinese family: the typical ideal family of pre-modern China is often equated with a large family with many children, several generations combined under one roof. This Confucian ideal, however, only applied to the wealthy elite. The majority of the Chinese population lived in the circle of a core family, on average containing no more than five to six people per household. Confucian regulations regarding the order within the family, the distribution of responsibilities between the sexes, and the relationship between man and woman, were ideals as well, and could only be put into practice by the families of the upper class. An image exists of the oppressed Chinese woman—as we perhaps know it from the novels of American Nobel laureate Pearl S. Buck—married against her will, crippled by bound "lotus feet" and, if failing to produce male offspring, bullied by the evil mother-in-law. This image might have corresponded to reality in individual cases, but cannot be generalized for all Chinese women. If we compared the living conditions of a peasant woman in China and Europe during the Middle Ages, they would be quite similar, except for the fact that the pressure to bear male offspring was most likely greater in China.

This pressure has continued until the present day and has even increased as a result of a rigorously practiced "one-child policy." We read of mobile ultrasound machines, used to determine the sex of the unborn fetus and resulting in intentional abortions of female fetuses. In this context, the following questions arise:

- Why this almost obsessive wish for male offspring?
- Why persisting until the present day?
- Surely there must be other reasons beyond merely the greater labor strength of men?

Answers to these questions are rooted in Confucian ethics, which provided a set of rules for heaven and earth, for state and family, more than 2000 years ago. Much of this system has been forgotten today, some virtues are considered once again, and plenty has outlasted all changes.

Nevertheless, this chapter is by no means meant to become an emancipatory men-defaming pamphlet. Rather, we have attempted to outline the conditions of family life and underlying ideology in imperial China. A certain amount of simplification and generalization is hereby unavoidable—especially in a time span of over 2000 years that was everything but homogeneous. This, of course, contradicts the common impression in the West that Qin Shi Huangdi united and standardized the country in the 3rd century BCE, and that China remained a stable empire without great changes up to the year 1911.

The Family

Like the social shape of the family, the character and role of women are not given by nature either, but are a product of socially dominant ideas.

Women and family symbolize order and peace—as is beautifully illustrated, for example, by the character *an* (安) for "peaceful," "content," "safe": a woman under a roof (of a house) meant peace, even though the actual condition of women in imperial China was often characterized more by violence and oppression.

Many researchers now believe that the existence of a matriarchal society in ancient China is a fact that can no longer be doubted.[1] What is still disputed, though, if we accept the existence of a matriarchy, is the time when this matriarchy transformed into a patriarchy; speculations range from 4500–1000 BCE.[21] The terms "matriarchy" and "patriarchy," often defined as "mothers' rule" and "fathers' rule" or as "mother-right" and "father-right," can be problematic in their usage. Most importantly, they should never be used as a pair of direct opposites because "matriarchies are social organizations that are created, shaped, and supported in all their features by women," while patriarchy also includes a certain ruling structure, social hierarchy, authority of a minority, etc.[15] That is, people knew their mother but not their father because the relationship between sexual intercourse and reproduction was not realized for a long time. Evidence for this is provided by the oldest clan names, which include the character for woman, as does the character for "family name" *xing* (姓), a combination of "woman" and "to give birth." In ancient religion as well, female shamans *wu* (巫) played a key role, and mother worship was the earliest form of Chinese ancestor worship. Hence, female deities like the "Queen Mother of the West" Xi Wang Mu (西王母), the "Goddess of Compassion" Guanyin (觀音), or the "Goddess of the Sea" Ma Zu (媽祖) are still of primary importance in popular religion.

Transition to Patriarchy

With the evolution of patriarchy, women lost their pre-eminent position in society. A drastic and far-reaching step in this process was the abolishment of "matrifiliation" in favor of "patrifiliation," that is, the fact that children were no longer assigned socially and legally to the family of the mother but to that of the father. At the same time, women lost their economic and social supremacy, a change to which Confucianism contributed substantially

from the middle of the first millennium BCE. In this context, the concept of the two eternal cosmic powers *yin* (陰) and *yang* (陽) was fundamental in framing the relationship between man and woman. The pair of opposites *yin* and *yang* originally did not include any value judgment, it merely represented two opposites that always complemented each other. *Yin* as the negative element stands for:

- darkness
- the moon
- water
- earth
- receiving
- what is concealed
- femininity

Yang as the positive element stands for:
- brightness
- the sun
- mountains
- heaven/sky
- giving
- what is obvious
- masculinity

Significantly, the female element *yin* always preceded the male *yang*. This cosmic world order was transferred onto the state and society, as a result of which the spheres of activity for men and women were clearly separated: women in the dark, in the concealment and isolation of the house, on the inside, and men in brightness, in public, on the outside. Hereby, the role of women also came to be sanctioned by the cosmic world order.

Legitimization by the Philosophers

Eventually, a hierarchical order was established for the state and family that incorporated the Confucian system of superiority and inferiority in the "five relationships":
- ruler–subject
- father–son
- man–woman
- older brother–younger brother
- friend–friend

In this order, the relationship between friends can either be seen as equal or can subliminally imply an unequal one between older and younger friend.

Already in the 6th century BCE, Mencius formulated the rules of the "three obediences" (*san cong* 三從). These state that a woman must revere and obey her father and older brothers in her youth, her husband during marriage, and her sons when she is widowed. In practice, however, the mother–son relationship turned out to mean that mothers commonly spoiled and pampered their sons during childhood, as a result of which the son remained more attached to his mother than to his wife for the rest of his life. Mothers were thereby often able to exert great influence in politics and society through their sons.

In the Confucian classic *Liji* (禮記), the *Book of Rites*, which was probably composed around the 2nd century BCE, we find the following statement: "Women shall not participate in public affairs, their words shall not penetrate past the threshold, and their sphere of influence shall be limited to the home." In addition, simplicity and lack of education was regarded as a female virtue and ideal (*wu cai jiu shi de* 無才就是德).

As such, it was not only the society, but also the family in China that were subject to strict order: "Wishing to let virtue shine on earth, the ancient [rulers] first brought order to the state. Wishing to bring order to the state, they first regulated the family" (古之欲明明德於天下者，先治其國；欲治其國者，先齊其家). This famous quotation from the Confucian text *Daxue (大學 Great Learning)* illustrates how important order was already in the small things, that is, in one's own family, with nothing being worse than chaos (*luan* 亂). The head of the family made all decisions including the choice of spouses, for which financial and political considerations were primary and the partners were generally not consulted.

Rules for Women

Rules regarding the conduct of women towards men were numerous, but rules of behavior for men towards women were sparse. It was only towards his mother that a man had certain obligations, among them the care of his parents in their old age. In the 1st century CE, the social constraints for women became even stricter when the historian and author Ban Zhao (班昭) (45–116 CE) in her book *Nu Jie (女誡 Precepts for Women)* set down in writing the perfect female attributes. Furthermore, the rules of the "four virtues" (*si de* 四德) applied to women within the family, which required the following:

- Proper behavior: Act with moderation. Do not draw attention to yourself, and act in accordance with the transmitted rites.
- Proper speech: Do not talk too much, and if so, only when asked.
- Proper appearance: Look feminine, that is, make yourself look beautiful for your husband and serve him.
- Proper work: Willingly complete all housework.

In spite of all these rules of conduct, women enjoyed relative freedom up to the Tang period (618–907 CE). Poems and paintings have come down to us that depict women as self-confident, happy, and sensuous. The indispensability of women's work capacity was also obvious and women hence enjoyed a certain independence, especially in the countryside. Towards the end of the Tang dynasty, though, increasing urbanization reduced the value of women's labor, and women became more or less economically useless beings, at least in financially better-off families. Servants and maids were in charge of housework and childrearing, and the only functions of "higher" ladies were therefore to satisfy the husband's sexual desires and to bear children. It was also due to the influence of neo-Confucianism during the Song dynasty (960–1276 CE) and even more so during the Ming dynasty (1368–1644 CE) that the rather liberal Tang ideals were completely replaced. The new puritanism straightened out the alleged immoral habits of women and from then on restricted them exclusively to house and home. A multitude of psychological and moral taboos confined women to the "inside" that had been assigned to them. Thus, women were expected, for example, to take their own life after being raped, because death was considered the lesser evil in comparison with the loss of chastity.

Physically Tied by Bound Feet

Since the 10th century, women's small feet were regarded as the ideal of beauty. Dainty feet that obtained their unnatural size by tying, binding, and finally breaking the bones were seen as the culmination of female elegance. Unable to move about normally on their deformed feet, women were now tied to the home; unable to carry out productive work, such women became pure objects of prestige for wealthy families. Their bound and thereby crippled feet prevented women from stepping outside the bounds of the domestic horizon. The history of Chinese women's liberation is hence also the history of "foot-binding" and of the fight against it.

Nevertheless, the custom of foot-binding was not practiced in all parts of China. Thus, foot-binding was more widespread in the North than in the South, and in some provinces this bad habit never became common at all; additionally, the poorer classes of society who depended on women's labor were unable to follow this custom. It is interesting in this context, for example, that the Mongolian conquerors, whose women had not bound their feet previously, regarded Chinese culture in many areas as superior during the time of their rule in China (Yuan dynasty, 1279–1368 CE) and adapted to it—including the habit of foot-binding. Mongolian women hereby lost their freedom of movement.

The Manchu conquerors who united China for the last time into an empire during the Qing dynasty (1644–1911 CE) acted similarly. They also originally regarded the custom of foot-binding as foreign and absurd. Without much success, they attempted to prohibit the Han Chinese to bind their feet, with the result that the Han Chinese now held on to the practice precisely as a symbol of rejecting the foreign rule. At the same time, some Manchu women accepted this practice because they were able to thereby demonstrate the wealth of their family. Only a wealthy man, after all, could afford the luxury of having a wife who was disabled for work by her bound feet and could therefore only serve his erotic entertainment.

The Life of a Girl

The ideal upbringing of girls from the upper echelons of society (referring to the class of officials, merchants, and big landowners) took place in strict isolation in a particular sequence: at the age of 7, a girl was separated from her brothers

and male relatives. From now on, she lived in the inner chambers, surrounded only by her wet nurse, maid servants, and female relatives.

After the practice of foot-binding had been introduced, girls began at this age at the latest to have their feet bound. At the age of 10, they were instructed in the various female household tasks, among these in particular sewing, weaving, embroidery, and the supervision of the household. This training ended when they were married at the age of 14–17 years. Marriage occurred so early because on the one hand this allowed families to take full advantage of the whole span of female reproductive capacity, and on the other hand because younger women were not as contradictory but better able to adjust.

To give birth to a male descendant was the first and foremost obligation of a young wife after marriage because sons remained in the family, functioned as labor in the household, brought an additional worker into the house in the person of the daughter-in-law, and ultimately contributed to the preservation of the family. Only sons were able to continue the family line, and only they could perform the ancestral sacrifices after the death of the parents; it was only through them that the family lived on.

Continuation of the Family in the Afterlife

The ritual of ancestor worship is the most important aspect of religious practice in China and has been maintained as long as anyone can remember. According to Chinese beliefs, death was like sleep or unconsciousness, a state from which a person could wake up (even if not as a living human being but as a soul with certain needs). The dead were therefore given articles from everyday life in the grave, and the surviving relatives "provided for them" with food and drink on the home altar. The souls were supplied with *qi* and *jing*, so to speak, and could thereby outlast death.

In this context, we should also mention one of the oldest notions of the "soul" (*hun* 魂), which leaves its physical cover after death but continues to remain with it in the grave and leaves the grave only during the performance of sacrifices. During sacrificial rituals, the soul settles temporarily in a "representative," usually a grandchild of the deceased. This belief formed the basis for the ideal of an uninterrupted line of descendants that was not to be broken under any circumstances by the lack of a male descendant in the family to "bring sacrifices." Such a prospect evoked the horrible possibility that an ancestor who was not worshiped would wander about as a "hungry ghost" (*e gui* 餓鬼) and bring misfortune on the entire family. Without sufficient "nourishment," that is, *qi*, an ancestor was forced to lead a life of deprivation in the netherworld, to gradually fade into insignificance and die in agony. As such, he was unable to request assistance from the gods for his descendants and to ward off otherworldly curses and attacks.[19] Dutifully performing sacrifices and worship, on the other hand, brought great benefits for the family. The reason for this is that a person who had been powerful alive became a powerful ancestor after death, protector of his family and clan. As such, we can say that ancestor worship ultimately benefited the descendants because they received the protection and support of their deceased ancestors.

The Economic Aspect

More sons at the same time also meant better financial security for the family since the highest obligation of filial piety was to provide for one's parents in old age (*duo nan duo fu* 多男多富). Girls, on the other hand, were unable to fulfill these tasks because daughters left their family of origin with marriage (*chu jia* 出家) and became members of the husband's family. To marry their daughter, moreover, cost the parents a dowry as well as the girl's labor in the house and on the farm. Girls were therefore more expensive but less valuable in economic terms; they were moreover not entitled to any inheritance and generally did not possess any property other than their jewelry and clothing. Hence, they were neither able to sustain their own parents nor to assist them in old age, and could not continue the family tradition of ancestor worship in their own family either. The only exceptions were particularly attractive daughters because as imperial concubines or mistresses of rich men, they were able to gain prestige and special favors for their parents.

Originally, Chinese law of inheritance was designed to divide inheritances equally among all sons, without privileging the firstborn. In practice, though, this was not feasible because the increasing division of landed property would have made it impossible for any of the heirs to farm the land profitably. The land was therefore in practice passed on to the oldest, while the younger sons looked for work outside the family. The parents (or the widowed mother) stayed with one of the sons and his family. Ideally, this was the eldest son who thereby continued the ancestral line (but it was also often the youngest son because he was particularly close to his mother). For these reasons, it is not surprising that women could only raise their status in the family and in society by giving birth to many sons. A daughter-in-law who became pregnant shortly after marriage and then gave birth to a healthy son henceforth became a respected member of her new family and was accepted with kindness by her parents-in-law into the family unit.

Who Would Want Girls?

The birth of a daughter, on the other hand, was only greeted with joy when healthy sons already existed. In times of famines, girls were often the first to be sacrificed, abandoned, or sold as household slaves or into prostitution. In poorer families, it was not uncommon to kill newborn girls because the family could not afford another "useless mouth to feed." Especially when the firstborn was a girl and the family did not want to deter the mother from a second pregnancy and debilitate her by prolonged breastfeeding, they often got rid of the child.

For this reason, the position of the (still) childless daughter-in-law was very low; under the most unfavorable conditions she was treated worse than a maid. It was only as mother of a son that she was able to improve her status in the patriarchal family structure and become a full member of the family. To have no male descendants or to be childless altogether signified a tragedy for the husband's family, but for the woman herself it meant that her exclusion from the family and unprotected status continued. The daughter-in-law had failed to fulfill the expectations and elementary obligations of a wife. For the childless woman, this was the beginning of an endless time of humiliation. When we take this centuries-old social pressure into consideration, the modern Chinese practice of aborting female fetuses in the context of the "one-child policy" becomes easier to understand. Until now, no social reforms—especially in rural areas—have been able to lessen this unconditional desire for male descendants effectively.

Men's Special Privileges

Wealthy men had the option in such cases to take one or more mistresses to ensure the continuation of the family and increase their chances for a son. In addition, families had the option to adopt a son (*guo ji* 過繼, literally "continuing the past"). If parents who lacked a son of their own did not want to do without ancestor rituals, they had to adopt a youth or adult (usually coming from relatives) in their child's place. According to traditional law, there was no difference between adopted and natural sons, especially with regard to inheritance law. By the same token, the adopted son assumed responsibility for the same drawn-out and lavish mourning rituals as a natural son.

The man possessed an additional freedom: the right to divorce, or in other words, he could expel his wife if she was found guilty of any of the "seven reasons for dismissal" (*qi chu* 七除):

- inability to give birth to a child (or better "inability to give birth to a son")
- loose lifestyle
- lacking efforts in serving the parents-in-law
- talkativeness
- stealing
- jealousy
- incurable diseases

There were only three exceptions (*san bu chu* 三不除), under which the wife could not be expelled from the husband's family:

- if the wife had observed the prescribed mourning period of 3 years for the parents-in-law
- if the husband's family had become rich in the meantime
- and if the wife did not have any relatives to return to

No Escape for the Woman

For the woman, there was no possibility, even under the most obvious circumstances possible, to leave an unhappy marriage; suicide was therefore often the last and only resort of a desperate wife. In addition, chastity was promoted as a key ideal virtue for women. Included in this was virginity before marriage, unconditional fidelity during marriage, and lastly a life as a virtuous widow after the husband's death. Even if the husband died early or even already during the engagement period—and this could begin in infancy or childhood—remarriage was frowned upon for women.

All these proscriptions and restrictions were, of course, only feasible in the narrow circle of official and other wealthy families, but nevertheless served as model for all classes. Still, the more the woman had to help her husband in making a living outside the home, the less she was able to approximate the female ideal. The wife was often in charge of small business enterprises or within the family, but the husband's authority had to be maintained towards the outside. Still, a woman was not able to gain public prestige by her own efforts, but only by means of an honorary title that she received in accordance with the husband's or son's rank. The only exception were honorary stone arches that were erected in particular for chaste widows, that is, when they did not remarry or chose suicide after the death of a husband or even of a fiancé at a young age. This recognition was connected with tax relief for her family and in theory applied to all levels of the population.

■ Causes of Childlessness

People in China looked for the causes of childlessness in the magico-religious, the medical, and the personal realms. The only thing people could change was their behavior and, if they were lucky and had a good doctor, their physical inadequacies. The influence of the gods, on the other hand, was not calculable.

The early religions but also today's popular religions start out from the fact that there are beings who are fundamentally more powerful than humans. In addition to deities, spirits, and demons, these are the manifestations of powers that are active in nature (lightning, thunder, earthquakes, floods). They also influence people's lives directly (children, wealth, illness, etc.).[20] It is practically impossible to give a generally valid definition of "religion." The Danish ethnologist Birket-Smith, for example, coined as a working definition for religion the "belief in a dependency on higher powers." It is this dependency in particular, which he derived from the Latin *religio* whose root appears to mean "binding," that is of great significance for the context of Chinese religion.[2] This state of being bound, or in other words dependency, does not always have to be interpreted only as a one-sided subjugation of humans to higher powers, but can also mean the possibility that humans influence these higher powers.

The foundations of religion in China, such as ancestor worship, oracle and divination, and conceptions of deities and sacrifices to them, can already be found in the state religion of the Shang dynasty (2nd millennium BCE). It would however, be wrong to speak of *one* religion in China; Confucianism, Daoism, and Buddhism all coexist, so to speak, on equal terms. The individual does not have to profess one direction exclusively either, a pragmatic approach that we can see, for example, in the attitude towards death:

"The Confucian ancestral cult requires that the deceased are included in the life of the living descendants; you are responsible for your actions to your ancestors and can expect protection and blessings from them in return. A key goal of Daoist practices is the lengthening of life, in the ideal case immortality. And for the actual death, it is comforting to know that Buddhism promises rebirth and a future paradise."[20]

Suiting the need of any given situation in their life, people could appropriate the opportune teaching and sacrifice to the particular gods. In this way, nobody took offense when a childless Confucian scholar family of the elite prayed at the home altar for children to Guanyin, strictly speaking a Buddhist goddess, and when the husband attempted to increase his *jing* with Daoist sexual practices. If all these efforts proved in vain though, people sought the cause of fertility among the following:

- The influence of malevolent spirits and demons who wanted to take revenge on the wife or family. Especially frightening were one's own deceased ancestors as "demons" (*gui* 鬼). People feared that their own originally benevolent ancestors, the "good spirits" (*shen* 神) would transform into vengeful ones if, for example, the grave site was unfavorable or if the funeral or the periodic sacrifices and care were insufficient. The revenge of the deceased could express itself as illness, impoverishment, or even childlessness.
- Unfavorable astrological constellations—childlessness as fate, so to speak. In this context we should add that the stars were believed to have great power to influence fate in imperial China. Not only the rise and fall of dynasties, but also the fate of the individual were controlled by the stars. Marital unions were considered with care: did the partners match and was the wedding day "auspicious"? Compromises in these areas could quite easily have negative effects on the descendants.
- Punishment by heaven because the rules of the cosmic order had been violated. People attempted to win the gods over with sacrifices and "pilgrimages."
- Individual fault of the wife, either due to a morally corrupt lifestyle in the present or as delayed guilt from events like abortions or miscarriages in previous lives.
- Physical inadequacy (most commonly the wife's) that should be addressed with fertility medicinals.

Occasionally, the attribution of blame even went as far as regarding the birth of healthy sons as a reward for the mother's virtuous behavior (in the Confucian, but also in the Buddhist sense of the doctrine of *karma*). And parallel to this, childlessness, the birth of girls only or of deformed children, or the premature death of children were then seen as proof of the mother's lack of virtue and as her punishment. Prayers and sacrifices to Guanyin, the Goddess of Compassion, were supposed to function as remedies. Even today, clay figures of children, children's shoes made of red silk, or red eggs are still given to Guanyin as expressions of gratitude for a successful pregnancy. Women who wish for a child then take these symbols of fertility, to make use of this positive blessing.[17]

Conception and Sexuality

In light of this social background, we can understand why physicians and midwives were greatly concerned with conception, pregnancy, and childbirth. The medical literature on this subject area is old and extensive. Especially in the context of conception, we find not only advice on how to become pregnant but also how to best produce a son. For this purpose, the exact timing of sexual intercourse was decisive:

"Only the relation between husband and wife is appropriate. Under no circumstances can it be compared to illegitimate love. Even though we speak of 'heavenly union,' the reason for sexual intercourse is the continuation of the family line, not pleasure. The couple should control their sexual passion. Only when sexual passion is restrained will it be 'auspicious.' Without restraint, sex is pure debauchery. In such cases, the 'taboo days' are violated and the gods and spirits become angry. The following 'taboo days' (days on which no intercourse should take place) must be observed:

- *the 3 'yuan days' (the 15th each of the 1st, 7th, and 10th month)*
- *the 5 'wu la days'*
- *the birthdays of gods and saints*
- *the day of the mother's labor (presumably their own birthday), and*
- *the days of the parents' birth and death*

In addition, there are:
- *the four divisions (1 day each before the summer and winter solstices, as well as the equinoxes)*
- *the four interruptions (1 day each before the beginning of the seasons)*
- *the crossing of heaven and earth (most likely the 15th day of the fifth month)*
- *the 9 poisoned days (certain days in the fifth month)*
- *the days of forgiveness*
- *as well as the first and 15th of each month*

Of course you should also observe:
- *the birthdays of the ancestors*
- *the 'geng shen' and 'jia zi' days (the first and 57th day of the 60-day cycle)*
- *and all 'ping' and 'ding' days of the four seasons and eight periods of the year*

In addition:
- *days of great cold or heat*
- *of strong winds or rainfall*
- *during earthquakes*
- *thunder and lightning*
- *during solar and lunar eclipses*
- *and intercourse exposed to the light of the sun, moon, or planets*

Furthermore, intercourse should not take place in the vicinity of:
- *wells*
- *fireplaces and hearths*
- *coffins*
- *tombs*

Likewise not when intoxicated or after eating too much or when the person was:
- *enraged*
- *depressed or*
- *frightened*

Nor when returning from traveling or exhausted, when one hasn't bathed yet after a trip, or soon after an illness. All these proscriptions are intended to preserve the body, and the first proscription for a filial son is to keep his body intact. Whoever fails to observe these taboos, shortens the length of his life."[4]

In the course of time, the prohibitions grew more and more numerous and became so confusing to the lay person that you could buy lists on the street for learning the "permitted" days. If a couple observed all these prohibitions related to time, location, and climate, there were maybe 100 days left in the year for sexual activity. Since this reduces the number of fertile days enormously, it is really a miracle that China did not suffer from permanent underpopulation. It is precisely the disappearance of these limitations in the 20th century with the rejection of tradition and superstition, and, of course, medical progress that has made the enormous increase in births possible.

When the woman at last became pregnant, a new, often frightening period of time began. The woman was responsible for her smooth pregnancy and the optimal growth of the embryo. The great number of proscriptions and rules for virtuous behavior during this time illustrates the great responsibility placed on the pregnant woman. Again, it was the woman who was held responsible for a potential miscarriage as well as for a deformed or sickly child. In addition to all these obligations, pregnant women, who were considered impure, had to observe many prohibitions, such as participating in weddings, funerals, sacrifices, or temple visits. Pregnant women supposedly had a certain power with which they could "suck" the life force of other people and places dry, so to speak, in order to use it for the benefit of their growing child.[17]

■ Couldn't It Have Been Different?

Today, people often ask why Chinese women did not rebel against these constraints and rules but seem to have submitted willingly to male authority. Were these constraints really that great or were women simply too lethargic? Thus, people have discussed, for example, why women did not react with a "refusal to give birth." Tradition shows that women in matriarchal societies knew means and methods for contraception and abortion. Nevertheless, it is likely that childless women were outcast from society, which was equivalent to a death sentence because it was almost impossible to survive without the protection of society. Bearing children was hence presumably the lesser of two evils.

People have often criticized the passivity of women, or even sometimes implied that women should be blamed for their own situation. Nevertheless, as we have already mentioned repeatedly, these prescriptions, misogynistic from our modern perspective, were only put into practice by a very small part of the population. The majority of women was integrated into the processes of agricultural production and therefore certainly no less content with their fate than women anywhere else in the world.

There were also some Chinese women from the educated elite who resisted their lot; nevertheless, they remained exceptions and were not always judged positively by Chinese historians. The concubine Wu (624–705 CE) may serve as an example: after getting rid of the emperor, she proclaimed herself empress in the year 655 CE and ruled long past the death of the prince (683 CE) until shortly before her death. As such, she was the first and only empress in Chinese history. In the two decades of her reign, she consolidated the empire, for example by instituting an entrance examination system for prospective officials (destroying the influence of the ruling families and surviving as an essential part of imperial power until 1905), and led the empire into a time of cultural flourishing. In spite of these achievements, Empress Wu Zetian is today mostly mentioned negatively in the context of her extravagance and bigoted favoritism of the Buddhist religion. It is doubtful that a male ruler would have received this much criticism.

Additional examples are the Empress Dowager Cixi who ruled China from behind the scenes during the entire second half of the 19th century, or Mao Zedong's wife, Jiang Qing, who played an infamous key role in the Cultural Revolution.

In Chinese historiography and literature, women appeared, if at all, always as stereotypes. As positive model of the filial daughter (*xiao nu* 孝女) and as "virtuous mother and good wife" (*xian mu liang qi* 賢母良妻), or as a deterrent example, such as the ruinous lover (e.g., Yang Guifei) or the female ruler (such as the above-mentioned Empress Wu Zetian or the Empress Dowager Cixi). The fact that it was extremely rare for women to gain fame as scholars or poets (Ban Zhao and Li Qingzhao are the most famous) supposedly proved women's inadequacy in the fields of literature and science. In addition, we find the model of the female warrior (e.g., Mulan), situated between history and myth. The most frequently encountered female image in literature, though, is that of the evil mother-in-law, the oppressed daughter-in-law, the tyrannical wife on the one hand, and the fox fairy transforming into a lover or a female spirit in fairytales and legends. In this way, the acknowledgment of women and their achievements was constantly neglected in the male-dominated world of Chinese officials. It was only as the mother of many sons or by means of her exceptional virtue and chastity that a woman could achieve honor and recognition; literary or intellectual achievements, on the other hand, were neither expected nor recognized.

Bibliography

1. Bauer W. *China und die Hoffnung auf Glück*. Munich: Hanser; 1971.
2. Birket-Smith K. *Geschichte der Kultur. Eine Allgemeine Ethnologie*. Zurich: Orell Füssli; 1948.
3. Chiu Vermier Y. *Marriage Laws and Customs of China*. Hong Kong: The Chinese University Press of Hong Kong; 1966.
4. Eberhard W. *Guilt and Sin in Traditional China*. Berkeley: University of California Press; 1967.
5. Ebrey Buckley P (editor). *Chinese Civilization and Society. A Source Book*. New York: Free Press; 1981.
6. Elisseeff D. *La Femme au Temps des Empereurs de Chine*. Paris: Stock; 1988.
7. Freedman M. *Lineage Organization in Southeastern China*. London: Athlone; 1958.
8. Fricker U. *Schein und Wirklichkeit. Zur Altchinesischen Frauenideologie aus Männlicher und Weiblicher Sicht im Geschichtlichen Wandel*. Hamburg: MOAG; 1988.
9. Furth C. *A Flourishing Yin. Gender in China's Medical History 960 – 1665*. Berkeley: University of California Press; 1999.
10. Gernet J. *Die Chinesische Welt*. Frankfurt: Insel; 1979.
11. Granet M. *Die Chinesische Zivilisation. Familie, Gesellschaft, Herrschaft. Von den Anfängen bis zur Kaiserzeit*. Frankfurt: Suhrkamp; 1985.
12. Gulik RH van. *Sexual Life in Ancient China. A Preliminary Survey of Chinese Sex and Society from ca. 1500 BC till 1644 AD*. Leiden: Brill; 1974.
13. Hemm D. *Wege und Irrwege der Frauenbefreiung in China*. Munich: Edition Global; 1996.
14. Kristeva J. *Die Chinesin. Die Rolle der Frau in China*. Frankfurt: Ullstein; 1982.
15. Kuhn A (editor). *Die Chronik der Frauen*. Dortmund: Chronik; 1992.
16. Leutner M. *Geburt, Heirat und Tod in Peking*. Berlin: Reimer; 1989.
17. Linck G. *Frau und Familie in China*. Munich: Beck; 1988.
18. Meyer C. *Histoire de la Femme Chinoise, 4000 Ans de Pouvoir*. Paris: Lattès; 1986.
19. Milanowski T. *Die Magischen Körper-Geistübungen Chinas und deren Verbindung zum Schamanismus*. Uelzen: ML Verlag 2005.
20. Müller C (editor). *Wege der Götter und Menschen. Religionen im Traditionellen China*. Berlin: SMPK; 1989.
21. Schon J. *Frauen in China. Eine Studie über die Stellung der Chinesischen Frau vor 1949*. Bochum: Brockmeyer; 1982.
22. Schottenhammer A (editor). *Auf den Spuren des Jenseits. Chinesische Grabkultur in den Facetten von Wirklichkeit, Geschichte und Totenkult*. Frankfurt: Lang; 2003.
23. Skinner W. *The Study of Chinese Society. Essays by Maurice Freedman*. Stanford: Stanford University Press; 1979.
24. Sommer MH. *Sex, Law and Society in Late Imperial China*. Stanford: Stanford University Press; 2000.
25. Wandel E. *Frauenleben im Reich der Mitte. Chinesische Frauen in Geschichte und Gegenwart*. Reinbek: Rowohlt; 1987.
26. Watson RS, Ebrey Buckley P (editors). *Marriage and Inequality in Chinese Society*. Berkeley: University of California Press; 1991.

5 Advice on Successful Sexual Intercourse from the Medical Classics

Dagmar Hemm

"Non-action" (*wu wei* 無為), or in other words, non-purposive action, is a popular philosophy of life in China; allowing things to flow and develop on their own as the highest premise of life. Targeted intervention would certainly contradict this maxim, as would sexual intercourse by the numbers and targeted seminal emission. Nevertheless, we will see that Chinese people acted extremely "intentionally" particularly with regard to (male) offspring. A contradiction? On this subject, here is a quotation from François Jullien that describes how Mencius qualified these behavioral guidelines in the 6th century BCE:

"One evening, a farmer from Song returned home exhausted and said to his children: 'Today I did good work, I pulled up all the seedlings in my field.' When the children ran out to the field to look at the result, they of course discovered a devastated field in which all seedlings were drying out. Mencius draws the following conclusion from this story: There are two types of mistakes in the world. One is to want to achieve the effect (zheng) immediately, as if effectiveness were only a question of purpose and will—a question of the project, the means, and the effort; the other error is to do nothing and to neglect one's field. But if we may neither directly pull on the seedlings nor give up intervening altogether, what are we supposed to do, according to Mencius? Every farmer knows the answer: We have to hoe and weed around the base of the plant. This might appear insignificant, but here we touch on one of the most subtle traits of Chinese thought: How to combine the artificial and the natural in such a way that they fit; or how to assist in something that is happening anyway on its own."[2]

The medical classics demonstrate in abundance how we can assist in the conception of children and making this ground fertile.

■ How Often is the Man Allowed? Containing the Damage in Spite of "*Jing* Loss"

In the *Secrets of the Jade Chamber (Yu Fang Mi Jue* 玉房秘訣*)* we can read the following conversation:

"Huangdi asks Sunu: 'It is the will of the Dao to avoid losing jing (shi jing 失精) but to treat one's bodily fluids (ye 液) with care. Nevertheless, if you desire to have descendants, how can you not have seminal emission (xie 瀉)?' Sunu answers: 'There are strong and weak, young and old men, depending on each person's life force. Under no circumstances should seminal emission be forced or rash; this would only cause damage.'"[5] *

The *Yu Fang Mi Jue* is one of the first collections on this topic. In addition to other quotations, this text contains the well-known *Su Nu Jing (*素女經 *Classic of the Plain Maiden)*, probably the first treatment of the art of the bedchamber in early China. Sunu—as befits the Daoist ideal—the plain maiden (sometimes translated as virgin), is presented like an immortal fairy, explaining to the legendary Yellow Emperor Huangdi (2698–2598 BCE) the importance of the correct relationship between *yin* and *yang*, that is, sexual union. The *Su Nu Jing* was obviously not written in the 3rd millennium BCE (but rather in the 3rd century CE), but the Yellow

---

* All translations come from the *Ishimpo* (in Chinese *Yi Xin Fang* 醫心方), compiled by the Japanese physician Yasuyori Tamba (丹波康賴) around 982 CE, but not printed until 1854. Comprising 30 volumes, this text contains the essential writings on TCM from that time. In this way, many medical classics that had been lost in China were "rediscovered" in the beginning of the 20th century indirectly via Japan. The translations used here are based on the 1996 edition (華夏出版社 *Hua Xia Chu Ban She*, Beijing).

Emperor was regarded as the ideal typical ruler, serving as an example in all areas of life. The conversations between Sunu and the legendary Yellow Emperor are written as dialogues. Sunu advises Huangdi on the topics of longevity and the preservation of vitality into old age. In this context, the notion of an original endowment of potential life energy played a key role: humans are born with a certain prenatal potential (*xian tian zhi jing* 先天之精) that is exhausted in the course of a person's life and must be continuously replenished with postnatal potential (*hou tian zhi jing* 后天之精). These essential energies are exhausted, for example, by hard physical labor, illness, but also by frequent seminal emission (*shi jing*, literally "loss of life essence"). For this reason, retaining semen was such an important aspect of sexual intercourse. Nevertheless, the semen should not only be held back but transformed with specific techniques into valuable life energy and conducted upwards along the spine–*du mai*–to nourish the brain (*huan jing bu nao* 還精補腦) and thereby also increase the *shen* (神).[3]

At the same time, sexual intercourse also dealt with ways in which the man was able to utilize the woman's *jing* for his own benefit. The union of *yin* and *yang* as a path to nurturing and prolonging life (*yin yang yang sheng zhi dao* 陰陽養生之道).

The sought-after *jing* of the woman refers to her vaginal fluids, formed during sexual arousal. Because the abundant flow of these fluids is directly related to the woman's state of arousal, men paid such great attention to sexually satisfying the woman. In this context, we might better understand advice that at times seems excessive, to have nightly intercourse with a large number of women without ejaculating but only to absorb their *jing*. Huangdi, for example, is reported to have slept with hundreds of women (virgins) every night to increase his strength. Any seminal emission therefore had to be considered with care, so as not to harm the man and ideally to create a (male) child:

"A strong 15-year-old man may ejaculate twice a day, a frail one only once; a strong 20-year-old twice a day, a weak one once; a strong 30-year-old once a day, a weak one only every two days; a strong 40-year-old every three days, an exhausted one only every fourth day; a strong 50-year-old every five days, an exhausted one only every tenth day; a strong 60-year-old every ten days, an exhausted one only every twentieth day; a strong 70-year-old every 30 days, an exhausted one may not have any seminal emission at all."[5]

If a man obeyed these recommendations, seminal emission should not cause any appreciable loss of *jing*. You were even safer when you furthermore conformed with the seasons and hence with the course of the world, the *dao*. In the *Yang Sheng Yao Ji* (養生要集 *Collection of Important Texts for Nurturing Life*), one of many Daoist texts on this subject, Liu Jing (劉京) advises:

"In the spring, you may ejaculate every third day, but in the summer and fall only twice a month, and in the winter you should preserve your jing and not allow the semen to drain out at all. The heavenly dao intends for the husband to preserve his yang in winter. If he follows this principle, he will achieve longevity. The reason for this is that seminal emission in winter consumes a hundred times more yang than one in the spring."[5]

If seminal emission does occur, it must not happen in passionate thoughtlessness. On this topic, here is a passage from the *Dong Xuan Zi* (洞玄子 *Master of the Dark Cave*), a Daoist text from the *Tang* period:

"When the man has reached the point where he wishes to ejaculate, he should absolutely wait until the woman has reached her orgasm before allowing his semen to drain. The man's movements should then become more superficial, playful between the woman's strings (qin xian 琴弦, Frenulum clitoridis) and the wheat grain (mai chi 麥齒, Labium minus pudendi), like an infant sucking on the breast. When emission occurs, the man closes his eyes, directs his thoughts inward, presses his tongue against the palate, raises the spine, stretches the head, widens the nostrils, pulls the shoulders back, closes the mouth, absorbs the qi, and can thus allow the jing to rise upward on its own. In this way, the amount can be regulated, even in seminal emission, and only 20 to 30% escape."[5]

The vital life energy *jing* (精), used as a synonym for semen, is so valuable that the man is urgently advised against consuming it frivolously. For this reason, it is important for the man to wait for the moment of greatest arousal in the woman and therefore of her greatest production of *jing*, and then finally to allow his own *jing* as well as that of his partner to rise upward through the spine by means of the above-mentioned breathing technique, posture, and concentration. This replenishes the stores of postnatal *jing* and can prolong the lifespan beyond measure. In addition, the retention of semen makes the man's *yang* and the force of his seminal emission so powerful that it will produce a male child with great certainty.[3]

At this point, we should mention the fear Chinese men had of "*jing*-sucking" women or fox spirits who were able to appear to the man in dreams, seduce him to emit semen, and thereby increase their own *jing*. There are hundreds of variations on a story in which a beautiful maiden appears to a young scholar studying at night. The maiden seduces him and mysteriously disappears in the early morning, only to reappear every evening thereafter. The scholar becomes weaker and weaker until a Daoist monk informs him that the maiden is a fox spirit who is sucking him dry to get his *jing*, which eventually will grant the fox spirit eternal life. Thus, the Daoist monk realizes the cause of the scholar's loss of vital energy and warns the young man.

These female spirits could also be deceased female family members who had suffered an injustice, who had not had a proper burial, or who were not receiving sufficient sacrifices. Predestined to become such restless spirits were women who had committed suicide out of unfulfilled love or protest. This could be related to an unwanted (because extramarital) pregnancy or occur before an arranged wedding, but also in an unhappy marriage or out of despair because of childlessness, intensified by pressure from the family and especially the mother-in-law.

■ Foreplay—Only the Excited Woman Increases the Man's *Jing*

How could the man be certain that the woman was truly aroused and that her *yin* and *jing* were at his greatest disposal? We learn this information from the already mentioned *Yu Fang Mi Jue*:

"Huangdi asks: 'How do I recognize whether a woman is aroused?' Sunu answers: 'Observe the five signs, the five desires, and also the ten movements of the woman and how they change. Then you will know. The man then responds to the five signs of the woman:
1. *Her face turns red; now approach her slowly.*
2. *Her breasts become firm and beads of sweat appear on her nose; now enter her slowly.*
3. *Her throat becomes dry and she swallows her saliva; now begin to move slowly.*
4. *Her yin becomes moist; now slowly penetrate more deeply.*
5. *Her fluids (ye 洞) spread over her buttocks; now slowly withdraw.'"[5]*

Almost like in an instruction manual, the man is advised on how to respond to specific signs of the woman. All this information appears to be only for the benefit of the man, so that he can receive as much *jing* as possible from the woman. In another paragraph, however, the text also emphasizes the importance of arousing the woman for her own benefit. Thus, the man is responsible for the woman's orgasm (*kuai* 快) and also for any damage that he causes her if he sleeps with her without having aroused her sufficiently. For this purpose, he must have stimulated the woman's nine energies (*nu zhi jiu qi* 女之九氣):

"Huangdi says: 'Very well! But how do you recognize the woman's nine energies?' Xuannu, the dark mysterious girl (玄女) answers: 'Observe her nine energies, then you understand her:
- *The woman breathes deeply and swallows her saliva; this shows the flow of lung qi.*
- *She moans and kisses the man; now the heart qi is flowing.*
- *She embraces him and holds him tight; now the spleen qi is flowing.*
- *Her Jade Gate becomes moist and slippery; now the kidney qi is flowing.*

- *Passionately, she bites the man; now the bone qi is flowing.*
- *Her legs clinch him firmly; now the muscle qi is flowing.*
- *She caresses his Jade Stalk; now the blood qi is flowing.*
- *She fondles the man's nipples; now the flesh qi is flowing.'* *

If intercourse lasts longer and the man cares about the woman and fulfills her desires, the nine energies flow. If there is no flow, this harms (the woman). If the energies do not flow, you can repeat the foreplay to rectify this problem."[5]

To increase desire, the text also describes in detail the different positions in sexual intercourse. The variations are manifold; Dong Xuanzi describes 30 different possibilities alone. But for conception, the "normal" positions, with the woman lying flat on her back and the man above her, seem to have been preferred. The reason for this is that this position best maintained the "natural" order: the man/the male/heaven above the woman/the feminine/earth.

■ "The Soldier is not Ready for Action"

But now the big question: what do you do when the man can't perform as he wants to? For before the man concerns himself with the flow of female energy, he has to have reached the right energetic state himself:

"Huangdi asks: 'If you feel the desire for intercourse, but the Jade Stalk will not rise, should you force it?' Xuannu responds: 'No, you should not. The dao of the desire for intercourse calls for the man to fulfill four conditions. Only then can he arouse the woman's nine energies.' Huangdi asks: 'What are these four conditions?' Xuannu answers:
- *'If the Jade Stalk is not enraged (erect), harmonious qi does not flow.*
- *If it is enraged but not enlarged, the flesh qi does not flow.*

- *If it is enlarged but not firm, the bone qi does not flow.*
- *If it is firm but not warm, the shen qi does not flow.'*

This means that the erection opens up the jing, the enlargement moves the jing, the stiffening brings the jing to the door, and the warming makes the jing step on the threshold. When the four qi flow and are regulated by the dao, nothing opens that should not be opened and no jing is drained."[5]

The *qi* of the four conditions hence refers to:
- the erection—liver *qi*
- the size—spleen *qi*
- the firmness—kidney *qi*
- the blood flow—heart *qi*

Lung *qi* appears to be missing, but since it is regarded as the source of all *qi*, it nourishes the other four *qi* and is, so to speak, the precondition for the existence of any *qi* at all.

The text offers a number of formulas to allow the man to fulfill these four conditions, for example, from the *Fan Wang Fang* (范汪方 *Formulas by Fan Wang*), a collection of formulas compiled by Fan Wang (ca. 305–370 CE):

"The 'Pill for Opening the Heart' with shu yu *for kidney* qi *(Kai Xin Shu Yu Shen Qi Wan 開心薯蕷腎氣丸) treats the 'five taxations' and 'seven damages' of the man. This includes the following signs: His bone marrow cannot tolerate any cold at all. When he goes to bed, he feels so bloated that his heart is confined by all the intestinal rumbling. He has no desire to drink or eat, and when he eats, it all stagnates under the heart and he cannot get rid of phlegm. In spring and summer his hands are unbearably hot, while in fall and winter his legs are cold as ice. The emptiness makes him forgetful, the kidney qi does not flow any more, and the union of yin and yang does not take place. He is exhausted like an old man. Taking this formula strengthens the center, nourishes the bone marrow, fills the emptiness, regenerates the will, opens the heart, calms the viscera, stops tearing eyes, clears the vision, relaxes the stomach, increases the sexual urge, expels wind, and protects from cold."*[5]

There is really nothing that this formula does not treat:
- rou cong rong *(cistanches herba 肉蓯蓉), 1* liang
- shan zhu yu *(corni officinalis fructus 山茱萸), 1* liang

---

* The ninth *qi* is missing—this is most likely the liver *qi*.

- gan di huang (Rehmanniae viride radix 干地黃), 6 fen
- yuan zhi (Polygalae tenuifoliae radix 遠志), 6 fen
- she chuang zi (Cnidii fructus 蛇床子), 5 fen
- wu wei zi (Schisandrae chinensis fructus 五味子), 6 fen
- fang feng (Ledebouriellae sesloidis radix 防風), 6 fen
- fu ling (Poriae cocos sclerotium 茯苓), 6 fen
- niu xi (Achyranthis bidentatae radix 牛膝), 6 fen
- tu si zi (Cuscutae chinensis semen 菟絲子), 6 fen
- Ddu zhong (Eucommiae cortex 杜仲), 6 fen
- shu yu (Dioscoreae rhizoma 薯蕷), 6 fen

[1 liang at the time corresponded to roughly 12.5 g; 1 fen to roughly 3.15 g]

These 12 ingredients are ground in a mortar, sifted, and then formed with honey into pills the size of Sterculia platanifolia seeds (wu zi), ca. 5 mm in diameter. One dose is 20 pills. Take two doses in the course of the day, and one in the evening. If you are depressed, either stop taking them altogether or reduce the dosage to 10 pills. After taking these for 5 days, the Jade Stalk (i. e., the penis) becomes hot and fiery; after 10 nights, the body is glistening and smooth; after 15 nights, the facial expression is rejuvenated and the hands and feet are always warm. After 20 nights, the man's reproductive power is strengthened, and after 25 days, the channels are full. After 30 nights, the hot qi is clear and free-flowing, the face becomes tender like a blossom, the veins of the hands turn into fine blood vessels, the heart opens, and you won't forget anything any more. You are free from sorrows and memory loss. Even if you sleep alone, you will not feel cold. You do not have to get up at night to urinate any more, and the yin is harmonized.

One course of treatment is sufficient for men until (the end of age) 40. From age 50 on, you should take two rounds. As a result, even a man over 70 can still produce children. There are no contraindications, with the exception that you should not consume large amounts of spicy or sour foods while taking this formula.

A similar formula with slightly less ingredients furthermore advises kneeling facing east, that is, in the direction of yang, when taking the pills. In cases where the Jade Stalk is very weak, double the amount of she chuang zi. If you need more strength, double the amount of yuan zhi. If the amount of semen is too small, doubling wu wei zi is advised. If you wish to lengthen the Jade Stalk, double rou cong rong. If the patient suffers from back pain, twice the amount of du zhong is necessary. And if you want to lengthen the duration of intercourse, add 12 fen of Xu duan (Dipsaci asperi radix) to the formula.[5]

But formulas could not only be taken internally, but could also be applied directly on the affected regions. Here, for example, is a recommendation from the Xin Luo Fa Shi Mi Mi Fang (新羅法師秘密方 Secret Formulas of the Buddhist Master from Xin Luo):

"In the middle ten days of the 8th lunar month, collect honey comb, place a flat object on top, and press for one night. After this night, wrap in a pouch made of fine raw silk and let hang on a pole in the shade. After a period of ten times ten days, you have a wonderful medicine. As soon as the man expects that he will have sexual intercourse, cut off a piece the size of six copper coins and boil it without any other ingredients in an earthen vessel until it has changed color from black to whitish grey. Now drink half of this dissolved in warm wine and take the other half in your hand, mix it with your saliva, and spread it on the hip bones and from the root to the tip (of the Jade Stalk). As soon as (the medicine) is applied, it will dry, and as soon as it has dried, you can begin with intercourse to your heart's content.

After 40 days of uninterrupted application, you will gradually see obvious results, after 100 days the positive changes in the body are so great that they will continue for the rest of your life. Harm is averted, good fortune will multiply, physical strength increases sevenfold, whatever you desire will come true, diseases stay far away, and life is prolonged. Cooling at the height of summer, warming in the deepest winter, and protective against counterflow qi, in this way, harm (to your health) is avoided. This preparation is also called 'Increaser of Positive Effects.' You have to apply it widely in the area of the hip bones, every time about 180 zhu. [Zhu is an old unit of measurement. At the time when the text was composed, 1 zhu corresponded to 1/24 liang, that is, 0.52 g. Hence 180 zhu are roughly 94 g, the amount to be rubbed in.] As a result, [the Jade Stalk] becomes strong like an iron hammer, its length increases by three cun, and its secretions become fragrant. The thoughts of the man and the woman become calm, but their hearts are stimulated, their vision and hearing improve, and the smells from mouth and nose become fragrant again.

If you desire more strength in the Jade Stalk, drink this preparation frequently, dissolved in warm wine. If you desire an increase in length, rub the preparation on the tip of the Jade Stalk. If you desire an increase in size, rub it all over the Jade Stalk.

While taking this preparation, you should avoid the following: Great worries, excessive joy, great fright, strong resentment, excessive fear, strong sweating, throwing yourself into torrents of water, climbing to dangerous heights, indulging (to an extreme) in the five flavors, cold and raw food, and strong alcohol."[5]

These formulas most likely came from a Buddhist priest from Korea, because Xin Luo was the name of the two largest states of Korea during the Tang period.

Besides these formulas for improving the quality of the Jade Stalk and the quantity of intercourse, we also find advice on how to achieve the opposite, that is, how to make the Jade Stalk weak and small. One formula recommends mixing mercury, Cervi parvum cornu (*lu rong*, normally *yang*-strengthening) and Croton tiglium (*ba dou*, croton oil, in the West a constituent of Baunscheidt oil) with deer tallow and applying this on the penis and scrotum. Another method for weakening *yang* is repeated moxa treatment on the point *san yin jiao.*[5]

The purpose of these formulas is not entirely clear. On the one hand, they could, of course, have been intended to dampen excessive sexual desire, hence, for example, for monks or during mourning periods. On the other hand, they could almost have been medicines for intentional castration. We only need to think of the eunuchs at the imperial court, who may not have been highly respected in society but were often very influential. Suppressing the man's desire was not propagated in general, since, as we have already mentioned, sexual intercourse was not equated with seminal emission, and frequent intercourse (without seminal emission) was therefore desirable up until old age. And because of polygamy there were no times (except during the period of mourning) in which the man would have had to restrain himself, such as due to the wife's illness, pregnancy, or lying-in period.

▪ When She Can't Do as She Wants

Up until now, the man has been the focus of the above formulas, but the (erotic) needs of the woman were also dealt with, if not in as much detail. This includes injuries sustained during defloration, pain or bleeding during sexual intercourse, or an excessively large Jade Grotto (i. e, the vagina), which lessens the sexual pleasure of the woman and the man. To address this condition, a formula from the already mentioned Dong Xuanzi:

"This formula treats the wide and cold yin of the woman, making it narrower and causing joy during intercourse. Take 2 fen each of:
- *shi liu huang (Sulfur 石硫黄)*
- *qing mu xiang (Aucklandiae radix 青木香)*
- *shan zhu yu (Corni officinalis fructus 山茱萸)*
- *she chuang zi (Cnidii monnieri semen 蛇床子)*

Rub and sieve the four ingredients into a fine powder and place a small amount of it into the Jade Grotto. Under no circumstances should she take too much, otherwise it is possible that the opening will close completely.

Another formula advises to dissolve three pinches of ground sulfur in 1 sheng [approximately 1 L] of warm water. If the woman washes her yin [i. e., her genitals] with this mixture, it will soon again be like that of a 12–13-year-old."[5]

▪ The When and Where Must be Heeded as Well

With this advice, all conditions should be set for the best possible execution of sexual intercourse, and nothing else should stand in the way of conceiving a child. But not so! Prohibitions concerning specific days, locations, or climate conditions were numerous. Here are a few exemplary passages from the above-cited *Yu Fang Mi Jue:*

"In the union of yin *and* yang, *seven prohibitions must be observed:*

1. *On the first day of the lunar month (that is, on the new moon) as well as on the full moon (around the 14th) and on the 'half-moons' (around 7th and 21st days of the month), the union of* yin *and* yang *causes a weakening of qi. Children that were conceived on such days are certain to have sustained physical damage; therefore you should observe this prohibition under all circumstances. [Here we should quickly note that the Chinese lunar year counted 354 days and was divided into 12 months of 29 and 30 days. Every few years, a 13th month was inserted. The beginning of the month always fell on a new moon.]*

2. *If a union of* yin *and* yang *takes place during a thunderstorm, when heaven and earth are jolted, the blood vessels will swell up. If a child is created from this, it will suffer from pain and swelling.*

3. *A union of* yin *and* yang *right after the consumption of alcohol or a heavy meal, when the* gu qi (谷氣, *literally: grain qi) has not dispersed, causes stagnation in the abdomen and turbid urine. Children conceived then are certain to be mentally disturbed.*

4. *The union of* yin *and* yang *right after urinating consumes the* jing qi (精氣). *This makes the channels impassable. Children conceived at this time are certain to be malicious.*

5. *If the union of* yin *and* yang *occurs after exhausting work or great exertion, the* zhi qi (志氣) *[the willpower—relation to the kidney!] has not calmed down, and the muscles and the back will be affected. Children conceived in this situation will die young [deficient kidney qi and not enough prenatal jing].*

6. *If the union of* yin *and* yang *takes place shortly after bathing and the hair and skin have not dried yet, this leads to a shortage of qi (*duan qi 短氣, *literally: short qi). Children conceived then will be physically incomplete (*bu quan 不全).*

7. *If the weapon is hard and ready for action but there is pain in the channel of the Stalk, there should never be a union. Otherwise, internal damages and illnesses will result (for the child as well as the man)."*[5]

The text continues:

*"Some children are born deaf or with a darkened spirit. These are children that were conceived after sunset on the sacrificial days of the 12th lunar month (*la 臘). *On this evening of sacrifices, all the spirits gather and do not settle down for the whole night. The wise man (*jun zi 君子, *literally: 'the gentleman, the man educated after the Confucian model') restrains himself on this night, only the simple man (*xiao ren 小人, *literally 'the small man,' i.e., the uneducated man) secretly abandons himself on this night to the union of* yin *and* yang. *This will invariably produce blind and deaf children."*[5]

La (臘) is explicitly the eighth day of the 12th lunar month, the day on which the winter sacrifices are performed. On this night, however, not only the malevolent souls of the deceased ancestors were active, but also malevolent demons (*gui* 鬼), who were able to overpower the sensory organs or the entire body of newly conceived fetuses. Even one's own, normally benevolent ancestors could turn into demons if they felt neglected: if the location of the tomb was not auspicious or if the sacrifices had been neglected. Besides this inauspicious time, there were also baleful locations, such as cemeteries or temple compounds, where malign influences could be particularly strong. In general, virtuous conduct was seen as immunization against demons and bad influences. Therefore, always the distinction between the *jun zi*, the virtuous Confucian "gentleman," and the *xiao ren*, the simple man who follows his urges.

The warnings in the *Yu Fang Mi Jue* continue insistently by describing what can happen with the descendants when certain commandments are not observed:

"Some children are born with injuries or dead, they are called 'fire children' because they were conceived before the candle had burned down. Such children arrive in this world with injuries or dead, or die soon. Fire children are in a sense burned and injured by sun- or daylight."[5]

According to this passage, sexuality was an activity of the night and of darkness, especially when practiced for the sake of conception. Associated with *yin*, it was supposed to take place during the time of *yin*, that is, at night, when the candle had been blown out. In this way, conception could not only be successful at that time, but was even a guarantee for healthy children. Would this mean that sex for the purpose of increasing *jing* (of the man) and prolonging life, that is, without seminal emission and without the intent of conceiving, was a *yang* and therefore daytime activity? And, by contrast, that the purposeful union with the intent of conceiving sons was a *yin* and therefore night-time activity? In general, the time around midnight is recommended as the most favorable moment for conception, since *yin qi* is strongest at that time. Laozi already stated: "Children conceived at midnight have the greatest longevity, the ones conceived before midnight have medium longevity, and the ones conceived after midnight, the smallest longevity."[5]

"Some children are born mentally disabled. These are 'thunderstorm children' because they were conceived during the great rains and thunderstorms of the 4th and 5th lunar month. The wise man practices restraint at this time, only the simple man secretly abandons himself to the union of yin and yang. This invariably results in the creation of mentally disabled children."[5]

The idea that conception was a union of heaven and earth implied that disturbances of these two elements could therefore also impede the creation of new life. A "lack in heaven," that is, thunder and lightning, storms and tempests, but also solar and lunar eclipses, were as inauspicious as a "lack on earth," that is, disease, emotional imbalance, or overexertion. These conditions could not produce healthy descendants.

"Some children are born but then become the prey of tigers or wolves. These are the children of 'mourning clothes.' The reason for this is that the filial son only wears plain hemp clothes during the period of mourning and does not eat meat. The gentleman puts all business activities aside during this time while the simple man secretly abandons himself to the union of yin and yang. If children are conceived during the mourning period, they invariably become the prey of tigers and wolves."[5]

Mourning rituals varied considerably depending on one's social status and clan membership. In general, the parents were to observe a 3-year mourning period.

"Some children are born and then die by drowning. This is the mistake of the parents. The reason is that they have placed the placenta in a bronze vessel and buried it upside down seven chi *deep on the (shaded)* yin *side of the courtyard wall. This is also called 'to enclose the son,' and these children invariably die by drowning."[5]*

Placenta burial was a common practice in which the placenta of a son was supposed to be buried in a hole under the bed and that of a daughter outside the house. If the placenta of a son was buried in an inappropriate location, this was bound to lead to problems. Thus, the text also states:

- *"Children conceived during a storm will suffer from many illnesses."* [Wind as a pathogenic factor that enters during conception and later causes wind diseases, that is, highly varied and "wandering" problems.]
- *"Children conceived during a thunderstorm will be confused or mentally disabled."* [Atmospheric turbulences confuse the child's clear shen.]
- *"Children conceived when inebriated are certain to be mentally deficient."* [This refers to alcohol and drugs (opium).]
- *"Children conceived in states of great exhaustion will die early."* [The child thereby receives an insufficient amount of prenatal jing. The "five taxations" (wu lao 五勞) and "seven damages" (qi sun 七損) of the parents negatively affect the life expectancy of the child.]
- *"Children conceived during the menstrual period will die as soldiers."* [The time of menstruation was regarded as impure. These children therefore died a useless and not very desirable death as soldiers.]
- *"Children conceived during dusk will experience much injustice."*
- *"Children conceived during the time of sleeping at night will certainly be deaf."*
- *"Children conceived during broad daylight will be at a disadvantage in verbal arguments."*
- *"Children conceived at noon will suffer from mental illness."*
- *"Children conceived in the afternoon will injure themselves."[5]*

But then when could you conceive a child? We are beginning to ask ourselves this question. If they had observed all these rules, the Chinese would have become extinct a long time ago. But we must not forget that all these rules were, if at all, only observed by the educated elite.

■ No Offspring Even Though Everything Was Done Correctly?

This question could stimulate a discussion on whether the early Chinese were aware of the relevant connections between the menstrual bleeding and the woman's fertile days. We can answer this question with a unanimous yes. Concerning this question, there is very concrete advice from Dong Xuanzi on the topic of fertile days and conception:

"If you wish to have a child, you should hold off on sexual intercourse until after the end of the menstrual period. Intercourse from the first to the third day afterwards will produce a son; on the fourth and fifth day afterwards, it will produce a daughter. Seminal emissions from the fifth day on only weaken the jing and strength and are of no use whatsoever. You should wait with ejaculating until the woman has reached her climax, and then orgasm should take place for both partners simultaneously, with the man emitting all his semen completely. It is best if the woman lies on her back facing up, focuses her thoughts, closes her eyes, and concentrates exclusively on receiving the semen."[1]

For exactly this moment, the imperial advisor Sunu additionally recommends the following for increasing the success of a conception:

"If a married woman has remained childless, during intercourse she should hold 27 red beans (xiao dou 小豆) in her left hand while introducing the tip of the man's yin (tip of the penis) into her yin. At the same time as the man's penetration, she takes the beans from her left hand into her mouth. As soon as she feels that the man's jing (semen) is descending, she swallows the beans. This method has never failed."[5]

The *Bing Yuan Lun* (病源論 *Treatises on the Causes of Diseases*), a reference to the *Zhu Bing Yuan Hou Lun* (*On the Origins and Symptoms of the Various Diseases*) by Chao Yuan Fang, further elaborates on the problem of childlessness:

"When a married woman fails to bear children, this can have three causes. First, the tomb is not properly cared for. Second, the fates of the two partners stand

in a relationship of mutual opposition (astrological incompatibility). Third, man or woman is ill. All of these lead to infertility. If the tomb has not been taken care of and the sacrifices have not been performed, or if the birth horoscopes do not match, in these two cases, medicine cannot redress the situation."[5]

In imperial China, people generally did not enter into marriage out of love, and the choice of partner was not left to chance. For this purpose, the matchmaker existed, a profession that was not well respected but frequently used. Usually older women, matchmakers made suggestions to families with matching social status on which connections might be beneficial for both families. Obviously, the financial and social compatibility were of primary importance, but the birth horoscope of the engaged partners also needed to be harmonious and suited to guarantee an abundance of children, health, and survival.

The *Bing Yuan Lun* continues:

"If the man or woman are sick, they have to ingest medicinals to achieve success. If the woman does in fact suffer from infertility, this has different causes. Overexertion (wu lao and qi sun) harms the blood and qi, and the woman is no longer able to perfectly adapt to cold and heat. Consequently, wind and cold can penetrate. This causes the embryo (ke yu zi gong 客于子宫, *literally 'guest in the uterus') to develop diseases, or the menses become lumpy or stop, or discharge occurs. In that case, the energies of* yin *and* yang *are no longer in harmony, the menses run counterflow, and infertility results."*[5]

The "five taxations" (*wu lao* 五勞) refer to the following:

- Excessive sitting harms the flesh and therefore the spleen.
- Excessive lying harms the *qi* and therefore the lung.
- Excessive standing harms the bones and therefore the kidney.
- Excessive walking harms the muscles and sinews and therefore the liver.
- Excessive seeing harms the blood and therefore the heart.

The "seven damages" (*qi sun* 七損) refer to the following:
- *qi* expiry (*jue qi* 絕氣)
- spillage of semen (*yi jing* 溢精)
- robbed vessels (*duo mai* 奪脈)
- discharge of *qi* (*qi xie* 氣泄)
- reversal and damage of the bodily functions (*ji guan jue shang* 机關厥傷)
- the "hundred blocks" (*bai bi* 百閉)
- exhaustion of the blood (*xue jie* 血竭)[5]

The *Bing Yuan Lun* further elaborates:

"If the man is responsible for the lack of children, the reason is that his semen is clear like water and [the penis is] cold like ice. Alternatively, if the semen is not discharged during the emission but gets stuck in the tip of the penis (yin head), this also leads to childlessness."[5]

Formulas for these problems fill whole volumes; we can cite here the *Qing Yun San* (慶云散 Blessing Clouds Powder) from the text *Seng Shen Fang* (僧深方 *Effective Formulas of [Buddhist] Monks*). The poetic name of this formula stems from the highly symbolic name for sexual intercourse as "clouds and rain" (*yun yu* 雲雨):

"Blessing Clouds Powder is a formula to be used for the husband's insufficiency of yang qi, *inability to emit semen, or lacking amount of semen:*
- tian men dong (*Asparagi cochichinensis tuber* (僧深方), *without the inside, 2* liang
- tu si zi (*Cuscutae chinensis semen* 僧深方), *1* sheng
- sang shang ji sheng (*Loranthi seu visci ramus* 僧深方), *4* liang
- zi shi ying (*Fluoritum* 僧深方), *2* liang
- fu pen zi (*Rubi fructus* 僧深方), *1* sheng
- wu wei zi (*Schisandrae chinensis fructus* 僧深方), *1* sheng
- tian xiong (*Aconitum carmichaeli tuber* 僧深), *roasted, 1* liang
- shi hu (*Dendrobii herba* 僧深), *3* liang
- [Cang] zhu (*Atractylodis rhizoma* [僧] 僧), *3* liang

(Prepare a decoction until the color changes. If the patient cannot tolerate cold, leave out the ji sheng and replace with 4 liang *of wild ginger root, Asari cum radice herba [xi xin* 僧深方*].)*
Thicken and strain these nine ingredients. Twice a day, take a square-cun spoon in wine before meals. If the

yang qi *is too small and this is the cause of childless-ness, leave out the* shi hu *and instead take 15 betel nuts (*bing lang 僧深).*"*[5]

And for the woman:

"The Cheng Ze Wan (承澤丸 *Pill for Holding Moisture) treats women's 36 diseases of the lower burner. It is a formula for infertility and unfulfilled wish for children:*
- mei he *(kernel of Pruni mume fructus* 梅核*), 1 sheng*
- xin yi *(Magnoliae liliflorae flos* 辛夷*), 1 sheng*
- gao ben *(Ligustici sinensis rhizoma et radix* 稟本*), 1 liang*
- ze lan *(Lycopi lucidi herba* 澤蘭*), 15 ge*
- sou shu *(Deutzia scabra* 溲疏*), 2 liang*
- ge shang ting zhang *(Puerariae radix* 葛上亭長*) grown large and straight, seven pieces*

(1 ge corresponds to 0.1 L)
*Melt and strain these six ingredients and form with honey into pills the size of a chan bean (*蟬豆*). Take two pills three times a day before meals, no more and no less."*[5]

■ Pregnant at Last—Now How to Avoid Mistakes?

People believed that the child's gender could be changed up to the third month of pregnancy. In the *Ru Yi Fang* (如意方 *Good Fortune Scepter Formulas*), a collection of formulas for difficult cases, we find folk advice on what to do to give birth to a son:

"Place 20 feathers from the left wing of a black hen under the woman's mattress; then it will be a boy." Or: *"Place two tail feathers of a male duck under the woman's kang without her noticing; then it will be a boy."*[5]

Instructions are numerous on which foods a pregnant woman should consume in which year in order for her to give birth to a healthy, long-lived, successful son. Chinese astrology counts time in 60-year cycles, divided into 12 years each (12 animals of the zodiac), with five influences of the five phases of transformation each. Hence we

have a year of the water snake, one of the wood snake, fire snake, and so on. After 5 × 12 years = 60 years, the cycle repeats itself. Each of these 60 years has its own name that can be looked up in the appropriate almanacs. As an example, we can look at the dietary advice with regard to the 60-year cycle from the *Chan Jing* (產經 *The Classic of Childbirth*):

"To ensure that sons born in the year Jiazi *live a long life until 90, you have to eat wheat. To ensure that those born in the year* Yichou *reach the age of 96, you must eat foxtail millet. To ensure that sons born in the year* Bingyin *reach the age of 95, the pregnant woman must eat rice."*[5]

This way of thinking implies a certain given life span that can be reached (it spans from 63 years for persons in the year *Bingzi* to 105 years for those born in the year *Dinghai*) if the person has received enough prenatal *jing* as a prerequisite. The future mother can contribute to this by consuming certain foods. She can and should, however, do far more than that in order to not only experience a smooth pregnancy and problem-free birth, but also to provide the child with its fullest congenital potential and thereby ensure a successful start in life for him or her. We can find an example of advice on prenatal education in the writings of Dong Xuanzi, who we have already mentioned several times above:

"After the woman becomes pregnant, she should only do nice things, she should not see or hear anything bad, she should curb her sexual desires, and she should neither curse nor argue. Additionally, she should not experience any fright or physically over-exert herself. She should be neither talkative nor gloomy. In her diet, she should avoid any cold or raw foods, as well as vinegary, oily, or spicy foods. She should no longer go out by carriage, climb great heights, or get close to precipices. She should not walk down steep slopes or walk too quickly. In addition, she should neither consume medicinals nor receive acupuncture or moxibustion. She should continuously hold good feelings and proper thoughts and she should frequently listen to the classics. If she does all this, her child will be smart, intelligent, loyal, and honest. This is what is called prenatal education."[1]

Bibliography

1. Hemm D. Stress und Zufriedenheit im kaiserlichen China. In: Noll A, Kirschbaum B (editors) *Stresskrankheiten*. Munich: Urban & Fischer; 2006.
2. Jullien F. *Der Umweg über China. Ein Ortswechsel des Denkens*. Berlin: Merve; 2002.
3. Needham J. *Science and Civilisation in China. Vol. II. History of Scientific Thought*. Cambridge: Cambridge University Press; 1956.
4. Noll A, Kirschbaum B (editors). *Stresskrankheiten. Vorbeugen und Behandeln mit Chinesischer Medizin*. Munich: Urban & Fischer; 2006.
5. Tamba Y. *Yixinfang*. Beijing: Huaxia; 1996.

Fertility Treatment and Pregnancy— Reproductive Medicine and TCM in Meaningful Cooperation

2

6 Fertility Treatment and Pregnancy—Reproductive Medicine and TCM in Meaningful Cooperation

Karin Kielwein, Fransiscus X. Sulistyo-Winarto, Kerstin Friol, and Christian Gnoth

■ Introduction

When we consider the modern options of reproductive medicine in the holistic care of couples, the question arises whether Western scientific medicine and TCM might not be able to complement and approach each other with regard to the different medical theories underlying both systems. By now, solid scientific studies exist that indicate the successful results of such cooperation. The necessity of combining biomedical reproductive medicine and TCM makes sense even on the most basic level since the principle of individualized treatment in TCM complements the normative approach of biomedical treatment.

The following paragraphs therefore shed light on the one hand on those areas where the strengths and therefore indications of the biomedical approach are situated, and on the other hand on those areas where TCM offers advantages to couples in regard to diagnosis and treatment of reproductive disorders.

Requirements for a Successful Pregnancy

The goal of a successful pregnancy requires a whole series of preliminary conditions:
- in the woman
- in the man
- during conception
- during implantation

Requirements in the Woman

In biomedicine, the "quality" of the gametes (reproductive cells with half the set of chromosomes) is seen as being of paramount significance. We now know that a hormonal disturbance with an elevated level of male sex hormones (hyperandrogenism, often so-called polycystic ovary syndrome [PCOS]) in women drastically reduces the quality of eggs and therefore the likelihood of pregnancy. Such hormonal disturbance is partly related to the patient's state of being considerably overweight. The quality of a woman's eggs is furthermore limited—as we know well—particularly by increasing age. The loss of quality is primarily because a woman's supply of eggs is limited. This supply peaks during the woman's own fetal stage. At the time of birth, it consists of approximately 500 000 primordial follicles (immature egg cells in the ovaries). With the exception of the 400–500 oocytes that reach ovulation during the course of a woman's fertile years, all others will spontaneously perish throughout her life. Furthermore, the development from primordial follicle to pre-ovulatory follicle takes almost a year (see **Fig. 6.1**); it is only in approximately the last 4 weeks before ovulation itself that the follicle is controlled by hormones via the female cycle.[29]

In a process called meiosis (reduction division of reproductive cells), the set of chromosomes in the cells is cut in half, into a single chromosome set. It is significant here that the oocytes remain arrested in this so-called first meiotic division during the entire time (longest period of cell division in humans up to ca. 50 years). This makes the oocytes particularly susceptible to damaging factors such as:
- nutritional state in the ovaries
- effect of cellular and environmental toxins
- nicotine abuse
- bodyweight
- ionizing radiation

As such, the rate of aneuploidy in oocytes increases with advancing age (> 50% of oocytes). As we know today, genetic disposition is also particularly significant in that it determines the number of initiated oocytes in the ovaries and influences the spontaneous decrease of eggs in the course of the woman's life. Additional factors that affect egg quality in women from a biomedical perspective are inflammations of the ovaries or autoimmune diseases (thyroid glands, the so-called antiphospholipid syndrome, autoimmune disorders, hereditary coagulation disorders).

In this short and obviously incomplete presentation of biomedical notions regarding the significance of oocyte quality, we can already see the importance of bodyweight (especially at the time of puberty!) and lifestyle. In this context, TCM and biomedical strategies can be used together preventatively, in which case TCM surely offers more varied and individual treatment concepts: from lifestyle advice, nutritional therapy, and *qi gong* to medicinal therapy, a multiplicity of options exist for influencing gamete quality and quantity.

Requirements in the Man

For the man, the situation is more complicated. We know today that excess weight and smoking have a considerable influence on sperm quality. In addition, biomedicine recognizes a multitude of factors that are said with more or less certainty to contribute to a decrease in semen quality. For some of these factors, the influence on sperm quality is only temporary; hence it makes sense to have a control spermiogram done after a so-called completed sperm cycle of 3 months or possibly even later (e. g., in cases of low sperm quality due to anabolic therapy related to bodybuilding). It has become apparent that spermiogenesis is characterized by considerable inter-individual sensitivities that may be genetically determined. There is also a connection here to undescended testes as a cause of reduced sperm cell formation (testicular dysgenesis). Biomedicine recognizes that after puberty, viral infections in particular can gravely affect spermiogenesis, with a possible complete destruction of the sperm-forming tissue. Many of these different factors have in common that they ultimately harm spermiogenesis by elevating the level of extra- and intracellular free oxygen radicals and can thereby even trigger point mutations. Biomedicine attempts to counteract this action with high dosages of vitamin E and zinc. In this area, TCM also offers options.

For successful fertilization, the ratio between egg cells and sperm cells is also decisive. At the site of natural fertilization, namely the ampulla of the fallopian tubes, an estimated ratio of one ovum (still encapsulated by the surrounding tissue) (**Fig. 6.1**) and ca. 100 000–150 000 motile spermatozoa is needed. It is only in the woman's inner genitalia that the spermatozoa reach their full functionality, that is, the penetration of the surrounding tissue to reach the ovum itself, the penetration of the zona pellucida that encases the ovum, and the fusion of the cell membranes of the sperm and egg. This process is called capacitation. Success is possible only for quickly moving and normally formed spermatozoa. We can assume a normal probability of fertilization when a man's sperms exceed the minimum values (**Table 6.1**).

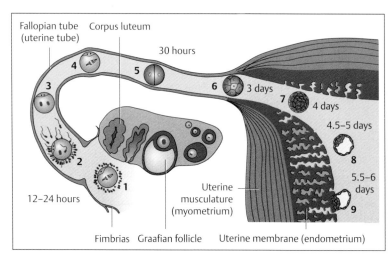

Fallopian tube (uterine tube)   Corpus luteum

30 hours

3   4   5

6   3 days

7   4 days

4.5–5 days

8

5.5–6 days

9

2

1

12–24 hours

Uterine musculature (myometrium)

Fimbrias   Graafian follicle   Uterine membrane (endometrium)

Fig. 6.1 Fertilization, fallopian tube transport, and implantation. Schematic presentation of the developmental processes in humans in the first week: **1** ovum directly after ovulation; **2** fertilization within 12–24 hours; **3** stage with male and female pronucleus; **4** zygote, 1st cleavage; **5** two-cell stage; **6** morula stage; **7** entry into the uterine cavity; **8** blastocyst with blastocyst cavity; **9** early stage of nidation (implantation).

43

Table 6.1   Normal sperm values as outlined by the WHO

Criteria	Values
Ejaculate volume per ejaculation	> 2.0 mL
pH	7.2–8.0
Sperm concentration	> 20 million spermatozoa/mL
Total sperm count	> 40 million spermatozoa
Motility (mobility)	> 25% rapidly progressing sperm of category a, or > 50% forwardly motile sperm of category a + b
Morphology	> 30% normally formed sperm
Viability (proportion of living sperm)	> 75% vital spermatozoa (eosin test)
MAR test (spermatozoa—autoantibody determination)	< 10% spermatozoa with particles
Leucocytes	< 0.5 million/mL
Round cells	< 1 million/mL
Alpha-glucosidase	> 11 mU/ejaculate
Fructose	> 13 µmol/ejaculate
Zinc	> 2.4 µmol/ejaculate

Requirements During Fertilization

If these requirements are met and a mature oocyte has emerged in the cycle (i. e., the first maturation division of meiosis is completed all the way), the gametes must come together. From the sperm deposit in the back of the vaginal cavity, rapid periovulatory penetration into the highly fertile cervical mucus occurs.

The sperm cells reach their full fertilizing capacity in this cervical mucus; a selection process takes place that effectively separates highly motile, normally formed sperm cells from less motile, morphologically conspicuous cells. The sperm do not swim into the fallopian tube completely on their own accord; rather, we now have proof of a targeted, uterotubal transport to the site of ovulation. Precondition for a normal transport of spermatozoa to the oocyte in the ampulla of the fallopian tube is, of course, that the woman's inner genitals are anatomically normal. Uterine deformities (partitions, complete bisection of the uterus) that disrupt this transport and can be responsible for repeated miscarriages later are not rare. In addition, myomas, polyps, and a dispersed uterine lining (endometriosis) can also disrupt this process considerably. Much more common in previous times than today were completely blocked fallopian tubes after inflammation (adnexitis).

Nowadays, especially chlamydial infections play an important role: they are often overlooked as the source of inflammation and remain undiagnosed and untreated because they produce few if any symptoms. In cases of uterine deformity or complete fallopian tube blockage, biomedical methods with microsurgical operations and, if necessary, subsequent assisted fertilization (in vitro fertilization) are certainly superior to the options of TCM.

Requirements During Nidation

Once the embryo has arrived in the uterus, it requires an endometrium prepared for implantation in the early secretory stage in order to implant there. Influencing uterine conditions to prepare for implantation is possible in both systems: on the part of TCM, by nourishing blood and *yin*, and on the part of Western biomedicine, by hormonally supporting the luteal stage. The options of modern reproductive medicine in this context consist specifically of supporting a synchronous proliferation of endometrial cells, mainly procured by estrogen. After ovulation, a marked increase in progesterone causes the so-called secretory transformation of the mucus and opens the implantation window. In humans, we can assume that the implantation window opens by about the second day of the progesterone increase and closes again about 7–9 days thereafter. Synchronization with embryonic development is essential. In humans, the embryo reaches the uterine cavity about 6 or 7 days post-conception. Strictly speaking, this is a capillary gap in which the embryo continues to move around in a layer of fluid due to peristaltic movements of the uterine muscles. Shortly before implantation, however, the human embryo must slip out of its cover (zona pellucida) when it reaches the uterine cavity (so-called "hatching").

We still do not understand the details of the process of implantation with all its contributing factors because the situation is completely different in other mammals. Of foremost importance is the viability of the embryo, as a result of which implantation is possible also in the periphery of the implantation window. Even implantation completely without endometrium (fallopian or abdominal pregnancy) is possible in humans, in contrast to the situation in animals. As we know from reproductive medicine, the human embryo (again, in contrast to the animal kingdom) can "wait" for the implantation window to open. This is of the greatest significance for the question on which day after oocyte punction the embryo transfer should take place. We know that vital embryos secrete typical patterns of growth factors for blood vessels and protein-splitting enzymes (so-called metalloproteinases) for optimal implantation. Apparently, implantation does not follow the rule of "all or nothing"; on the contrary, we nowadays assume that qualitative differences exist. Later pregnancy complications such as high blood pressure, retarded growth, premature detachment of the placenta, and intrauterine fetal death are sometimes attributed to early implantation problems. Some miscarriages are also caused by implantation mistakes, as we know, for example, in serious corpus luteum insufficiency with progesterone deficiency.

As a rule, highly targeted intervention, as is often desired by Western medicine, is very difficult in this complex event; at the same time, therapeutic effects are therefore also difficult to evaluate or prove. Herein lies the strength of TCM.

■ Causes of Subfertility and Infertility in Women and Men

The Four Phases of the Menstrual Cycle from the Western and TCM Perspective

The **first phase**, the menstrual period (day 1–5), is defined by a sharp drop in estrogen and progesterone levels, as a result of which the endometrium is deprived of nourishment, becomes necrotic, and is expelled with the blood. In TCM, we have to ensure in this phase that *qi* and blood flow freely, to guarantee the gentle shedding of old blood (**Fig. 6.2**).

In the **second phase**, the follicular phase (around day 6–11) the follicle grows under the influence of the follicle-stimulating hormone (FSH), the estrogen level rises, and the lining of the uterus is rebuilt. After blood and *yin* have been lost in the first phase, they must be nourished in this phase to allow the egg cells to mature and to build a well-nourished endometrium.

In the **third phase**, the ovulatory phase (around day 11–17), the release of luteinizing hormone (LH) causes the follicle to rupture and release the ovum. The corpus luteum is formed from the ruptured follicle. The *chong mai* and *ren mai* gradually fill up in this phase, and ovulation takes place. This dynamic process corresponds to the transition from the *yin* to the *yang* stage of the cycle.

In the **fourth phase**, the luteal phase (around day 18–28), the corpus luteum grows and secretes progesterone. The *yang qi* increases and liver *qi* is mobilized, in order to then be able to move the blood during menstruation. Treatment strategies should be designed in accordance with these phases.

Probabilities of Pregnancy

These days, it is not uncommon that women and men practice birth control sometimes for 20 years before they think of realizing their wish for children. The remaining 20% of the woman's fertile years are unfortunately also the ones that are least fertile. Thus, the biological clock begins to tick sooner or later. Today, about every sixth cou-

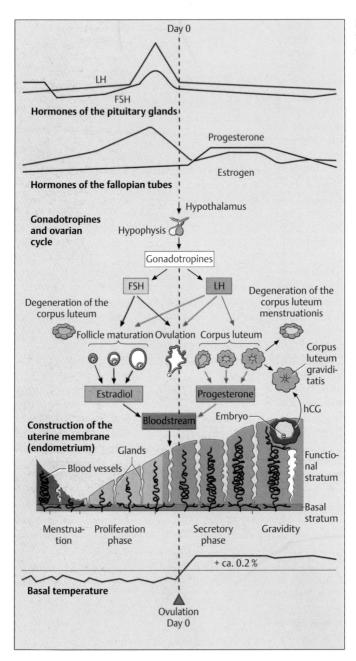

Fig. 6.2 Synchronized processes in the menstrual cycle (modified based on Faller).

ple suffers—at least temporarily—from the problem of unwanted childlessness. **Table 6.2** shows that the probability for a pregnancy is greatest 1–2 days before ovulation.

The maximum probability of pregnancy in a cycle with intercourse on every fertile day lies around 27%. For the definition of subfertility and sterility, the question of pregnancy probability is, of course, more interesting in a series of cycles (cumulative probability of pregnancy). Here, **Table 6.3** shows that after three cycles approximately 70%, and after six cycles approximately

Table 6.2 Probability of pregnancy on the different days of the cycle

Cycle Day	− 8	− 7	− 6	− 5	− 4	− 3	− 2	− 1	Rise in temperature	+1	+2
Probability (%)	0.3	1.4	2.7	6.8	17.6	23.7	25.5	21.2	10.3	0.8	0.35

Note: Study: 3175 cycles with 434 pregnancies. Reference point is the first day of elevated temperatures; ovulation itself usually occurs on the day before the rise in temperature.[5]

Table 6.3 Cumulative probability of pregnancy in successive cycles

Cycle	1	3	6	12
Cumulative probability of pregnancy in all unselected couples (%)	38	68	81	92
Cumulative probability of pregnancy in those who ultimately became pregnant (%)	42	75	88	98

Note: Number of subjects: total of 340 prospectively followed couples; among these, 304 couples who ultimately became pregnant.[17]

80% of all couples who had intercourse in the highly fertile time became pregnant. Of the successful couples, as much as almost 90% became pregnant within the first six cycles. In only 2% of couples, it took more than 12 cycles.

We can thus assume after six unsuccessful cycles with intercourse in the most fertile time that a mild impairment of fertility is already present and that in such cases every second couple could even suffer from an impairment of fertility. On the other hand, though, chances of a natural pregnancy are not bad either for couples who have not had success after 1 year. The reason for this is that approximately half of those couples can count on a child in the next 36 months. After 4 years of unsuccessfully trying to get pregnant at the latest, we can speak of a definitely sterile partnership. After that, only sporadic chances exist for a natural pregnancy (**Table 6.4**).

We know that the woman's age plays a significant role. With increasing age, the risk of fertility problems clearly increases. Nevertheless, differences between women increase with increasing age, that is, a growing percentage of women suffer from considerable fertility problems on the one hand, but there are still some women with very high fertility on the other. For this reason, it is very important for women over 30 and especially for women over 35 to know whether they can wait longer after six unsuccessful cycles or whether a personal fertility problem is reducing their chance for a natural pregnancy.

Causes of Subfertility and Infertility in Women and Men

Modern medicine by now possesses easily performed and dependable diagnostic methods for identifying couples with a possibly bad prognosis for a spontaneous pregnancy. This is very impor-

Table 6.4 Prevalence and definition of subfertility (limited fertility) and infertility (failed fertility)

Of All Couples Desiring Children		
After six unsuccessful cycles	ca. 20% at least mildly subfertile couples	i. e., 50% of these couples will conceive in the next six cycles; the other half is considerably subfertile or infertile
After 12 unsuccessful cycles	ca. 10% considerably subfertile couples (old clinical definition of sterility)	i. e., ca. 50% of these couples still have a chance of spontaneously conceiving in the next 36 months (!); the other half is infertile
After 48 unsuccessful months	ca. 5% definitely infertile couples	i. e., with only sporadic chances of conceiving

tant because in cases with a fertility problem, enough time must remain for utilizing the tools of reproductive medicine. For a woman past the age of 40, the chance of becoming pregnant with the assistance of reproductive medicine is only about 10–20% of that of a woman aged 30–35. The most important factor is here the declining function of the ovaries.

There are many reasons why a pregnancy does not occur. In the woman, we have to check for:

- hormonal disorders (disturbed hypothalamic regulation, hypophysic insufficiency, polycystic ovary syndrome, premature ovarian exhaustion, disturbed thyroid function, hyperprolactinemia)
- a declining reserve of ovarian function (age, previous surgery)
- anatomical changes in the female genital organs (e.g., tubal occlusion, uterine deformity, cervical sterility, e.g., after surgical intervention in conization or after inflammation)
- endometriosis

In the man, we have to check for:

- damage to the testicles resulting in insufficient semen production
- congenital or acquired blockage of the vas deferens
- ejaculatory disorders

The cause is also often found in both partners, such as, for example, in compatibility disorders (immunological sterility, often as a result of inflammation in the area of the inner genitals). Mild disturbances in both partners frequently add up, to the point where nature is no longer able to compensate. Western medicine nowadays fails in every fifth to 10th case to find the precise cause for infertility (so-called idiopathic sterility).

Diagnosis of Subfertility, Infertility, and Sterility

The diagnostic tools of **reproductive medicine** in subfertility, infertility, and sterility of men and women consist of:

- hormonal tests: especially gonadotropin (LH and FSH), examinations of the androgen metabolism, anti-Mullerian hormone, endometriosis

activity parameter (CA 125), thyroid hormones, prolactin
- ultrasound
- hysteroscopy and laparoscopy
- screening for infections

For TCM practitioners the so-called cervix factors (especially cervical mucus quality and quantity, opening of the uterine orifice, position and consistency of the portio uteri) and the basal temperature curve carry a high diagnostic value.

In contemporary scientific literature, the term "basic infertility workup" after six unsuccessful cycles has gained acceptance. In this basic examination, the levels of the gonadotropins LH and FSH, AMH, TSH, prolactin, testosterone, androstenedione, and DHEAS (dehydroepiandrosterone) are determined on the third to fifth day of the cycle to clarify the endocrinological environment, and a basic ultrasound is performed to count the number of small antral follicles (6–8 mm diameter) in both ovaries. In addition, a further ultrasound examination can be carried out around the time of ovulation at the peak of mucus secretion (see p. 49) as evidence for the development of a dominant follicle and synchronous development of the endometrium. At the same time, this examination can also determine simple uterine anomalies like an adenomyosis uteri. The basic ultrasound exam also serves to purposely eliminate the possibility of myomas, polyps, a hydrosalpinx, and uterine deformities. Also on the day of maximum mucus level, a postcoital test can be carried out to exclude the possibility of interaction disorders and of cervical sterility. This test has a high prognostic value in cases of idiopathic sterility (spontaneous conception probability). In cases of suspected uterotubal pathology, a hysteroscopy and hysterocontrastsonography, possibly also a laparoscopy with chromopertubation, can be performed in the first half of the cycle. Due to its invasive nature, though, the indication for a laparoscopy with chromopertubation should be given only under strict parameters and has on the whole declined in significance.

Six to 8 days after the rise in temperature, determining the level of estradiol and progesterone can prove the sufficient luteinization of the dominant follicle and eliminate a latent weakness of the corpus luteum.

Of course, the beginning of any check-up on subfertility and infertility also includes an examination of the man. After 3–5 days of rest, a basic spermiogram in accordance with WHO criteria should be carried out (see **Table 6.1**). In addition, in cases of suspected limited male potency (condition after undescended testicles, condition after infections, absence of male gametes in the sperm, ejaculatory disorders, condition after varicocele surgery, condition after surgery in the groins), an andrological examination should be carried out that includes determining testicular volume, checking testicular circulation, and a testicular sonography.

Due to the special significance in TCM, the examination of the uterine cervix is presented here in greater detail. The cervical mucus changes in quality in relation to the phases of the cycle (**Fig. 6.3**). Under the influence of estrogen, it becomes increasingly clear and stretchable (spinnbarkeit), which is an important precondition for the capacitation of the sperm.

In addition, the portio uteri becomes deeper and the external os of the uterus widens. This stage signifies the optimal point for conception. At the same time, scientific research has shown that the quality of the cervical mucus on the day of intercourse is more important for maintaining optimal conception chances than the distance in time between intercourse and ovulation itself.

An additional method of infertility diagnosis is the course of the basal temperature curve. The basal temperature is the body temperature measured in the morning after waking up. At the time of ovulation or shortly thereafter, the core body temperature rises slightly (basal temperature curve, BT), due to the effect of progesterone on the hypothalamus and the slowing down of skin circulation; the temperature does not drop back down until the end of the cycle. The rise in temperature is often relatively small, sometimes only 0.2 °C (0.4 °F). This rise is proof for the luteinization of the mature follicle, hence almost always also for ovulation itself. For measuring the basal temperature curve, the following is important:

- Measure in the morning: immediately after waking, before getting up, before any other activity.
- Measure for 5 minutes, orally or vaginally, not under the arm.
- Do not change the method of measuring within one cycle.
- After disturbed nightrest: sleep or relax in bed for about an hour before measuring.
- Begin measuring after the menstrual period when cervical mucus production starts.*
- You can stop measuring after the rise in temperature.

Cycle days		1	2	3	4	5	6	7	8	9	10	11	12	13	14	15	16	17	18	19
Mucus	Bleeding																			
	Sensation/feeling						Dry	Dry	Dry	Dry	Moist	Moist	Moist	Wet	Wet	Moist	Moist	Moist	Dry	
	Appearance						|	|	|	|	|	Whitish	Stretchable	Stretchable	Stretchable	Creamy	Thick	Thick	|	
Neck of the uterus	Position and opening						•	•	•	•	o	o	o	o	o	•	•	•	•	
	Firmness						h	h	h	h	s	s	s	s	s	h	h	h	h	
	Intercourse																			
	Fertile days																			
	LH test																			
	Medical findings																			

Fig. 6.3 Typical change in cervical mucus and portio uteri in the course of the cycle.

---

* This applies when the intention is to determine ovulation from the biomedical perspective. For TCM diagnosis, on the other hand, you should measure continuously.

The body temperature is subject to the biorhythm; it is lower in the morning than in the afternoon. In many women, though, deviations of 1.5 hours in the measuring time are insignificant. Different circumstances can elevate the temperature and perhaps even simulate a rise in temperature.

Possible factors that interfere with the temperature are:

- unusually late measuring time
- going to bed unusually late
- unusual alcohol consumption
- late partying
- stress
- emotional strain
- traveling
- climatic change
- short or interrupted night's sleep

Ideally, the temperature values are entered in a cycle sheet with 0.1 °C (0.2 °F) gradation. The temperature values are connected to each other. In addition, you should also enter symptomatic information on the cervical mucus and the pattern of bleeding.

Ignore any abnormal elevated temperature values that jut out upward from the usual range of variation among the low temperature values before ovulation and that can be explained by a potential interference factor; disregard these in the analysis of the curve in accordance with the rules of the **symptothermal method of natural family planning**. It is important to recognize the rise in temperature because this indicates whether and when ovulation has taken place.

Symptothermal Method of Natural Family Planning

The rules of the symptothermal method of natural family planning (STM of NFP) serve to identify the correct rise in temperature instead of wrongly identifying another elevation in temperature as the temperature rise. A temperature rise (**Fig. 6.4**) has taken place when three successive readings are higher than the six previous readings (the so-called "three-over-six rule").

In addition, the third higher reading must be at least 0.2 °C (0.4 °F) higher than the highest of the preceding six low temperature readings.

Note the following two exceptions:

1. If the third temperature reading is not 0.2 °C (0.4 °F) higher, you have to wait for a fourth reading, which merely has to lie above the six low values (**Fig. 6.5**).
2. In between the three higher values, a reading can fall below or on the imagined line through the preceding six low temperature readings. This value is then ignored in the analysis of the temperature rise (**Fig. 6.6**).

The rules of the STM of NFP have been validated in numerous studies; additional information on the rules of the STM of NFP can be found in the literature.[1]

Ovulation usually takes place 1–2 days before the first higher reading, occasionally also on the first day of the higher reading itself. For diagnostic purposes in biomedicine as well as in TCM, addi-

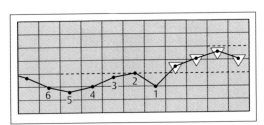

Fig. 6.4 Determining the rise in temperature.

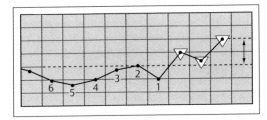

Fig. 6.5 Determining the rise in temperature; exception 1.

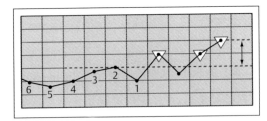

Fig. 6.6 Determining the rise in temperature; exception 2.

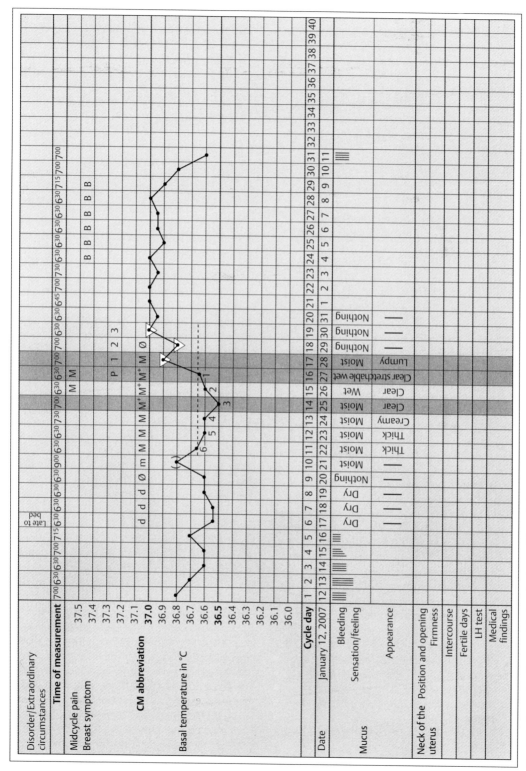

Fig. 6.7 Example of a completed cycle sheet with analysis.

tional symptoms can be entered on the cycle sheet, such as mid-cycle pain, mastodynia (pain in the breasts), ovulation bleeding, as well as consistency and position of the vaginal portion of the cervix.

Due to its special significance in TCM diagnostics, we discuss the interpretation of the basal temperature curve in more detail below (see pp. 59 ff). **Fig. 6.7** shows a typical BT curve of a healthy woman.

■ Biomedical Methods for the Treatment of Infertility and Sterility

The therapeutic strategies of TCM must be synchronized with those of biomedicine. In order to accomplish this, it is necessary to acquire a basic knowledge of modern reproductive medicine in addition to the suitable treatment strategies and principles of TCM. In this section, we explain the basic terms of reproductive medicine and its therapeutic techniques.

Depending on the cause of infertility, different therapeutic approaches are utilized. Here, we present a hierarchy of the various options for intervention by means of reproductive medicine—from less invasive to highly invasive methods. These are selected in accordance with the type of disorder:

1. **Hormone therapy for cycle optimization** (supporting follicular maturation and optimizing the luteal phase for intercourse at the optimal point in time):
   - oligomenorrhea
   - luteal insufficiency
   - for the timing of ovulation
2. **Intrauterine insemination (IUI)**:
   - mildly deficient sperm quality
   - interactive disorders in the area of the cervix (so-called immunological sterility)
   - cervical sterility
   - idiopathic sterility
   - impotentia coeundi (inability to complete intercourse)
   - uterotubal transport disorders (adenomyosis uteri)

3. **In vitro fertilization (IVF)**:
   - functional disorders of the fallopian tubes
   - mildly deficient semen quality
   - endometriosis
   - idiopathic sterility (infertility without known cause)
   - after hormone treatment and polyfollicular development to prevent multiple pregnancies
   - immunological sterility
4. **Intracytoplasmatic sperm injection (ICSI)**:
   - severely deficient semen quality
   - when fertilization fails in conventional in vitro fertilization

Hormone Therapy for Cycle Optimization

Provided that the woman has passable tubes and a partner with acceptable fertility, cycle-optimizing hormone therapy can be the first step (optimizing follicular maturation and supporting the luteal phase). In cases with delayed follicular maturation or luteal weakness but with an intact hypothalamus-hypophysis-ovarian axis, follicular maturation can be stimulated with Clomifen or subcutaneous injection of the gonadotropin FSH (follicle-stimulating hormone). Clomifen is an estrogen antagonist that blocks the hypothalamic and hypophysic estrogen receptors without triggering the following signal cascade. This simulates a peripheral estrogen deficiency. The body reacts by increasing the secretion of FSH, which stimulates follicle formation in the ovaries. The success of follicular recruitment and maturation can be evaluated by ultrasound. From a follicle diameter of about 18 mm upwards, administering human chorionic gonadotropin (hCG) will trigger ovulation. This process takes advantage of the fact that human chorionic gonadotropin has a strong LH effect. Especially due to its long half-life, 80% of all ovulations occur 36–48 hours after administering hCG. Shortly before the expected ovulation, the couple should engage in sexual intercourse.

When Clomifen is taken, insufficient proliferation of the endometrium is observed occasionally, due to its estrogen-antagonistic effect. This anti-estrogen effect can also change the cervical mucus so that it becomes more difficult for the sperm to pass. The negative effect on the endometrium is regarded as one cause for the low pregnancy rate in Clomifen-stimulated cycles. In addition, it is suspected to thereby cause a higher rate of miscarriage. Therefore, follicular stimulation with gonadotropines (controlled ovarian hyperstimulation) is a commonly used option. Disadvantages are the high costs and the danger of polyovulation (also possible with Clomifen) with increased risk of multiple pregnancies. Because of the higher success rate, gonadotropine stimulation should if possible be combined with intrauterine insemination (IUI).

Intrauterine Insemination

In deficient sperm quality, compatibility disorders, or as the first therapeutic step in unexplained sterility, intrauterine insemination (IUI) is indicated. After ovarian stimulation, prepared sperm are injected with a thin catheter into the fundus of the uterus and both tubes at the ideal point in time. Scientific data proves that especially intrauterine insemination after gonadotropine stimulation increases the chances of pregnancy by four as compared with the approach of simply waiting. Extensive analysis of the records shows, however, that pregnancy rates by means of intrauterine insemination are still disappointingly low with a total of 9–12%. Above the age of 35, they clearly drop even further. It is, however, essential that the indication for insemination is given correctly. Moreover, no more than three to four insemination cycles should be performed since further attempts hardly offer additional chances for a pregnancy. Modified insemination techniques like double insemination in the cycle or intratubal micro-insemination do not offer advantages either, since they do not make the method more effective. In combination with hormone treatment, on the other hand, intrauterine insemination also carries the risk of multiple pregnancies. Almost all high-grade multiple pregnancies (triplets and especially quadruplets) come from insemination cycles! One advantage of this treatment strategy that is important in our times is the low costs to insurance companies and patients.

In Vitro Fertilization

For in vitro fertilization (IVF), the woman should ideally be under 40 years of age; in addition, at least one ovary and the uterus have to be functioning properly. The typical IVF procedure looks like this:

In a pretreatment cycle, the follicle cohort ready for stimulation is synchronized by means of a special antibaby pill. Overlapping with this, the so-called down-regulation (long protocol) begins with the desensitization and complete emptying of the pituitary gland, as a result of which it no longer discharges any FSH and LH. This prevents premature ovulation and—for example, in women with hormonal disorders—improves the quality of the maturing egg cells. The retrieval of egg cells (follicle punction) can be planned in a relatively large window for the possible administration of hCG.

A new, additional option for suppressing premature ovulation consists of administering so-called GnRH antagonists, which competitively antagonize the effect of the hypothalamic regulatory hormone of the hypophysis. The specific selection of one or the other stimulation protocol must be reserved for the specialist and clinical experience.

Stimulation aims at bringing several eggs (around 5–20) to maturity. Nowadays, a variety of drugs are administered to stimulate the granulosa cells of the follicles (cells that surround the oocyte). These include:
- highly purified hMG (human menopausal gonadotropin, contains equal parts of FSH, LH, and some hCG)
- genetically produced recombinant FSH and LH

If the follicles have been able to mature long enough (at least 6 days), hCG injection induces ovulation. Of main biological significance is hereby the fact that this signal causes the oocyte to complete its first meiotic division and to halve its chromosome set (expulsion of the so-called polar body). It becomes clear that inducing ovulation and timing are of great significance for the quality of the oocyte and the success of the performed treatment.

After about 35 hours, the egg cells are sucked out of the follicles shortly before spontaneous ovulation in a minor surgery by transvaginal, ultrasound-guided punction (follicle punction). After a short period of incubation in special cell culture mediums, the egg cells are fertilized with the processed semen fluid. The fertilized eggs are first cultured for 16–18 hours and then examined to determine whether fertilization has taken place. But before this, the egg cells must be extricated from the surrounding tissue. At this time, a first quality check of the fertilized eggs (the so-called zygotes) can take place (**Fig. 6.8**).

Assessments about developmental potential and chromosomal integrity are possible. The most suitable two or at most three fertilized oocytes are cultured for an additional 2–3, sometimes 5 days. Surplus fertilized oocytes in which the nuclei are not yet melted together (syngamy) can be frozen for later cycles. For various reasons, transferring the embryo on day 2–3 has proven to be most favorable. At this point in time, the embryos are in the four- or eight-cell stage (**Fig. 6.9**). Very carefully, they are then transferred to the lower part of the uterus by means of a thin catheter. The following luteal phase must be supported hormonally (especially with progesterone), otherwise pregnancy is unlikely to occur. A pregnancy test can be performed reliably 11–12 days after the embryo transfer.

A complete IVF cycle from day 1 of the antibaby pill to the pregnancy test hence takes about 6–7 weeks (**Table 6.5**). The chances of pregnancy are, depending on age, 25–40% per initiated IVF cycle. Data from the German IVF Registry clearly indicates a marked decrease in chances of pregnancy by IVF treatment for women from the age of 35 on. From 40 years on, the chances are only 10–20% of those of a woman between 30 and 35.

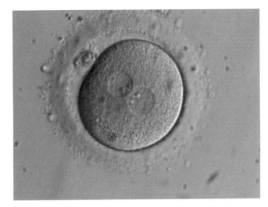

Fig. 6.8 Pronucleus stage. Sixteen hours after insemination and removal from the surrounding granulosa cells.

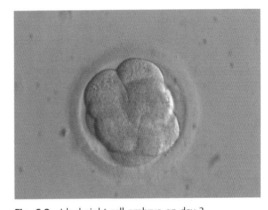

Fig. 6.9 Ideal eight-cell embryo on day 3.

Intracytoplasmatic Sperm Injection

The method of intracytoplasmatic sperm injection (ICSI, first introduced in 1992) has revolutionized modern reproductive medicine and has since given a child to many couples who would never have become parents otherwise. This method of microinjecting individual sperm cells into the mature egg cell is an additional measure within the framework of in vitro fertilization. It is indicated particularly in cases when very bad semen quality makes fertilization by means of conventional IVF doubtful. It is also used when a previous IVF resulted in no or only very few fertilizations. All steps—with the exception of inseminating the egg cells—are identical with the conventional IVF procedure. Under a special microscope, a single sperm is drawn up into a thin injection needle by means of micromanipulators and injected directly into the egg cell (**Fig. 6.10**). But the egg cell must previously have been extricated from the surrounding tissue (cumulus cells).

MESA and TESE

Both of these procedures are combined with intracytoplasmatic sperm injection (ICSI), especially in the most severe cases of male infertility with almost complete or even complete absence of sperm in the ejaculate (testicular damage or blockage of the vas deferens).

Table 6.5 Ultralong, programed stimulation protocol in the IVF area

Pre-cycle	PD	Mens	FSH (IE)						US				US	hCG	FoPu 35 hours	ET after 2–3 days
			200 or more						pot.	pot.	pot.	pot.			After hCG	
			150													
			100													
Pill			50													
	GnRHa															
1–	15(–21)		Injection day	1 Mi	2	3	4	5	6	7	8	9	10	ff		

Note: PD = pill day, US = ultrasound, Mi = begin of injections, mostly on a Wednesday or Thursday, ff = possible follow-up days, GnRHa = GnRH-agonist, pot. = potential dosis increase up to 400 IE FSH. FoPu = follicle punction, ET = embryo transfer.

MESA stands for microsurgical epididymal sperm aspiration. In this method, sperm is retrieved from the epididymis in cases where no sperm cells are present in the ejaculate. MESA is appropriate in:
- inoperable blockage of the vas deferens
- immotile sperm cells in the spermiogram
- ejaculatory disorders as a result of paraplegia or
- radical tumor surgery

TESE stands for testicular sperm extraction; in this technique, sperm is retrieved for ICSI in a testicular biopsy. Testicular biopsy is also a diagnostic procedure, as an initial test in cases of extremely limited spermiograms to see how high the chances of success are and to freeze testicular tissue for later IVF/ICSI therapy.

Methods to Complement IVF and ICSI

Methods to complement IVF and ICSI are:
- cryoconservation
- laser-assisted hatching
- spindle detection
- polar body biopsy

Cryoconservation

Often, more oocytes are fertilized than are used in subsequent culturing. To secure the "surplus oocytes" (we speak of fertilized zygotes or pronucleus stage), they can be frozen (cryoconserved). These fertilized egg cells are thawed in later cycles, cultured some more, and transferred as usual in the embryonal stage to the hormonally prepared uterus (so-called cryocycle).

The chance of pregnancy in a so-called cryocycle ranges between 20 and 25%. According to our experience up to now, fertilized egg cells (zygotes) can be kept frozen over many years.

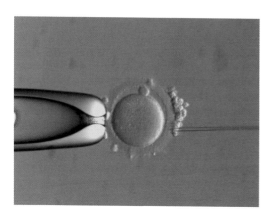

Fig. 6.10 Intracytoplasmatic sperm injection.

Laser-assisted Hatching

The egg cell and therefore also the embryo are surrounded by a protein cover, the so-called zona pellucida, until the sixth day. Before implantation, the embryo must "hatch" from the zona pellucida. For certain patient groups (women over 35, previous unsuccessful IVF attempts, women with an abnormally thick or dense zona pellucida), it has proven advantageous to assist the embryo in hatching by notching the zona pellucida with a diode laser (**Fig. 6.11**).

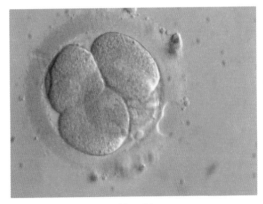

Fig. 6.11 Laser-assisted hatching.

Spindle Detection

Before an intracytoplasmatic sperm injection (ICSI), the spindle assembly, that is, the division assembly of the oocyte and the zona pellucida, can be visualized under computer-guided polarization microscopy (**Fig. 6.12**). For the first time, this has made possible a supravital quality and maturity check of the egg cells. Additionally, information about the localization of the spindle is important so that the spindle with the attached chromosomes will not be destroyed during ICSI, thereby avoiding a chromosomal maldistribution in subsequent cell divisions.

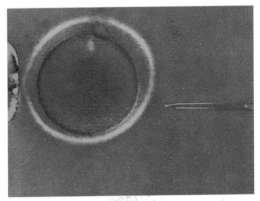

Fig. 6.12 Spindle detection by means of polarization microscopy prior to performing ICSI.

Polar Body Biopsy

In women from the age of 35 on, about 40% of all oocytes are chromosomally impaired; in women from age 40 on, about 50–70%. In order to identify oocytes with chromosomal maldistribution for chromosomes 13, 16, 18, 21, 22, and/or X and hereby exclude them from the transfer, a so-called polar body screening can be performed. The background for this procedure lies in the fact that the egg cell passes through two maturing divisions and thereby eliminates half of its chromosomes. These surplus chromosomes stay outside in the two polar bodies, which can be retrieved and examined for the above-mentioned chromosomes by means of a molecular genetic procedure, the so-called FISH analysis. Because the genetic material is distributed equally among the oocytes and the polar bodies, we can thereby draw conclusions on the chromosomes present inside the oocyte (**Fig. 6.13**).

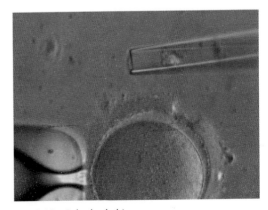

Fig. 6.13 Polar body biopsy.

Diagnostic certainty for this method lies at 90–95% when both polar bodies are retrieved, and at 80% if only the first polar body is retrieved. Nevertheless, this examination only makes sense when six to eight oocytes or five fertilized egg cells are available, because otherwise no embryo is left over for transfer after the selection. In addition, this method only provides information on the maternal set of chromosomes. This examination is therefore no substitute for a prenatal diagnosis.

Risks of Treatment with Reproductive Medicine

Risks to the Woman in the Stimulation Phase

In rare cases, hormonal treatment to stimulate the ovaries can lead to complications because the effective hormone dose varies considerably not only from one woman to another but can even vary substantially within the same woman from one cycle to another. The chosen hormone dose depends on the woman's age and hormonal preconditions. For a better estimation of the necessary dose, it is helpful to count the antral follicles by means of ultrasound and determine the so-called anti-Mullerian hormone (AMH). If the selected hormonal dose is too small, the stimulation cycle must sometimes be interrupted. No harm is done in this case. If the selected hormonal dose is too large, however, the stimulation effect on the ovaries can result in an overstimulation. A potentially triggered ovulation can then lead to an even greater enlargement of the ovaries, in extreme cases with accumulation of fluid in the abdominal cavity and chest. This results in blood coagulation with a risk of blood clots (thrombosis) and very rarely even in embolisms. In addition, the increased pressure in the abdominal cavity that is the result of considerable ascites formation decreases circulation in the kidneys, which can lead to kidney failure.

Nevertheless, severe overstimulation syndromes occur only in 1–2% of performed stimulation cycles. Careful supervision during treatment allows for an early detection of such complications. Treatment of an overstimulation syndrome consists of giving infusions and anti-coagulant medications; in exceptional cases, the woman must be treated in hospital.

Risks to the Woman during Punction

In less than 1% of all cases, complications occur during punction of the ovaries. Punction is performed via the vagina under visual control with ultrasound; organ injuries are therefore rare. It is, however, possible that blood vessels in the vagina, ovaries, bladder, or intestines are injured. In addition, inflammatory reactions in the area of the ovaries have been reported. Nevertheless, complications during follicle punction can be treated effectively and successfully if recognized early enough.

Risks to the Woman after the Embryo Transfer

Ectopic pregnancies (in ca. 3% of all cases) and miscarriages (in 15–20% of all cases) can also happen after an IVF treatment. The frequency of these unfortunate pregnancy results is, however, in general no greater than in any other pregnancies. Nevertheless, we must take into account the age of the woman during treatment, the source of sperm, the cause of the infertility, and also the duration of fertility treatment so far, all of which affect the rate of miscarriage.

Multiple Pregnancies

Treatments with reproductive medicine clearly lead to an increase in multiple pregnancies. Fortunately, more refined methods and the practice of transferring three embryos only in exceptional cases have clearly lowered this higher risk of multiples in the last few years. A higher rate of multiple pregnancies is therefore found today particularly after insemination treatments in which the number of mature egg cells could not be determined properly. The 2005 data on in vitro fertilization by the Center of Disease Control and Prevention (CDC) shows that one in three pregnancies resulted in the birth of twins, triplets, or higher (twins 28.5% and triplets 4.4%)[8]. Quadruplets are the exception, fortunately. Multiple pregnancy not only presents a health risk to the future mother but are also a considerable risk to the health of the unborn children.

Risks to Children Born after Assisted Reproduction

The risks to children born after assisted reproduction are initially caused primarily by the increased age of the future mother on the one hand and the above-mentioned greater risk of multiples and the related premature birth rate on the other hand. Premature birth is and remains the greatest risk factor for severe disabilities in children. We must count on neonatal deformities as the possible cause of later disabilities in about 3–7% of all births, of which 1% are severe.

After ICSI was introduced into the treatment of infertility in 1992, a discussion erupted regarding the safety of this method with regard to neonatal deformities. Different studies have reached greatly divergent results, largely due to methodology. A large German study with 3372 children born after ICSI found that the risk of deformities for these children increased by the order of 1035–1113, compared with children from spontaneous pregnancies. The adjusted risk calculation turned out to be statistically insignificant, which means that the ICSI method in itself apparently does not lead to an increased risk of deformities. It appears certain, though, that couples with an unfulfilled wish for children carry a risk for neonatal deformities that increases in correlation with the duration of this wish. This includes, for example, the proven increase in genital deformities in boys and the increased risk of number-related deviations of the sex chromosomes in all children produced by ICSI. Hereby, we must take into consideration that chromosome anomalies are 10 times higher in couples with fertility disorders than in the average population. From the genetic perspective, there appears to be no difference in whether the sperm used in the ICSI came from the ejaculate or was retrieved surgically (TESE or MESA). For more detailed information on these very important questions of the risks of assisted reproduction, see the literature.[22]

Summary of the Risks

In conclusion, our current state of knowledge suggests that it is not the method of IVF or ICSI itself that increases the rate of deformities, but rather that infertility presents a risk in itself. Ultimately, we cannot know which effects an intervention into reproduction has. The indication for a medical genetics consultation should therefore be given generously to all couples desiring children.

Pregnancies that occur following measures of assisted reproduction are burdened by two factors as risk pregnancies: first by the increased multiples rate, and second by the higher average age of the woman.

Multiple pregnancies are linked to a clearly increased risk of premature birth. Fertility centers in the United States therefore generally recommend not to transfer more than two embryos in women under 35 and to transfer three or four embryos in women over 35. With hormonal stimulation, no insemination should be performed and no intercourse at the optimal point for conception should be advised when more than three follicles can be verified sonographically.

For detailed numbers on assisted reproduction see the literature.[8]

Options of TCM in the Treatment of Infertility and Sterility

What role does TCM play in the optimization of biomedical therapy methods? The decision on whether to attempt to reach the goal by the sole use of TCM or whether a combination with increasingly invasive methods of reproductive medicine is necessary is influenced, among other factors, by the following data:
- age of the couple
- endocrinologic results
- condition of the sperm
- "tube factor" (passability/mobility of the fallopian tubes)
- anatomical changes

In this section, we explain the therapeutic options of TCM.

Special Characteristics of TCM Diagnosis and Therapy

The topic of infertility concerns couples who often do not manifest any of the typical TCM syndromes; that is, traditional TCM diagnosis does not necessarily supply all the information that is necessary to realize differentiated therapeutic consequences. An example is kidney vacuity, a common condition in infertility or sterility: affected couples do not always manifest the typical TCM symptoms for kidney vacuity (such as back pain, pollakiuria, nocturia, tendency to feel cold, cold feet, vertigo, tinnitus, lack of tongue fur). This means that terms and concepts from biomedicine such as basal temperature curve, cervical mucus, phase-specific therapy, or spermiogram must be included as well.

Women who undergo fertility treatment frequently have no other signs that point to a certain pattern of disorders; only the BT curve gives information that can be used for diagnosis and therapeutic consequences. With the BT curve, TCM practitioners have been given a simple tool to gain a large amount of information.

Scientific medicine has also recognized the diagnostic value of self-observation ("fertility awareness," cycle monitoring by means of the basal temperature curve and observation of the cervical mucus). "Fertility awareness" is a natural method of family planning that teaches us to distinguish fertile from infertile days in relation to the cycle, for the purpose of determining the optimal time for conception. But "fertility awareness" also means to become conscious of changes in your fertility and to consciously take these into consideration in designing your life ("reproductive competence"). This is particularly significant because in Western societies the desire for children has increasingly been deferred to the later years in life, resulting in a growing risk of becoming subor infertile. Here, TCM and biomedicine meet because "fertility awareness" also means awareness of the risk factors for fertility (e. g., tubular damage from inflammatory processes in the area of the internal genitals, age-related decrease in fertility) and promotes familiarity with possible protective measures ("fertility protection"). As such, both TCM and biomedicine pursue a preventative goal.

Diagnostic Procedures in TCM

The four diagnostic methods—inspection, inquiry, smelling, and palpation—that are normally used to acquire information on physiology and pathology in TCM are in this context expanded by a very important additional method: measuring and evaluating the course of the **basal temperature curve (BT curve)**.

Basal Temperature Curve and Chinese Pattern Diagnosis

During the first half of the cycle (days 1–13), when an increasing secretion of estrogen occurs, *yin* begins to grow—immediately after the onset of menstrual bleeding. This reaches its peak with ovulation, that is, around the time when estrogen concentration peaks as well. Now begins the phase of transformation from *yin* to *yang*. The progesterone level begins to rise and falls again towards the end of the cycle (see **Fig. 6.1**).

Typical Pathogenic Basal Temperature Patterns in the Follicular Phase

Basal Temperature in the Follicular Phase Below the Desired Value
On day 1 of the cycle, the temperature should fall to its basal level, measured rectally to values between 36.2 and 36.5 °C (between 97.16 and 97.7 °F). If the BT lies clearly below this range, for example, below 36.0 °C (96.8 °F) this is interpreted as a general lack of *yang*, here particularly as a lack of spleen and kidney *yang*. This results in the therapeutic necessity to support *yang* in the entire cycle.

Biomedical Opinion.[14] The basal temperature curve in the follicular phase is subject to considerable inter-individual and intra-individual fluctuations. The method of measuring is decisive. Here, we find a remarkable difference between (now no longer available) mercury thermometers and modern digital thermometers. Measurements with infrared thermometers are unsuited! In rare cases, hypothyroidism can certainly be accompanied by a lowered body temperature, when other factors have been excluded.

Extended Follicular Phase

An extended follicular phase, clearly lasting past the normal 14 days, can possibly be caused by an existing *qi* stagnation. In cases with a pronounced lack of kidney *jing*, ovulation can fail to take place at all. Accordingly, we must choose therapeutic measures to nurture kidney *jing, yin,* and blood, and implement these over a longer period of time (**Fig. 6.14**).

Biomedical Opinion.[14] Extended follicular phases (longer than 20 days) are a sign of disturbed follicle maturation, for example, in the context of hyperandrogenemic, hyperprolactinemic, or dysgonadotropic ovarian insufficiency (central regulatory disorder). Up to a total cycle length of 35 days, we cannot assume a considerable reduction in the probability rate for spontaneous pregnancy if the subsequent luteal phase (temperature peak) lasts for at least 10–12 days and no intermittent bleeding occurs. If the temperature peak is shortened or shows an arched course, this suggests a luteal phase insufficiency. Because of the clearly reduced chance of conception, follicle maturation disorders with consecutive luteal phase insufficiency or follicle maturation disorders with a follicular phase of more than 20 days require treatment (i.e., ovarian stimulation therapy) by an experienced physician.

Abbreviated Follicular Phase

In an abbreviated follicular phase (9–10 days), the phase must be prolonged because follicle and ovum must mature first. *Yin* and blood are lost during menstruation but are then needed directly for maturing the egg cell. The process of nurturing *yin* and blood must begin early enough, approximately from day 3 on.

Biomedical Opinion.[14] Abbreviated cycles (< 23 days, **Fig. 6.15**) are pathological and must be cleared up. We must question whether we are faced with real menstrual periods or with pathological intermittent bleeding. The combination of an abbreviated follicular phase with a subsequent corpus luteum insufficiency is critical and indicates a failing ovarian function. Shortly before the final tapering of the menstrual process, the cycles become longer due to follicular persistence and cyst formation, in which case we often do not notice any rise in temperature or notice only a mar-ginal rise, which is related to the spontaneous luteinization of the dominant follicle.

Basal Temperature in the Follicular Phase Above the Desired Value

An excessively high BT in the follicular phase (above 36.6 °C) (97.88 °F) can be a sign of hyperthyroidism. When there are signs of internal heat, you must clear the heat and strengthen *yin.*

Biomedical Opinion.[14] A rise in the basal temperature values can be caused by hyperthyroidism or by chronic inflammatory diseases. Nevertheless, most often the cause remains unknown. We do not have scientific data on the relevance of the basal body temperature for the prospects of a spontaneous pregnancy, but such data is certainly known for the above-mentioned diseases that can affect body temperature.

Basal Temperature Fails to Drop on Day 1 of the Cycle

If the basal temperature does not drop on day 1 of the cycle, that is, *yang* fails to transform into *yin,* this is a sign of blood stasis. In such cases, we must support the complete elimination of blood.

Biomedical Opinion.[14] Prolonged high temperatures and a slow return of the body temperature to its pre-ovulatory level is most likely caused by a biochemical pregnancy, that is, an early pregnancy that does not last and can only be proven by an hCG test. Occasionally we observe incomplete luteinization in very young women with cycles that are still maturing.

Unstable Temperatures in the Follicular Phase

A so-called unstable follicular phase, with temperature variations of more than 0.2–0.3 °C (0.3–0.5 °F) is interpreted as liver and heart fire. We must calm the spirit and clear liver and heart fire. Stress reduction, a more regular lifestyle, and a regimen of relaxation exercises are recommended to complement treatment.

Biomedical Opinion.[14] Unstable temperatures in the follicular phase are a common occurrence in the biomedical evaluation of the basal temperature curve. The interfering factors mentioned in the introduction affect the body temperature in different ways. Stress reduction and an appropri-

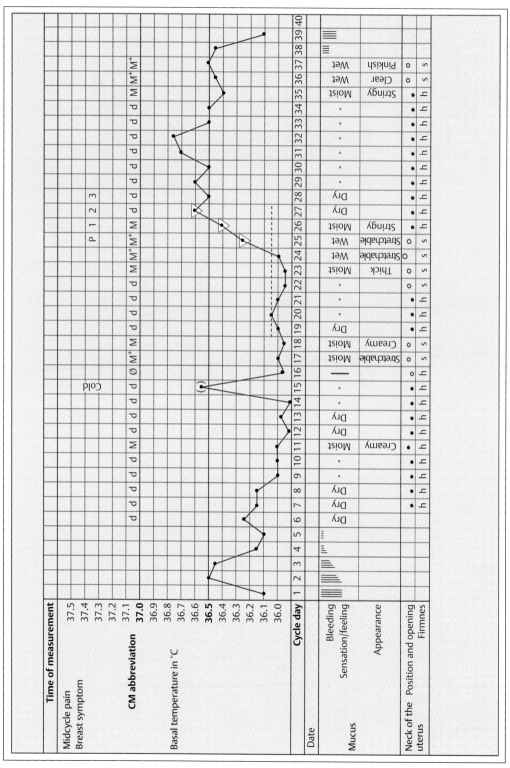

Fig. 6.14 Clearly extended cycle, but with stable corpus luteum phase.

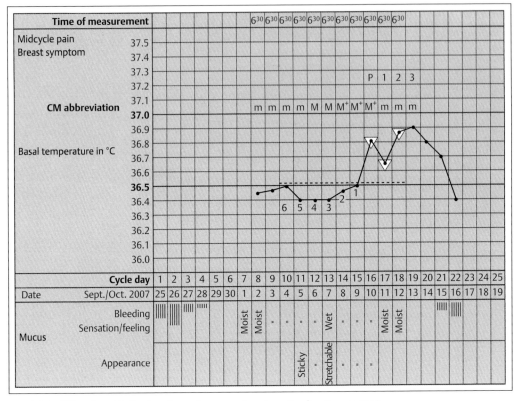

Fig. 6.15 Abbreviated follicular phase. *Beware:* reduced ovarian function reserve!

ate lifestyle are therefore advised also from the biomedical perspective. This is certainly one of the great strong points of TCM.

Typical Pathogenic Basal Temperature Patterns in the Luteal Phase

Delayed Basal Temperature Rise in the Luteal Phase

If the temperature rises too slowly after ovulation, this is a sign of kidney *yang* vacuity, related to spleen *qi* vacuity. The cause can be found in an original *yin* vacuity because a good foundation of *yin* is necessary for the formation of *yang*, or in *qi* stagnation, which prevents the transformation of *yin* to *yang*. Consequently, therapy can aim at supporting *yin* in the first half of the cycle and subsequently at assisting movement (liver *qi*) around the middle of the cycle.

Biomedical Opinion.[14] A delayed temperature rise in the luteal phase is found most commonly in cases of disturbed follicular maturation as an early sign of a beginning weakness in the luteal phase that should be addressed in further detail.

Premature Basal Temperature Drop in the Luteal Phase

If the temperature rises but cannot be sustained long enough (less than 12 days) on the higher level, this is a sign of kidney *yang* vacuity. In a clearly abbreviated luteal phase, we must prescribe medicinals in subsequent cycles that strengthen the kidneys to solve this problem.

Biomedical Opinion.[14] Typical sign of corpus luteum insufficiency.

Basal Temperature in the Luteal Phase Below the Desired Value

If the temperature fails to reach the desired height (less than 0.3 °C [0.5 F]), this indicates a clear kidney *yang* vacuity. You must support the foundation of kidney *yang*, namely kidney *yin*. Only a sufficient foundation of kidney *yin* can ensure the adequate formation of kidney *yang*. Depending on the symptoms, *qi* or blood vacuity can also play a background role.

Biomedical Opinion.[14] Typical sign of corpus luteum insufficiency.**Unstable Basal Temperature Values in the Luteal Phase (Sawtooth Pattern)**

An unstable luteal phase in which the temperature initially rises adequately with ovulation but afterwards oscillates widely points to an instability of heart and liver *qi*. Such a pattern tends to develop as a result of emotional imbalance and can usually be recognized already in the follicular phase. Stress reduction and relaxation techniques are necessary with concurrent nurturing of blood.

Biomedical Opinion.[14] Possible sign of corpus luteum insufficiency.

Unstable Basal Temperature Values in the Luteal Phase (Saddle Pattern)

In a saddle-type pattern, the temperature rises once approximately 1 week after ovulation and then drops back down to the desired value. This is a sign of an insufficiently functioning corpus luteum and a resulting lack of progesterone. In TCM, we can interpret it as a vacuity of spleen and stomach *qi*. Because this problem concerns a sensitive cycle phase (moment of implantation), supportive intervention makes sense.

Biomedical Opinion.[14] Possible sign of corpus luteum insufficiency.

Cervical Factors

Cervical factors like the amount of cervical secretions, their stretchability, and the cervix width are of particular importance as diagnostic information to TCM practitioners. In addition to the body temperature, the quantity and quality of the cervical mucus also change throughout the course of the cycle.

If fertility is optimal, the body secretes abundant clear mucus from the glands in the neck of the uterus before ovulation. This secretion should additionally be stretchable into 5–10-cm-long strings. After ovulation, the secretion again becomes thicker and is no longer clear. In addition, the cervix should be open at the moment of ovulation, and the mucus membranes should be hyperemic, that is, well-supplied with blood. We have already pointed out the special significance of the cervical mucus for sperm function and for determining the optimal conditions for conception.

The patient should pay attention to the amount and stretchability of her cervical mucus; deficient mucus formation is a sign of *yin* deficiency.

Therapeutic Options of TCM when Assisting Reproductive Medicine

Optimizing the Cycle and Timed Intercourse

The category of patients with the diagnosis of "idiopathic sterility," that is, infertility without any recognizable cause, includes many patients with a hidden disturbance of gamete interaction. In other words, these patients suffer from a disordered maturation of the ovum, with a high percentage of egg cells that are not fertilizable, or from disturbed sperm function in the partner, either of which would only become obvious in IVF treatment. Often, we also see the symptoms of premenstrual syndrome (PMS) and dysmenorrhea in this group. Such couples profit the most from the possibilities of TCM, for example, in the areas of cycle optimization and timed intercourse.

In addition to this group of patients, patients with anovulatory infertility who suffer from dysfunction of the hypothalamus-hypophysis axis in biomedical terms profit from the possibilities of TCM as well.

The most common diagnoses for these types of problems are:
- kidney vacuity
- blood vacuity
- *qi* stagnation
- blood stasis
- accumulation of dampness and phlegm

By evaluating the BT curve, cervical mucus, menstrual period (amount, color, consistency), accompanying symptoms (pain, emotional instability, disturbed sleep, sweating), pulse, and tongue, we can analyze and differentiate the individual condition of the patient. Necessary therapeutic measures can be chosen accordingly: acupuncture, medicinal therapy, nutritional therapy, and *qi gong*.

Assisting Intrauterine Insemination

When a specialist in reproductive medicine decides on intrauterine insemination (IUI), assistance with TCM therapy is no different from assistance with cycle optimization and timed intercourse.

Assisting In Vitro Fertilization

The following factors are important for determining the indication for IVF treatment:
- age of the couple
- tubal factor
- quality of the spermiogram
- individual attitudes of the couple

In relatively young couples (woman under 37 years), treatment with TCM only (medicinal therapy, acupuncture, nutritional therapy, *qi gong*) is recommended for the duration of six cycles. If pregnancy fails to take place in this time frame, the question of IVF must be discussed anew. When the indication for IVF is clear, the following course of action is recommended:

Preparatory Phase. A preparatory phase of three cycles with simultaneous treatment of the male partner is ideal.

Therapeutic Principle. Treatment should focus on regulating and harmonizing in accordance with the cycle (see Chapter 22). The IVF protocol can then be assisted by TCM as follows:

TCM Assistance to the IVF Protocol

Down-regulation (cycle before the start of stimulation in the IVF cycle): Emphasize supplementing treatment strategy (*bu fa, yin* and blood).

Menstrual phase: move *qi* and blood. "New blood can be formed when old blood has been

---

eliminated." Thus wrote already Sun Simiao (581–682).[13] This means that we promote a gentle harmonious menstrual period and ensure that the old endometrium is completely sloughed off, to facilitate the construction of an ideal new mucous membrane.

Stimulation phase (day 2 of the cycle up to follicle punction): nurture *yin* and blood. In this phase, a new endometrium is constructed in the uterus. In the Chinese view, this means that we must strengthen *yin* and blood for this purpose and in addition support follicular development. Our goal is here to support the formation of about six to eight mature follicles of good quality (the number is handled differently in individual IVF centers). For concrete measures, see Chapter 22.

Follicle punction and **embryo transfer**: in the literature, we find two opinions on the processes in this phase. On the one hand, the phase is seen as a dynamic process with the transformation of *yin* into *yang*, and nidation is regarded likewise (follicle rupture and the emergence of the egg cell, hatching of the egg from the zona pellucida, and penetration of the embryo into the endometrium; e. g., Paulus et al.[26]). This movement is assisted with acupuncture—for example, LR-3, SP-10—and medicinal therapy—for example, Bupleuri radix (*chai hu*), Cyperi rotundi rhizoma (*xiang fu*). On the other hand, we find the opinion that it is necessary to support this phase with calming therapies (e. g., Lifang[21]), such as acupuncture on HT-7, GV-20, and medicinals like Lilii bulbus (*bai he*), Albizziae cortex (*he huan pi*), Nelumbinis semen (*lian zi xin*), to assist in relaxation of the uterus and of the *shen* and thereby have a positive influence on fertilization.

Post-transfer, all authors pursue a very similar therapeutic concept.[20,21,30] In this phase, the practitioner should focus on nurturing, supplementing, and calming, with individual emphasis on *qi*, blood, *yin*, and *yang* (see Chapter 22).

Assisting Intracytoplasmatic Sperm Injection

Of central importance here is the treatment of the male partner for at least 3 months (complete spermiogenesis cycle) to achieve the best possible sperm quality (ICSI indication = low sperm quality). If fertilization has failed in a previous treatment course, treating the woman, of course, becomes the first priority, in which context either the quality of egg cells is limited or the egg cells cannot be fertilized. At this point, biomedical options are limited to exceptional cases. Here, however, TCM can contribute in the area of improving egg cell quality.

■ Cooperation between TCM and Biomedicine

Therapeutic measures in the treatment of infertility depend on the question of when the couple asks for help. After six cycles of unprotected intercourse during the fertile time and without pregnancy, we can already assume that fertility is mildly reduced (see **Table 6.3**). Nevertheless, affected couples still have a very good chance of conceiving spontaneously.

If the TCM practitioner is the first point of contact for a couple, before visiting a center for reproductive medicine, the practitioner should initiate a complete diagnosis, depending on earlier findings and attempted therapies, in order to eliminate the possibility of potentially essential measures of reproductive medicine.

It is absolutely necessary to check (especially in couples where the woman is older than 35 years):
- the ovarian functional reserve and androgen metabolism
- the quality of the spermiogram and, in certain cases, the tubal factor

Depending on the individual situation, a decision must be made on whether an initial course of treatment should be started with TCM alone for about six menstrual cycles or whether a center for reproductive medicine should be consulted as well.

If the couple enlists the help of a TCM practitioner only after having first visited a center for reproductive medicine, measuring and recording the basal temperature curve is initiated first. In light of additional findings like age, spermiogram, and tubal factor, a decision should be made in consultation with the center on whether an initial attempt should be made only with TCM (in the

sense of cycle-optimizing therapy) or in combination with measures of reproductive medicine.

It is important to synchronize the therapeutic steps of TCM with the measures of reproductive medicine by mutual information. For a perfect cooperation between the two methods (TCM and reproductive medicine), it would be ideal if the couple were asked during their first contact in the center for reproductive medicine to keep a basal temperature curve and to present relevant basal temperature curves to facilitate an appropriate TCM diagnosis. Scientific reproductive medicine profits greatly from presented basal temperature curves as well, since problems with follicular maturation are thereby easily identified and it becomes evident whether the conception potential has been utilized to its fullest in the past. From this information, the indication for additional diagnostic procedures is deduced.

■ Case Histories

The case histories presented below are examples of the possibilities of medical care with a combination of reproductive medicine and TCM. To protect patient privacy, we have changed the patients' names.

Case History 1: Female patient, 38 years (IUI)

Ms. Andrea H., a 38-year-old patient with a 35-year-old partner, came with the following biomedical diagnosis: "idiopathic infertility." Her partner's spermiograms had shown no abnormal results three times, spaced 4 weeks apart.

Medical History
No abnormal endocrinological findings and tubal factor. Occasional left-sided migraine attacks, most severe in the temple region. Frequent neck tension that could be relieved temporarily by massage. Important in her early history is a subjectively serious trauma at age 18 (the sudden death of her mother who was very important to her).

Cycle

Menstruation every 26–29 days, length 4 days, bright red blood without clots. From the age of 20 on, the patient has been suffering from dysmenorrhea, with particularly severe pain one day before the onset of her period. In addition, she complained of PMS with tension in the breasts, emotional instability, and disturbed sleep 3–4 days prior to her menstrual period.

Tongue

Normal in size, pale red, the edges slightly curled up, normal tongue fur, and mild stasis in the sublingual veins.

Pulse

Guan position on the left (liver position) tense.

Basal Temperature Curve

Biphasic, frequency 26–30 days with a rise in temperature around the 12th to 14th day. The evaluation of three cycles showed a sawtooth-shaped BT curve (**Fig. 6.16**).

TCM Diagnosis

Liver *qi* stagnation and blood stasis.

Treatment Plan

Primarily harmonizing (*he fa*), by means of a modified prescription of *Xiao Yao San* (Free Wanderer Powder) (plus Salviae miltiorrhizae radix, *dan shen*; Leonuri herba *yi mu cao*) from the 11th day of the cycle on to the onset of the period.

Result

After two cycles with this therapy, the patient stated that she did not feel any more menstrual pain. After six cycles with medicinal therapy, a successful intrauterine insemination was performed.

Commentary

A great number of female patients with the diagnosis of "idiopathic sterility" or "functional sterility" receive the TCM diagnosis of liver *qi* stagnation and blood stasis. Experience shows that these patients profit most from treatment with TCM.

Case History 2: Female patient, 42 years (IUI)

Ms. Monika W. did not meet her partner, with whom she now wants to have children, until very late in life. Their desire for children has therefore only been present for 2 years.

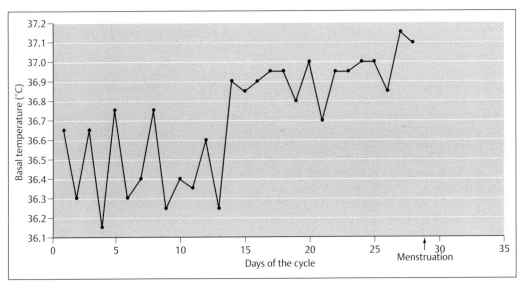

Fig. 6.16 Basal temperature curve of patient Andrea H.

Medical History

Myoma enucleation in the year 2000, furthermore three small myomas in the uterine wall. Subsequently, five failed attempts at insemination after prior hormone stimulation. As a result of the hormone stimulation, strong side-effects such as abdominal distention, headache, and general state of tension. The patient is, however, always a very tense woman, most likely primarily because of the urgency of her desire for children. At the time of her first patient contact, an additional hormone-stimulated insemination was planned. The patient desires support with TCM because she is hoping to thereby experience the time of stimulation and insemination as less straining.

Cycle

Shortened to about 23–25 days, severe menstrual complaints on days 1–3 with heavy dark periods with large clots. Premenstrually irritated, tension in the breasts 3 days before onset of menstruation.

Tongue

Bluish tongue with white fur, peeled in the area of the lower burner, clear stasis in the sublingual veins.

Pulse

Faint, especially in the kidney position.

Basal Temperature Curve

The BT curve shows a clearly abbreviated luteal phase (**Fig. 6.17**).

TCM Diagnosis

Blood stasis, kidney vacuity, liver *qi* stagnation.

Treatment Plan

Three months' preparation for a new stimulation. Elimination of the liver *qi* stagnation and therefore of the symptoms of tension that were experienced as so uncomfortable by the patient (e. g., feeling of a lump in the throat, upper abdominal pressure, general tension). Treatment of the obvious signs of blood stasis (myomas, dysmenorrhea with clotted menstrual blood). Support of kidney *yin* and blood.

Ms. Monika W. receives in accordance with her cycle and the phase:

- day 1–5: *Tao Hong Si Wu Tang* (Peach Kernel and Carthamus Four Agents Decoction) plus *Shi Xiao San* (Sudden Smile Powder)
- day 6–11: *Gui Shao Di Huang Tang* (Chinese Angelica, Peony, and Rehmannia Decoction)
- day 12–18: *Hei Xiao Yao San* (Black Free Wanderer Powder) plus *xiang fu, yi mu cao,* and *dan shen* Chinese Angelica, Peony, and Rehmannia Decoction
- day 19 –menstruation: *Jia Wei Shen Qi Wan* (Supplemented Kidney *Qi* Pill) minus *fu zi* (Aconiti carmichaeli praeparata radix)

On day 12 of the cycle, open *ren mai* (LU-7, KI-6), LI-4, LR-3, CV-4, *zi gong, yin tang.*

After this, her condition clearly improves. The pressure in the throat disappears and she feels more relaxed. Premenstrually, acupuncture to move blood (SP-10, LR-5) and support the kidneys (KI-7, CV-4), in combination with the relevant bladder *shu* points.

Result

After subsequent insemination, the pregnancy test is positive but unfortunately a miscarriage occurs only 14 days later. Ms. Monika W. decides with a

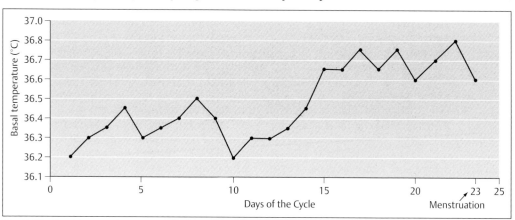

Fig. 6.17 Basal temperature curve of patient Monika W.

heavy heart that she does not want any further treatment for infertility.

Case History 3: Female patient, 38 years (IUI)

The first contact with Ms. Katharina E. took place when four intrauterine inseminations after stimulation with Clomifen did not bring the desired result. Because the partner's sperm cells clump together (agglutinate), an ICSI protocol is planned as the next step. With this type of problem on the male side, a traditional IVF procedure is often not successful, that is, no fertilization of the ovum takes place.

Medical History
Uterus myomatosus, endometriosis was diagnosed in 2004 and subsequently operated on in September of 2005. Since then, only mild pain during the period, blood continues to contain small clots. Premenstrually, when experiencing a lot of stress, and during weather changes, migraine-like headaches in the *shao yang* region.

Because the patient now wants to undergo the ICSI procedure, which she herself believes to be quite stressful, she wants to design all external conditions as ideal as possible and therefore to utilize simultaneous support with TCM. ICSI treatment is planned for the next cycle.

Treatment Plan
Acupuncture on the 13th day of the cycle (right LU-7, left KI-6, left LI-4, right LR-3, CV-4, *zi gong*, LR-14, and GV-20). Before needling, the patient complains of a headache. After the treatment, the headache has disappeared. Ms. E. receives the following prescriptions to support one cycle:
- day 1–4: *Tao Hong Si Wu Tang*
- day 5–10: *Gui Shao Di Huang Wan*
- day 11–18: *Xiao Yao San* (Free Wanderer Powder) plus *xiang fu* and *dan shen*
- day 19–menstruation: *Jin Gui Shen Qi Wan* (Golden Coffer Kidney Qi Pill) minus *fu zi* plus *dan shen*

On the 24th day of the cycle, needling of SP-4, PC-6, CV-4, ST-30, and GV-24. In addition, acupuncture on the partner: strengthening kidney *yang* and harmonizing liver *qi*. Prescription during

hormone stimulation: *Zi Shen Tiao Chong Fang* (Kidney-enriching Thoroughfare-regulating Formula) according to Professor Wu (see Chapter 22). Due to the small number of follicles from stimulation (only two follicles), ICSI treatment is called off and an additional insemination is performed.

From day 11 until 3 days after insemination, a variation of the formula *Xiao Yao San* On the day before insemination, needling of LI-4, LR-3, SP-6, ST-36, CV-4, ST-30, and *yin tang*, and 3 days after insemination: *si shen cong*, HT-7, KI-3, SP-10, ST-36; 4 days later to support implantation again GV-20, GV-24, KI-3, ST-36. Formula 3 days after insemination: *Yi Shen Gu Chong Fang* (Kidney-boosting Thoroughfare-securing Formula) plus Atractylodis macrocephalae rhizoma (*bai zhu*) and *fu ling* (Poriae cocos sclerotium) for 14 days (see Chapter 22).

Result
Much to her surprise, the pregnancy test comes back positive on the 14th day after insemination. In the 6th week of pregnancy, the patient comes to clinic with morning sickness without vomiting, experienced as troubling. This symptom is easily treated with two courses of needling on PC-6, LR-3, ST-34, CV-12, KI-21, and GV-24, and some nutritional advice. At the point of going to press, Ms. E. has not yet given birth to her child.

Case History 4: Female patient, 39 years (IVF)

Three years ago, Ms. Sabine S. had given birth to her first child by means of IVF. One year before that, laparoscopy had shown that both of her fallopian tubes were blocked. A first IVF attempt remained without success. On the second attempt a good year later, again no success was achieved with fresh embryos, but the following cryocycle was successful. At the calculated date, a healthy daughter was born by c-section.

Two years later, Ms. S. again attempted by means of IVF to have a second child, without success. Another year later, the couple wants to start a new attempt, before Ms. S. turns 40.

Medical History

The patient suffers from frequent upper abdominal complaints, frequent bitter taste in the mouth, is always rather constipated, and frequently suffers from a feeling of fullness and nausea. She perceived the first pregnancy as "torture" because she continuously suffered from severe nausea up to delivery. In addition, the patient suffers from lower back pain, a slipped disc on L 5/S 1, a weak and cold-sensitive lumbar spine, constant knee problems, and shoulder and neck pain. She is very sensitive to wind and cold, and, in spite of sufficient bedrest, frequently tired.

Cycle

The cycle fluctuates between 26 and 32 days. The menstrual period is very heavy and painful (before the onset and on the first day), with dark red blood with large clots. Premenstrually (ca. 3 days before the onset), she is very irritated and suffers from tension in the breasts and disturbed sleep (waking up around 2 a.m.). But she claims to have always been an easily irritated, quick-tempered woman.

Tongue

Pink, swollen, with dental impressions and a thin white fur, very strong stasis in the sublingual veins.

Pulse

In the liver position string-like, both kidney pulses vacuous.

Basal Temperature Curve

Biphasic with sawtooth-shaped course (**Fig. 6.18**).

TCM Diagnosis

Liver *qi* stagnation, blood stasis, kidney *qi* vacuity, spleen *qi* vacuity.

Treatment Plan

Three months' preparation by means of herbal therapy in accordance with the phase, parallel treatment of liver *qi* stagnation and blood stasis with acupuncture:

- day 1–4: *Tao Hong Si Wu Tang* plus *yi mu cao*
- day 5–10: *Gui Shao Di Huang Wan*
- day 11–17: *Xiao Yao San* plus *dan shen* and *xiang fu*
- day 18 –menstruation: *Jin Gui Shen Qi Wan* minus *fu zi*

Around the middle of the cycle from day 10 on as well as prior to menstruation, acupuncture treatment to promote movement. Single opening of *chong mai* on the 28th day.

Result

Already the second period is practically without pain, and the premenstrual tension in the breasts also disappears. During the next IVF attempt, seven egg cells are fertilized. In the following embryo transfer, the patient receives acupuncture before and after the transfer (before transfer: LI-4, LR-3, SP-6, ST-36, *yin tang*; after transfer: HT-6,

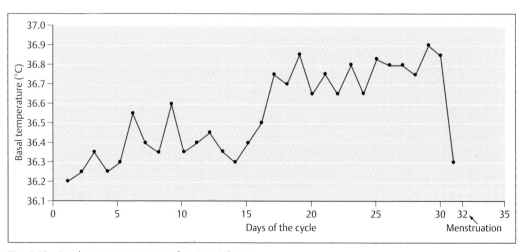

Fig. 6.18 Basal temperature curve of patient Sabine S.

KI-5, ST-36, *si shen cong*). Sabine S. becomes pregnant. She receives four more acupuncture treatments during the pregnancy for nausea, which is completely cured. After an otherwise normal pregnancy, Ms. S. gives birth at full term to a small healthy boy who is 3480 g (7.6 lbs) in weight and 53 cm (21 in) tall.

Case History 5: Female patient, 38 years (ICSI)

Four years ago, Ms. Jessica T. gave birth to her first son. Since then she has not practiced birth control because she wanted to have her second child as quickly as possible. When she came to her first consultation, she had been receiving fertility treatment in a center for reproductive medicine for 2 years.

Medical History

Three times optimized intercourse, that is, with hormonal stimulation with FSH and ovulation triggered by hCG, subsequently three times IUI, without success. Spermiograms of the partner: too few sperms with disrupted motility. No objectifiable causes for infertility found with Ms. T.

Subsequently, two ICSI cycles (in each of which three follicles were formed, of which two could be fertilized each time but failed to implant), without success. Ms. T. had been anorexic in her youth and is still very slender, 1.76 m height and 58 kg weight. In addition, she has been receiving treatment for high blood pressure for years.

During her third ICSI cycle, she came to a TCM consultation for the first time on the day before the embryo transfer. In this cycle, she develops six follicles, and four egg cells are fertilized.

Treatment Plan

Acupuncture before and after the transfer:
- before transfer: LI-4, LR-3, SP-6, ST-36, CV-4, *zi gong*, *yin tang*
- after transfer: KI-5, HT-6, ST-36, GV-24, GV-20

Four days after the transfer, the patient returns with very severe spasmodic lower abdominal pain, with a very tense lower abdomen. No explanation for this pain can be found in the gynecological examination. This attempt remains unsuccessful as well. From the TCM perspective, treat-

ment of the partner is recommended, to then start a better-prepared attempt at a time after about 70 days (time of spermiogenesis). But this never happens because two of the egg cells that were gained by stimulation, fertilized, and cryoconserved, are transferred in the following cycle and lead to the desired result.

During the cryocycle, the following formulas were used:
- day 1–4: *Tao Hong Si Wu Tang*
- day 5–11: *Gui Shao Di Huang Wan* plus *shen qu* (Massa fermentata), for upper abdominal pressure)
- day 12–17: *Xiao Yao San* plus *xiang fu* and *yi mu cao*

On day 10 of the cycle: acupuncture on LI-4, LR-3, SP-6, ST-36, LR-14, CV-4, *zi gong*. On day 13 of the cycle: opening the *ren mai*, plus LI-4 on the left, LR-3 on the right, CV-4, KI-13. One hour before the transfer on the 18th day of the cycle: HT-7, LR-3, SP-6, SP-10, *yin tang*; and 1 hour after transfer: GV-24, GV-20, KI-5, ST-36, CV-17.

Two days later, repeated acupuncture to support the implantation: GV-20, *yin tang*, KI-3, ST-36. At the same time to support implantation: *Yi Shen Gu Chong Fang* (see Chapter 22).

Result

Ms. Jessica T. becomes pregnant with twins. At the beginning of pregnancy, she suffers from light bleeding, but otherwise experiences an uneventful pregnancy. In the meantime, she has given birth to two girls. Jessica T. expressed sincere gratitude for the support with the "terrible teas."

■ Conclusion

In conclusion, we can state with regard to fertility treatment that cooperation between the two different medical systems—TCM and reproductive medicine—appears practical and important because TCM methods can affect the procedures of reproductive medicine on very different levels, at different times, and in different ways. Basic requirements for the joint solution of infertility problems are mutual respect and knowledge about the strengths and weaknesses of one's own and the other system. In addition, successful cooperation demands a willingness to also acquire the necessary familiarity with the other system, in order to be able to solve this very special problem together.

Bibliography

1. Arbeitsgruppe NFP. *Natürlich und Sicher.* Stuttgart, Trias; 2005.
2. Bensky D, Barolet R. *Chinesische Arzneimittelrezepte und Behandlungsstrategien.* Kötzting: VGM Wühr; 1996.
3. Bensky D, Clavey S, Stöger E, Gamble A. *Chinese Herbal Medicine—Materia Medica.* Seattle: Eastland; 2004.
4. Chen BY. Acupuncture Normalizes Dysfunction of Hypothalamic-Pituitary-Ovarian Axis. *Acupuncture and Electro-Therapeutics Research.* 1997;22.
5. Colombo, B. *Demographic Research.* 2000;3:5.
6. Deadman P, Al-Khafaji M, Baker K. *Großes Handbuch der Akupunktur.* Kötzting: VGM Wühr; 2002.
7. Englert S. *Großes Handbuch der Chinesischen Phytotherapie, Akupunktur und Diätetik.* Kötzting: VGM Wühr; 2002.
8. *Assisted Reproductive Technology Success Rates.* Centers for Disease Control and Prevention. http://www.cdc.gov/ART.
9. Flaws B. *Schwester Mond. Diagnose und Behandlung von Menstruationsstörungen mit Traditioneller Chinesischer Medizin.* Kötzting: VGM Wühr; 1994.
10. Focks C, Hillenbrand N (editors). *Leitfaden Chinesische Medizin.* Munich: Urban & Fischer; 2003.
11. Frank-Herrmann P, Heil J, Gnoth C et al. The Effectiveness of a Fertility Awareness Based Method to Avoid Pregnancy in Relation to a Couple's Sexual Behaviour During the Fertile Time: A Prospective Longitudinal Study. *Human Reproduction.* 2007.
12. Freundl G, Gnoth C, Frank-Herrmann P. *Kinderwunsch. Neue Wege zum Wunschkind.* Munich: Gräfe & Unzer; 2006.
13. Furth C. *A Flourishing Yin. Gender in China's Medical History.* University of California Press. 1999; 960–1665.
14. Gnoth C. Die Bedeutung der natürlichen Fertilität für Diagnostik und Therapie der Sterilität. Unpublished habilitation treatise; 2008.
15. Gnoth C, Frank-Herrmann P, Freundl G. Opinion: Natural Family Planning and the Management of Infertility. *Arch Gynecol Obstet,* 2002;267:67–71.
16. Gnoth C, Frank-Herrmann P, Freundl G. Angepasstes Management bei unerfülltem Kinderwunsch. *Geburtsh Frauenheilk.* 2003;63: 124–129.
17. Gnoth C, Frank-Herrmann P, Freundl G, Godehardt E. Time to Pregnancy: Results of a German Prospective Study and Impact on the Management of Infertility. *Human Reproduction.* 2003;18: 1959–1966.
18. Kirschbaum, B. *Atlas und Lehrbuch der Chinesischen Zungendiagnostik.* Vols. I and II. Kötzting: VGM Wühr; 2002.
19. Kirschbaum, B. *Die 8 Außerordentlichen Gefäße in der Traditionellen Chinesischen Medizin.* Uelzen: ML; 2000.
20. Lewis, R. *The Infertility Cure.* Boston: Little, Brown and Company; 2004.
21. Lifang L. *Acupuncture and IVF.* Boulder: Blue Poppy; 2003.
22. Ludwig, M. *Pregnancy and Birth After Assisted Reproductive Technologies.* Berlin: Springer; 2002.
23. Lyttleton J. *Treatment of Infertility with Chinese Medicine.* London: Churchill Livingstone; 2004.
24. Maciocia G. *Die Praxis der Chinesischen Medizin.* Kötzting: VGM Wühr; 1997.
25. Maciocia G. *Die Gynäkologie in der Praxis der Chinesischen Medizin.* Kötzting: VGM Wühr; 2000.
26. Paulus W, Zhang M, Strehler E, El-Danasouri I, Sterzik K. Influence of Acupuncture on the Pregnancy Rate in Patients Who Undergo Assisted Reproduction Therapy. *Fertil Steril.* 2002;77:4.
27. Raith E, Frank P, Freundl G. *Natürliche Familienplanung Heute.* Berlin: Springer; 1999.
28. Ross, J. *Akupunktur-Punktkombinationen.* Uelzen: ML; 2000.
29. Schirren C (editor). *Unerfüllter Kinderwunsch.* Cologne: Deutscher Ärzteverlag; 2003.
30. Wing TA, Sedlmeier ES. Measuring the Effectiveness of Chinese Herbal Medicine in Improving Female Fertility. *J Chin Med.* 2005;S0:22–23.
31. Wood V. Infertility and the Use of Basal Body Temperature in Diagnosis and Treatment. *J Chin Med.* 1999;61:33.
32. Wu YS. Infertility Treatment, IVF Aufzeichnungen. Seminar Prof. Dr. Wu. TCM Conference. Rothenburg/Tauber; 2006.
33. Xia Guicheng. Discussion of the Menstrual Cycle and the Cycle-regulating Treatment. *J Chin Med.* 2001;67:10.

Fertility Treatment and Pregnancy— Foundations of TCM

3

Physiology and Pathology of Fertility and Reproduction from the TCM Perspective

Dagmar Hemm

Prerequisites for the creation of new life include, on the one hand, "external" conditions like harmony and love in the relationship. On the other hand, everything must also be ready "internally" so that the fertile sperm finds a mature egg ready for implantation and a good environment—that is, a receptive uterus. From the perspective of TCM, all viscera, bowels, and channels participate in this process. Only their harmonious cooperation ensures that fertility disorders are prevented:

Shen

The heart *qi* ensures the necessary harmony between kidney *yin* and kidney *yang*, which is of fundamental importance for fertility. It is closely related to the *shen*, the radiance and consciousness of the person. The *shen* resides in the heart; it is an aspect of heart *yang* and is mirrored among other places in the eyes. The *shen* controls consciousness, thinking, memory, and sleep, and ultimately distinguishes humans from animals. As a result of the close relationship between heart and *shen*, disturbances tend to affect both of these at the same time. Good energy in the heart and permeability for the *shen* contributes to the smooth performance of all bodily functions. Disturbances in these functions can also affect fertility because at the time of sexual maturity, the heart and *shen* bring about the transformation of kidney essence into heavenly *gui (tian gui)*. This contributes to ovulation, menstruation, and sperm formation (see Chapter 23).

According to the biomedical definition, a woman is regarded as infertile if she fails to become pregnant within 2 years in spite of a normal sex life and healthy sperm from the man.[5] The search for causes should therefore initially turn to some general considerations. This includes a general constitutional weakness of kidney essence in the woman, that is, on the one hand a lack of prenatal essence because her own parents were already quite old or in bad health during conception, and on the other, a lack of postnatal essence due to overwork but also to excessive or too early sexual activity. Physical exhaustion from hard labor but also from excessive sports causes not only kidney *yin* but also spleen and kidney *yang* to fade. Too much sex, especially in one's younger years or during puberty, can have a negative effect on the kidney, *ren mai*, and *chong mai*.

Exposure to cold and moisture, but also insufficient clothing—for example, due the fashion of exposing the belly—can displace the uterus, *ren mai, chong mai*, as well as the channels, as a result of which fertilization becomes more difficult. Especially during menstruation, women should avoid cold and wetness and should not play sports excessively. Likewise, an excessive consumption of cold, fatty, and phlegm-forming foods or drinks can cause the fallopian tubes to shift because of the moisture that is formed in the lower burner.

The primary differentiation in the treatment of infertility lies in the distinction between patterns of vacuity and repletion. Do we have to supplement or do we have to eliminate pathogenic factors? In this context, let us first clarify some important terms.

■ The Energies *Jing, Qi*, and *Xue*

Jing, qi, and *xue* are vital substances that are essential for reproduction. Their unimpeded circulation guarantees the harmonious progression of all body functions.

The Essence *Jing*

The vital essence *jing* consists of two components: first, the congenital prenatal potential, the constitution so to speak, that was inherited from the parents. Second, it consists of the acquired *jing*, which a person can increase or at least maintain throughout the course of his or her life. In accordance with the laws of nature, *jing* runs out towards the end of life. The amount of prenatal *jing* that a person is born with is predestined by fate. We can try to use it sparingly and continuously replenish the store in the kidney with acquired *jing* by a correct lifestyle (*yang sheng*, "nurturing/cultivating life"). In addition to proper diet, lifestyle, and breathing and movement exercises, the preservation of *jing* also includes advice on sexuality.

Jing is stored in the kidney. When it is strong, it enables women to still bear children after their 40th birthday. In addition, strong *jing* is the foundation for a healthy *shen*. *Shen*, the spirit, the love of life, our social competence, our talents and skills, all of these can only develop if a good and sufficient supply of *jing* exists.

Couples seeking a child should not disregard their own age completely since the parents' advanced age and weakening health is one cause for a lack of prenatal *jing* in the child:

"The Yellow Emperor replied: 'But there were people who in spite of being old in years were able to engender descendants. How is this possible?'
Qi Bo replied: 'These are people whose natural end of life should be set higher. The beat of their pulse remains active, and an excess of semen remains in their testicles. Even though they beget children, their sons will not survive past the age of 46 and their daughters will not grow older than 49, because at this time the strength of heaven and earth will be exhausted.'"[8]

Lack of *Jing*

Weak *jing* leads to weak, sickly children, delayed puberty, and partly to underdeveloped primary and secondary sexual characteristics. In women, we often find not only menstrual irregularities, but also eggs of lower quality, which can then be fertilized only with difficulty and often produce weak embryos. In the man, a lack of *jing* causes low-quality sperm or a reduced sperm count. Generally speaking, a lack of kidney *jing* has a complicating effect on reproduction.

The Moving Force *Qi*

Qi has many diverse functions; without its moving attributes, for example, ovulation would not take place, the egg would not migrate, and the sperm would not move either.

The functions of *qi* are:
- **movement**: reproduction, physical and mental movement
- **transformation**: metabolism, digestion, separating the pure and the impure
- **warming**: maintaining the body temperature
- **protection**: guarding the body against external pathogenic influences
- **transportation**: bodily fluids, food, waste products
- **stimulation**: growth and development, bodily fluids (sweat, urine, tears, saliva, semen)
- **containment**: containing blood and fluids in the channels
- **lifting**: keeping the organs in their place

Lack of *Qi*

Any state of *qi* vacuity is usually rooted in the spleen or lung, since the lung directs the *qi* and the spleen, by its moving and transforming activity, is the source of *qi*. Lack of *qi* manifests in shortness of breath, fatigue, a weak voice, lack of appetite and strength, and sometimes diarrhea and spontaneous sweating. The pulse is weak and vacuous, the tongue pale with a whitish fur.

Qi Stagnation

Qi can wane in its movement and cause stagnations. Frequently, the decisive is an insufficient regulatory function in the liver. These stagnations can be felt as palpable abdominal "knots" that change their location and can even disappear altogether. They are accompanied by painful, pulling feelings of tension and pressure in the entire abdominal region, with irritability, emotional instability, and periods of mental depression. In men with sterility, we often find enduring *qi* stagnation, commonly accompanied by a lack of *jing*. The pulse is stringlike or tight, the tongue mildly purple-colored.

The Blood *Xue* and the Special Characteristics of the Menstrual Blood *Jing Shui*

A direct translation of *xue* as "blood" does not do justice to the Chinese understanding of the function and attributes of blood. Rather, blood is the material form of *qi*, it constitutes the substantial foundation of the *shen*, and it nourishes and moistens the body. With the help of the spleen, the blood of the body *xue shui* (blood-water) is formed from *ying qi* (constructive *qi*) and bodily fluids; spleen *qi* also contains it in the blood vessels. The blood is stored in the liver, especially in the muscles (uterus!). The liver thereby also regulates the volume of blood. Ultimately, though, heart *qi* dominates the blood, while the lung is also involved as the source of *qi*.

The menstrual blood, on the other hand, the *jing shui* (menstrual water), is produced from kidney water and is transformed with the help of the heart, liver, and spleen. Kidney water or kidney *yin* is hence the foundation for the formation of menstrual blood. The kidney is the storehouse of prenatal *jing* and *yuan qi* (original *qi*). It is also the source of menstrual blood and of sexual maturity, the so-called *tian gui*. *Tian* means heaven, and *gui* is the 10th heavenly stem from the old Chinese calendrical system that ordered the macrocosm. It is associated with the element water. This "heavenly water" is present in the human body from birth on, but only manifests with sexual maturity. In the man, the *tian gui* regulates the transformation of blood into semen; in the woman, it starts the menstrual period and provides for the moistening of the vagina. Thus, girls begin menstruating at the age of 14 because this is when the heavenly water has arrived. The *ren mai* opens and fills with *qi*, the *chong mai* fills with blood, and the girl is ready to conceive. In the man, the *tian gui* manifests in the form of sperm at age 16—as is described in the *Huang Di Nei Jing (The Yellow Emperor's Inner Classic)* (see below).

The number 7 is attributed to women: At age 7, the essence rises; at 14, it is present in abundance. Then, the heavenly *gui* arrives, the *ren mai* is open, the *chong mai* blooms, and the menstrual period begins. Men are associated with the number 8; their ability to reproduce will begin at age 16.

The material foundation of the menstrual blood is thus the heavenly *gui*, manifesting as menstrual fluid. This is therefore not formed from regular blood, but from prenatal essence that is stored in the kidney and materialized with the assistance of the heart. Kidney essence thereby has a profound influence on female physiology (and, of course, equally on male physiology), from puberty through pregnancy up to menopause.

Functions of the heavenly water *tian gui* are:
- regulating sexual development
- producing the menses
- producing and secreting *yin* water
- facilitating pregnancy
- producing sperm, transforming *jing* and *xue* into sperm
- Forming the secondary sexual characteristics. In women, *yin qi* sinks heavily downward; in men, the *qi* of heaven and earth rises upward via the *ren mai* and *chong mai*; *qi* and *xue* are transported upward, the voice changes, the body hair and pubic hair grow, the breasts form.
- It is comparable to reproductive hormones.

Lack of Blood

General lack of blood causes insufficient nourishment of the mucous membranes of the uterus and ultimately also of the embryo. Nidation of the fertilized egg is impeded because the endometrium is insufficiently formed. A lack of liver blood in particular supplies the uterus with an insufficient amount of blood, the menstrual period is scant, and the cycle can become irregular or even cease altogether.

A weak menstrual period with rather pale blood and in general a longer cycle are typical of this pattern. Such women are pale, they feel tired, without energy, often dizzy, and generally rather depressed. Often, the vision is also impaired, the skin is dry, and we find constipation. The tongue is pale and thin, the pulse rough or else fine.

Lack of blood on its own is more common in women; in men, we are more likely to find *qi* disorders with stagnation of *qi*, blood, or fluids instead.

Lack of *Xue* (Blood) and *Qi*

This combination manifests in a general state of exhaustion, palpitations, paleness, shortness of breath, dizziness, and tinnitus. Erections are weak, and the more exhausted and overburdened the patient feels the more problematic they become. The pale tongue shows a thin whitish fur, the pulse is weak and vacuous.

Blood Heat

Typical of Blood heat are such symptoms as a short cycle, sometimes up to twice in 1 month, accompanied by a feeling of heat, thirst, and unrest. The tongue is red, the pulse is rapid and surging.

Blood Stasis

In patients with Blood stasis, the menstrual period is irregular and painful with dark and often clotted blood because the *chong mai* is unable to drain completely. Such patients feel irritated, nervous, and restless. The tongue is purple, possibly with macules and blocked sublingual veins, the pulse is stringlike or rough.

> The Interplay of *Qi* and *Xue*:
> * *Xue* nourishes the body as the substance of *qi*.
> * *Xue* moistens.
> * *Xue* is the material basis of the spirit.
> * *Qi* engenders *xue*.
> * *Qi* moves *xue*.
> * *Qi* contains *xue*.
> * *Xue* nourishes *qi*.

Blood and *Qi* in Men and Women

Female Physiology

Women's physiology is determined by blood; it is the source of fertility, conception, and pregnancy. In contrast to men, whose orgasms depend primarily on *qi*, women's bodily functions are controlled by blood, clearly visible in the blood of menstruation, which prepares their body every month.

TCM refers to that part of the female sexual organs that is encircled by the liver channel as the actual sexual organs *yin qi*. The uterus—which also includes the fallopian tubes and ovaries—is the key reproductive organ in women and the point from which menstruation originates. In the *Huang Di Nei Jing Su Wen*, the uterus is referred to as "woman's protective cover," *nu zi bao*, and is included among the six "extraordinary organs" because it fulfills both the function of a *yang* organ (menstruation and childbirth as elimination) and of a *yin* organ (blood storage and nourishing the embryo). It "transforms" the fetus from the man's essence (his sperm) and the mother's blood, and protects and nourishes it until childbirth:

> The six "extraordinary organs" *qi heng zhi fu* are the brain, marrow, bones, blood vessels, gallbladder, and uterus. In contrast to the six bowels (small intestine, large intestine, stomach, bladder, gallbladder, *san jiao*), which are responsible for intake, transformation, and elimination, the "extraordinary organs" are in charge of *yin* functions but resemble *yang* organs in shape.

Anatomically speaking, the uterus, which corresponds to the *dan tian*, lies in the lower burner between the bladder and rectum. It is a structure of circuits that is linked to the abdomen through the points CV-3, CV-4, and CV-6 and to the kidney channel through an internal branch. Via the uterine network vessel *bao luo*, the uterus is linked to the kidney below; above, it connects to the heart via the uterine vessel *bao mai* (**Fig. 7.1**). Kidney *jing* and heart blood are therefore also responsible for a normal menstruation and for fertility. If heart blood is lacking, heart *qi* fails to descend into the

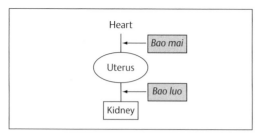

Fig. 7.1 The connection of the uterus to the heart and kidney.

abdomen; if kidney *jing* is lacking, the menses fail to arrive.

The *bao mai* and *bao luo* connect the heart and kidney to the uterus and transport *jing* and menstrual blood from the kidneys as well as blood from the heart to the uterus. In addition, heart and kidney *qi* direct the opening and closing of the uterus:

The opening of the uterus is initiated by the heart. The uterus opens during ovulation to let the egg in, during sexual intercourse for the sperm, and also during menstruation to allow the blood to drain out. A stagnation or blockage in this area—for which emotional and mental factors play an important role—prevent the egg or sperm from entering the uterus. Likewise, the menstrual blood can no longer drain out freely.

The kidneys regulate the closing of the uterus after menstruation and after ovulation, when the egg has arrived in the uterus, and, of course, also after fertilization, to keep the embryo safe. A weak kidney *qi* would hence contribute to a miscarriage because of a failure to close the uterus. Similarly, intermenstrual bleeding and dribbling of blood after the end of the actual menstrual period can be attributed to a weakness of the kidney in this area.

After experiencing shock or great stress, the heart and kidney can be practically traumatized. This often leads to heart heat, which causes heart *qi* to stagnate and, if the uterus opens suddenly, can cause a miscarriage or intermenstrual bleeding.

"When a girl turns 7, the energy of her kidneys increases, her teeth change, and her hair grows longer. When she turns 14, menstruation starts, the girl can get pregnant, and the pulses in the great thoroughfare channel* beat strongly. The girl menstruates regularly

and hence can bear children. When the girl turns 21, the energy of her kidneys is normal, the last teeth have emerged, and the body is fully grown. At the age of 28, the woman's muscles and bones are solid and strong, her hair growth has reached its full length, and her body flourishes and is fertile. At the age of 35, the pulse in the area of the sunlight** wanes, her face becomes wrinkled, and her hair begins to fall out. At the age of 42, the intensity of the pulse in the area of the three yang regions*** in the upper half of the body wanes, her whole face is covered with wrinkles, and her hair begins to turn white. At the age of 49, she can no longer become pregnant, and circulation in the large thoroughfare pulse wanes. The gates of menstruation are now closed. Her body declines, and she can no longer bear children."[8]

Male Physiology

The man's physiology is primarily determined by *qi*. In the place where the uterus is located in the woman in the *dan tian*, we find the "sperm chamber" in the man. The testicles and the scrotum are the "palace of *jing*"; here, the man stores the essence *jing* in the form of sperm.

Sperm, which is generally *yin*, from an energetic perspective consists of a *yang* part, namely the rapidly moving sperm, and a *yin* part, the nourishing seminal fluid. Thus, we must, for example, supplement *yang* or *qi* in cases with slow sperm cells, but supplement *yin* or essence in cases with low sperm quality.

"When a boy turns 8, the energy of his testicles is fully developed; his hair grows longer, and his teeth change. At the age of 16, the energy of his testicles increases, and he thus begins to discharge semen. He has a surplus of semen, which he strives to get rid of, and if the male and female element unite in harmony at this point, a child can be conceived. At the age of 24, the energy of the testicles is normal in the man; his muscle [sic!] and bones are solid and strong, the last teeth have emerged, and the body has reached its full size. At the age of 32, the muscles and bones develop their

---

* An old collective name for the pulses of the *ren mai* and *chong mai*.

** These are the pulses of the stomach, large intestine, and small intestine.

*** That is, the *tai yang, yang ming,* and *shao yang* channels.

full splendor, the man's flesh is healthy, he can with-stand physical strain, and he is fertile. At the age of 40, the man's testicles become smaller and his hair and teeth begin to fall out. When the man turns 48, his male strength is exhausted or decreases, wrinkles mark his face, and his hair turns white at the temples. At the age of 56, the energy of the liver wanes, his muscles no longer move faultlessly, his eliminations of sperm are exhausted, his vital strength decreases, his kidneys de-cline, and the physical strength comes to an end. At the age of 64, he loses his teeth and hair. The kidneys regulate the water flow and store energy that is sup-plied by the five viscera and six bowels. Semen can only be discharged if the five viscera are filled with energy. But if they are dry and empty at this time, the muscles and bones degenerate, the sperm for conception is ex-hausted, and the hair at the temples therefore turns white, his body fills up and becomes heavy, his gait is no longer straight, and he is no longer able to produce offspring."[8]

■ The Extraordinary Vessels

The eight extraordinary vessels, also called "mira-cle channels," are reservoirs of energy, with a spe-cial significance for embryonic development and reproduction. They distribute *yin, yang, qi,* and blood outside of the system of the main channels and viscera and bowels.

Chong Mai (Thoroughfare Vessel) and *Ren Mai* (Conception Vessel)

For conception and pregnancy, the *chong mai*—the thoroughfare vessel—and the *ren mai*—the concep-tion vessel—are the most important channels. For the time after ovulation and for menstruation, the *chong mai* as the "sea of blood" is the most impor-tant extraordinary vessel. It regulates the blood supply and the movement of blood in the uterus. The *ren mai* is highly significant for a woman's ability to conceive and for supplying the internal and external genitals. Disorders in the cervix, va-gina, and vulva can be influenced through the *ren mai*.

Nan Jing 66: "The 'moving qi between the kidneys is what creates human life, and the root of the 12 chan-nels. Therefore [this location] is called 'source' yuan."[2]

The *ren mai* and *chong mai* originate in the area of the "moving *qi*" (*dong qi*) between the kidneys and from there run downwards through the uterus to CV-1. Here, the *ren mai* emerges to the surface and runs upward to CV-24, encircles the mouth, and enters the eyes at ST-1. The *chong mai* emerges to the surface at ST-30 and runs along the kidney channel up to KI-21 or KI-27, then crosses the throat, encircles the mouth, and seeps "into *yang* and moistens *yin*" at the forehead. Other branches of the *chong mai* run through the legs and back.

The *ren mai* is also called the "sea of the *yin* channels" because it provides all *yin* substances (blood, essence, fluids) that are involved in the hormonal changes in a woman's life: puberty, con-ception, pregnancy, and menopause. After meno-pause in particular, we can nourish *yin* through the *ren mai* to alleviate the symptoms of vacuity heat.

The *chong mai* as the "sea of blood" provides the blood for menstruation, moves it, and moist-ens the essence. Vacuity in the *chong mai* causes amenorrhea or prolonged cycles; *qi* stagnation or blood stasis cause premenstrual syndrome (PMS) and dysmenorrhea.

Du Mai (Governing Vessel)

The *du mai*—the governing vessel—also originates in the space between the kidneys, runs downward through the uterus, and emerges to the body's sur-face at CV-1. Its main branch runs through the spinal column to the head, enters the brain, and ends on the upper lip at GV-28. Several classical sources define the *du mai* as a branch of the liver channel; others see the *du mai* and *ren mai* as two branches of one channel: *du mai* with *yang* char-acteristics, *ren mai* with *yin* characteristics.

Of clinical relevance, though, is primarily the fact that one of the side branches of the *du mai* encircles the vagina. Hence, we treat not only the *ren mai* in vaginal problems but also the *du mai*, especially in cases with pronounced kidney *yang* vacuity. The reason for this is that the *du mai* re-presents the influence of the *ming men* (see also p. 87) and ministerial fire.

The *du mai* and *ren mai* connect the uterus (blood) with the kidney (essence), heart (blood), and brain ("sea of marrow"). With this axis, we can also explain the influence of emotional and mental problems on menstruation and ovulation. From the Western perspective, this corresponds to the axis hypothalamus–hypophysis–ovaries.

Su Wen, Chapter 60, explicitly defines the cause of infertility in women as a *du mai* disorder:

"Du mai *disorders can cause stiffness of the spinal column and pulling pain in the back. The* du mai *originates in the center of the bones below the lower abdomen*; in women, it penetrates to the inside and connects with the* ting kong *(obscure term associated with the external opening of the urethra),* kong *being the external opening of the urethra. A network vessel circumvents the genitals and connects to the area between the front and back of the pubic region, another branch circumvents the buttocks ... The branch that runs upwards in a straight line from the lower abdomen crosses the center of the navel, ascends, crosses the heart, enters the throat, runs upward to the cheek, circumvents the lips, and connects with the center below the eyes. When disorders originate here, the* qi *surges upward from the lower abdomen straight against the heart and causes pain, and the patient is unable to urinate or defecate. This is* chong shan, *pain from surging [qi]. In women, [we see] infertility, inhibited urination, hemorrhoids, incontinence and dry throat. When the* du mai *is diseased and you want to treat the* du mai, *treatment is applied above the pubic bone, in serious cases at* qi xia ying***."*[7]

Dai Mai (Girdling Vessel)

The *dai mai*, the girdling vessel, which—as the name implies—encircles the body like a girdle at the level of the waistline, plays a harmonizing role, due to its connections to the leg channels. Through LR-13, it affects the smooth flow of liver *qi*, a good starting point in liver *qi* stagnation. At the same time, LR-13 is also the *mu* point (alarm point) of the spleen; hence, you could, for example, also

---

* This is a reference to the pubic bone.
** This is a reference to CV-2, the point from which the *ren mai* and *du mai* originate and where the liver channel meets the *ren mai*.

treat vaginal discharge, that is due to damp-heat in chronic spleen vacuity, via the *dai mai*.

The *dai mai* influences the rise and fall of the energies of the spleen, liver, and kidney. It must be relaxed and stretched, so that the *qi* of the uterus and the essence can flow but at the same time are also supported. If the *dai mai* is too slack, this can lead to liver, spleen, and kidney vacuity. *Qi* is unable to rise, the organs become feeble (prolapse), and the fetus does not receive the necessary stability either, which can result in miscarriage.

Yin Qiao Mai (Yin Springing Vessel)

Starting at KI-6, the *yin qiao mai*—the springing vessel—runs along the inside of the legs through the external genitals and the thorax up to the inner corner of the eyes. It influences the organs of the pelvis and is used in states of repletion in the lower burner (feeling of pressure in the abdomen, myomas, retained placenta). Repletion patterns of the external genitals can also be treated through the *yin qiao mai*.

In the context of pregnancy, the extraordinary vessels determine the growth of the physical shape during embryonal development from the biomedical perspective as follows:
- *du mai*: bone marrow and brain
- *yin* and *yang qiao mai*: motor nerves
- *chong mai*: adrenal cortex and marrow
- *ren mai*: ovaries[5]

The Energetic Interplay of the Extraordinary Vessels

The **ren mai, du mai**, and **chong mai** originate in the kidney, run downward through the uterus to CV-1, and separate there to run upward—on the stomach, on the back, and inside the body. Because they originate from the *yuan qi* (original *qi*) between the kidneys, they are closely linked to essence, blood, and the heavenly water *tian gui*.

The *yin qiao mai* and *yang qiao mai* harmonize the left and right sides of the body as well as the lateral and medial bodily structures (e.g., inside and outside of the leg). Beginning at BL-62, the *yang qiao mai* carries *yang* energies upward to the eye. The *yin qiao mai* transports—beginning at KI-6—*yin* energies upward. Herein it supports the *ren mai* by removing, for example, *yin* repletion in the lower abdomen.

The **yin wei mai** and the **yang wei mai**, the *yin* and *yang* linking vessels, link the *yin* and *yang* channels to each other. They have a balancing effect on the inside and outside, as well as on *gu qi* (grain *qi*) and *wei qi* (defense *qi*). From a gynecological perspective, it is significant that they complement the *chong mai* and *dai mai*—which regulate the horizontal energies—because the opening point of one is the central hub of the other.

The Viscera and Bowels

The viscera store the energies of the human body and play a key role in the intake, production, and transformation of *qi*, blood, and fluids. The bowels always have the function of conducting substances to and from the viscera. The bowels therefore do not play such a significant role in this context.

Physiology and Pathology of the Kidney

The kidney plays a key role in reproduction because as the storehouse of *jing* it is the root of all life. The essence *jing* can transform into *qi*, but *qi* can also produce essence as well. In addition, the *qi* produced from kidney essence controls the heavenly water *tian gui*, which regulates the sexual functions of the human body.

The kidney as "source of *yin* and *yang*" and as the storehouse of *jing* is hence of primary importance for sexuality and fertility. According to TCM, it is also the origin of the libido, and disturbances therefore affect not only fertility but also the perception of sexual desire as such. Kidney *yang* vacuity would therefore lead to lack of desire or in the worst case, frigidity—in either sex. Kidney *yin* vacuity, on the other hand, commonly manifests in excessive libido, often coupled with premature ejaculation.

Even worse, dual vacuity of kidney *yin* and kidney *yang* causes not only physical and emotional symptoms *per se*, but is also often the source of disharmonies in the other viscera and bowels.

On the one hand, the kidney as the source of water is the origin of the menstrual blood, that is, kidney *yin* supplies the essence. By means of the *ming men* fire, on the other hand, kidney *yang* warms the uterus, which in turn stores the blood. In women, kidney vacuity manifests both as a weakening of *yin* (water—and therefore "hot uterus") and as a weakening of *yang* (fire—and therefore "cold uterus").

In general, men need kidney energy for maturing the sperm, and women need it for maturing the egg cells. In men, the kidney controls the "essence gate," which should only release a small amount of semen, that is, essence, in order to preserve as much vital *jing* as possible. For this reason, spermatorrhea as such is in China regarded as a condition that requires medical treatment.

Kidney *Yin*

Kidney *yin* represents the substance and reserve that is necessary for conception. As the storehouse of prenatal *jing*, it stores the energy reserves, so to speak. If these reserves are depleted immoderately without being refilled, infertility is often predictable.

Kidney Yin *Vacuity in Women*

In kidney *yin* vacuity, infertility tends to have persisted for a long time already because of problems related to ovulation. How can an exhausted, overworked, drained woman have extra energy available for conceiving and growing new life? A life governed by *yin* vacuity is marked by restlessness, hectic rushing, and heat states. Further symptoms are dry mucous membranes, little or no stretchable mucus during ovulation, but also a malnourished endometrium in which a fertilized egg can implant only with difficulty. In addition, the menstrual period is often scant, as if dried out. TCM calls this a "hot uterus."

Kidney Yin *Vacuity in Men*

In men, the internal heat of kidney *yin* vacuity dries up the fluids, noticeable, for example, in scant semen and low sperm count. If no changes in the amount of sperm are found, we can still see the heat of kidney *yin* vacuity reducing sperm motility and the ability to penetrate into the egg, or causing a higher rate of sperm deformity. The semen can become viscous or show changes in color. Additionally, heat—mostly in connection with dampness—can cause prostatitis.

Regarding the libido, we often see increased desire but coupled with reduced stamina. Premature ejaculation or inability to sustain an erection over a long period of time are additional symptoms of kidney *yin* vacuity. In general, all symptoms worsen after sexual intercourse because this exerts *yin* even further.

General symptoms are signs of dryness (mucosa, parched skin), heat in the five hearts (palms of the hands, soles of the feet, sternum), and night sweating, often accompanied by dizziness and tinnitus. The tongue is red and without fur, the pulse is superficial and vacuous, but often also rapid and thin.

Kidney *Yang*

Yang as a warming force is indispensable for the processes of fertilization, nidation, and maturation. At the same time, kidney *yang* supplies the "warmth" and energy in the uterus that make nidation successful.

The *ming men* fire warms the uterus, facilitates conception, influences sexual desire, and regulates *yin* influences. The heat of the *ming men* fire can, in repletion, lead to hypermenorrhea, infertility, or miscarriage. If it becomes vacuous, on the other hand, it is no longer able to warm the uterus. This cold can result in infertility, dysmenorrhea, or lack of libido. TCM refers to such kidney *yang* vacuity as "cold uterus"; Western medicine speaks of a progesterone deficiency that causes the body temperature to drop lower than in women with normal progesterone levels.[4]

Kidney Yang *Vacuity in Women*

Kidney *yang* vacuity often results in hypothermia and physical exhaustion. Especially during men-

struation, the body is very sensitive to cold because the *chong mai* is open and susceptible to pathogenic energies. During this time, women should therefore perhaps avoid swimming in cold water or consistently having cold legs. Cold food and drinks can weaken kidney *yang* over time as well. Overwork, immoderate sports, excessive sexual activity, miscarriages, and abortions also damage kidney *yang*.

In women, vacuity cold in the uterus often develops as a result of existing kidney *yang* vacuity. It is commonly found in young women. Menstruation is delayed, often with scant bleeding only and small clots in dark red blood. The women complain of menstrual pain that is relieved by warmth. In general, such women suffer from chills especially during their menstrual period, the face appears pale, and the patients complain of a frequent urge to urinate, as well as of back pain and dizziness. The mood is rather depressed. The fertilized egg has problems during nidation, and infertility is more likely a problem of implantation.

The tongue is pale, partly enlarged, and moist, the fur is thin and white. The pulse is slow, deep, and weak.

Kidney Yang *Vacuity in Men*

In men as well, feeling cold is the primary symptom. Erections are weak and often do not last long. Furthermore, loss of libido is a typical symptom. Few sperms with low motility in often watery ejaculate.

The tongue is pale and moist, possibly swollen (in simultaneous dampness), often with a thin white fur. The pulse is deep and slow.

In men, kidney *yang* vacuity leads to the most common disorders of sexuality and reproduction:

- reduced sperm motility
- watery ejaculate
- impotence
- erectile dysfunctions, especially concerning the duration
- loss of libido

Dual Vacuity of Kidney Yin *and Kidney* Yang *in Men and Women*

Because kidney *yin* and kidney *yang* complement each other, a weakness of one can cause damage to the other. As such, chronic kidney *yin* vacuity can also have a detrimental effect on kidney *yang*. Likewise, chronic stagnation of liver or heart *qi* can impede kidney *yang* in its moving and transforming properties.

In China, the treatment of male infertility is seen as easier than that of women, but also as requiring more time. A treatment that stretches over 2–3 years is still considered appropriate. As far as formulas are concerned, we mostly prescribe medicinals that strengthen kidney *yin* at the same time as medicinals that strengthen kidney *yang*.[4]

Kidney *Qi*

Kidney *qi* is the mobilizing force that distributes *yin* and *yang* and is closely linked to kidney *yang*. Kidney *qi* also has an uplifting and containing function that affects the bodily fluids, including urine, sperm, and vaginal secretion.

Kidney Qi *Vacuity in Men and Women*

Similar to kidney *yang* vacuity, general exhaustion and overexertion are of primary significance here. In addition, though, kidney *qi* vacuity is accompanied by general lack of strength, and often incontinence. The uplifting strength—the *qi*—weakens, which results in shortened erections, nightly (dreamless) seminal emissions, or in women in watery discharge. In conjunction with these, patients often complain of dizziness, impaired vision and hearing, pain in the lumbar and knee areas, and vacuity headaches.

The cause of kidney *qi* vacuity can also be found in a weakness of the lung, when the lung is unable to supply the kidneys with sufficient *qi*. The tongue is pale and limp, the pulse deep and weak. In women, we find amenorrhea or irregular cycles with bright scant blood.

Kidney *qi* vacuity means:
- complete or partial impotence
- frequent spontaneous seminal emissions

- dizziness
- tinnitus
- pale appearance
- cold extremities
- defective hearing
- weakness and lack of strength
- pain in the lower back and legs
- frequent urination
- watery vaginal discharge

Physiology and Pathology of the Liver

Besides the kidney, the liver is the most important viscus for reproduction. Liver *qi* stagnation or liver blood depletion have far-reaching effects in men and women.

From the TCM perspective, the liver facilitates the regular and uninhibited flow of *qi*. *Qi* as the driving and self-actualizing force is also necessary for the actual practice of sexuality. Disorders in this area—as the result of stress, fears, or exaggerated expectations—lead to stagnation, first of *qi* and then also of blood.

When the liver no longer supplies the muscles and sinews with sufficient *qi* and blood, this can lead to blockages especially in the channels or their *luo* network vessels. In men, the penis as the "sinew of the liver" can be directly affected, causing erectile dysfunctions and inability to penetrate.

Erectile and ejaculatory dysfunctions:
- **kidney *qi* vacuity**: lack of strength, nocturia, and general weakness
- **kidney *yang* vacuity**: listlessness
- **liver *qi* stagnation**: sexual desire but inability to perform intercourse
- **spleen *qi* vacuity**: heaviness and dampness
- **heart *qi* vacuity**: fear of failure

In women, the small pelvis is supplied energetically with *qi* and blood also by the liver channel and the *luo* network vessels. Any obstruction in this area can lead to problems during ovulation and also on the path of the ovum to and through the fallopian tubes. In this context, the liver is eminently important due to the relationship between the uterus and blood in particular, since the uterus stores the blood that comes from the liver.

Liver blood as the *yin* part and liver *qi* as the *yang* part influence each other because if *yin* fails to nourish *yang*, vacuity results; if *yang* fails to move *yin*, stagnation results.

Liver *Qi* Stagnation in Men and Women

In women, stagnation of liver *qi* commonly arises in conjunction with blood stagnation. Liver *qi* is essential for menstruation as the mover of blood. Especially in the premenstrual phase, liver *qi* stagnation leads to PMS and in general to menstrual irregularities, with dark red, clotted blood, in combination with tension in the chest, irritability, and dysmenorrhea.

In men, liver *qi* stagnation is often connected with insufficiency of *jing*. Such patients feel irritable, depressed, have a tendency to forgetfulness, and their knees and lower back hurt and seem weak. Erections are weak and often accompanied by a loss of libido, because liver *qi* stagnation prevents the blood and muscles from being filled as time and situation require. Sometimes, men are no longer able to ejaculate at all (mostly when combined with kidney *yang* or spleen *qi* vacuity).

The tongue can be inconspicuous or bluish purple with blood macules (blood stagnation). Sometimes the margins are slightly reddened, sometimes pale when the stagnation arose as a result of blood vacuity. In such cases, the pulse is rough, otherwise more stringlike.

> Liver *qi* stagnation has the following effects:
> * temporary sexual weakness
> * periods of impotence or premature ejaculation
> * in women, cycle-related lack of desire
> * disquietude and liver disharmony

Physiology and Pathology of the Spleen

The spleen is the source of postnatal *jing* because it takes in nourishment and energy from the environment, assimilates these, and thereby transforms them into postnatal *jing* that can be utilized by the kidney. With nourishment, we, of course, mean food but also emotional and spiritual nourishment—a person can become depleted in this area as well. If the spleen can no longer carry out these tasks, this in turns leads to a depletion of kidney *jing*.

The spleen is the producer of blood, which is then stored in the liver. We can therefore attribute every case of liver blood vacuity in women also to spleen vacuity. The spleen produces blood. In men, it transforms it into sperm; in women, into menstrual blood and breastmilk. Hence, the heart controls the blood and the liver stores it, but the spleen produces it.

Spleen *qi* with its ascending movement is important for lifting organs and tissue and thereby for holding the human body in its center. A spleen *qi* vacuity would lead to sagging disorders and to prolapse. We can also use spleen *qi* vacuity to explain menorrhagia of the vacuity type because the spleen is no longer able to contain and collect the blood.

Phlegm-Dampness in the Lower Burner

These patients, often overweight, feel heavy and phlegmatic; in addition to excessive phlegm production, soft stools and edemas are common symptoms. Infertility has often persisted for a long time already. We commonly see vacuity in the center, namely weakness of spleen *qi* and kidney *yang*, which can disturb the *jin ye* (bodily fluids) mechanism and prevent them from lifting and warming sufficiently, combined with *qi* stagnation and blood stasis.

Women tend to complain of abundant vaginal discharge. A long but irregular cycle with midcycle pain and scant thin red blood characterizes this pattern. Men suffer from erectile dysfunctions, often in combination with a feeling of heaviness or lack of strength in the lower abdomen. The tongue is pale and enlarged with a whitish sticky fur, the pulse is slippery and rather slow.

> Phlegm and dampness in the lower burner have the following effects:
> * premature ejaculation or inability to achieve an erection
> * lethargy

- lack of appetite
- feeling of fullness in the chest or abdomen
- cloudy secretion in the urine
- urinary retention or dribbling at night
- edemas

To treat such conditions, we must resolve the dampness and remove the obstructions, especially those that can change the course of the *ren mai* and *chong mai*. In this context, the significance of a proper diet cannot be overemphasized. Foods that are difficult to digest, including fat but also raw foods, make the unfavorable combination of spleen *qi* vacuity (i.e., dampness) plus kidney vacuity (i.e., lack of strength) even worse. If this is further compounded by alcohol, nicotine, sugar, gratins, and deep-fried foods, this can lead to damp-heat with inflammatory and destructive changes.

Damp-Heat in the Lower Burner

Damp-heat in the spleen and/or liver—aggravated by fatty foods and alcohol—can lead to dampness and phlegm formation in the genitals. An original *yin* vacuity (heat) and persistent stagnation of *qi* and dampness (phlegm, moistness) can also cause this pattern as a result of the simultaneous occurrence of dampness (spleen vacuity) and liver *qi* stagnation. As a consequence, damp-heat sinks down and collects in the liver channel as well. Pathological accumulations of dampness arise: edemas, swellings, and tumors can appear (prostate hypertrophy, cysts, carcinomas). Inflammations in the genital area such as orchitis, prostatitis, adnexitis, vaginitis, or bartholinitis also result from damp-heat in the small pelvis. Yellow discharge from the vagina or penis is a common accompanying symptom. We can also see obstructions of the vas deferens (or the fallopian tubes). Ejaculatory or erectile dysfunctions with weak, sometimes impossible erections, reduced sperm count, limited motility, and sperm antibodies, thick ejaculate, spermatorrhea, and premature ejaculation can occur as well. The tongue is red with a yellow slimy fur, the pulse is rapid and slippery.

Damp-heat sinking into the lower burner has the following effects:

- premature ejaculation
- erectile dysfunctions
- sweating in the genital area
- inflammations in the small pelvis
- yellow discharge
- dark yellow and cloudy urine

Physiology and Pathology of the Heart

Heart fire initiates new life and unites *yin* and *yang*. Love, friendship, and joy in sexuality are affairs of the heart. The heart controls the blood and distributes it—unlike the lung and liver—in dependence on emotions and feelings.

As the kidney's *ming men* fire strengthens the fire of the heart, heart *yang* likewise provides powerful support to kidney *yang*. If it dries up, the result is erectile and ejaculatory dysfunctions and in addition to the associated feeling of cold also general exhaustion, especially after sexual intercourse.

In its function as the ruler of blood, the heart also has a direct influence on menstruation. Kidney essence forms menstrual blood with the assistance of heart *yang*. Heart blood reaches the uterus via the *bao mai* (uterine vessel), and the heart thereby influences the downward flow of menstrual blood. Emotional strain can disrupt this function and lead, for example, to heart blood vacuity, just as an experience of shock can cause amenorrhea. On the other hand, though, heart blood vacuity can also have emotional consequences; here we can think of postpartum depression, caused by blood vacuity after delivery.

Heart *Qi* Stagnation

Heart *qi* stagnation most commonly occurs in conjunction with a disturbance of the *shen*, often following a traumatic event or long-lasting emotional conflicts. Through the axis heart—*bao mai*—uterus, irregular ovulation and menstruation result. The tongue shows a red tip, the pulse is replete and rapid.

Heart Heat

Heart heat is characterized by general overexcitement, accompanied by hypertonicity, tachycardia, and heat sensations with a red face. We often see pain during sexual intercourse.

Physiology and Pathology of the Lung

The lung is the source of *qi* and as such essential for supplying especially the kidney with *qi*. *Qi* gives the person and his or her activities strength, it is responsible for the movement of blood, and it provides support and stability. *Qi* vacuity in the lower burner in particular not only causes listlessness but also a weakening of the muscles in this region. A slack pelvic floor, short strengthless erections, and an insufficient supply of the kidneys in general are the long-term results of lung *qi* vacuity.

The mother's **corporeal soul** *po* is of great significance for conception as well. It would in fact be more correct to speak of *po* souls since there are seven corporeal souls that die together with the body at death. The *po* souls enter the body of the fetus at the moment of conception and thereby supply the new life with essence. With the *po* souls, essence enters the body (conception) and exits it (death). In this process, the embryo's *po* souls are formed from those of the mother; the father has no influence in this area. Because the *po* souls reside in the lung, the congenital constitution of the child is affected by the energetic condition of the mother's lung—and hence not only by the condition of both parents' kidneys.

■ The Physiology of Menstruation from the TCM Perspective

As explained above, the heavenly water *tian gui* is responsible for regulating the human sexual functions and therefore also for menstruation. In a sexually mature woman, whether menstruation occurs and whether the menses flow depends on the fullness of the sea of blood—*chong mai*. The liver ensures that the *chong mai* is supplied with blood. When the sea of blood is full, everything is ready for the nidation of the fertilized egg. If no implantation takes place, on the other hand, the blood is discharged by the distributing function of the liver. The sea of blood is empty after menstruation; it fills back up with blood after ovulation, in order to be ready again for the fertilized egg.

The phases of the menstrual cycle are:

1. Menstrual phase (ca. 5 days). The blood is moving, for which purpose liver *qi* and liver blood must be able to flow freely.
2. Follicular phase (ca. 7 days). Blood and *yin* are relatively vacuous, the *ren mai* and *chong mai* are drained.
3. Ovulatory phase (ca. 7 days). Blood and *yin* gradually fill the *ren mai* and *chong mai* back up. Switch from *yin* to *yang* phase.
4. Luteal phase (ca. 7 days). *Yang qi* increases and liver *qi* moves.

During the phase of discharging blood, the body temperature drops to a physiological level. After menstruation, the body must again be nourished by the function of the spleen and warmed by the function of the kidney. With the assistance of the triple burner (*san jiao*), the absorbed *gu qi* (grain *qi*) is transformed into blood and transported to the sea of blood. In the middle of the cycle, ovulation takes place, which requires energy and thereby causes a short drop in body temperature, to be followed by a rise to a higher level on the next day. This rise in body temperature is a function of *yang*. The sea of blood fills back up completely between the time of ovulation and menstruation or implantation of the fertilized egg. The relative balance between *yin* and *yang* has been restored.

A regular menstrual cycle is therefore a basic requirement for any successful treatment of female infertility. In this context, Chinese doctors attach much more value to what they see as the optimal length of 28–29 days. Regarding the length of the menstrual cycle, the classical texts also describe exceptions that were seen as unusual but not pathological. The *Mai Jing (Pulse Classic)* from the 3rd century CE, for example, reports that some women menstruate only once every 3 months or even only once a year. Li Shizhen (16th century) recognized a menstrual period that occurred regularly every 2 months as a physiological phenomenon.[7] Western biomedicine, on the other hand, considers anything between 25 and 35 days as normal.[4] A prolonged cycle could thus suggest blood vacuity: the follicle would need longer to mature and build up enough substance; this delays ovulation and decreases fertility.

The quality of the menstrual blood is another important source of information for diagnosis in TCM. Clots or mucus, for example, would point to a stagnation of *qi* or blood, manifestations of a disturbance in the flow of *qi* and blood.

In the treatment of female infertility, TCM therefore recommends harmonizing the menstrual cycle first. Ideally, this treatment is carried out parallel to the phases of the menstrual cycle described above. In concrete terms, this means:

1. **Menstrual phase**. Transition from *yang* to *yin*. The blood moves downward. While menstruating, we can regulate the cycle, that is, stop the bleeding in hypermenorrhea or quicken the blood in hypomenorrhea. Stasis and stagnation can be eliminated by supplementing *qi*.
2. **Follicular phase**. The *yin* phase with the build-up of *yin* and blood. After menstruation, the time is opportune for nourishing blood (in liver blood vacuity) and supplementing the kidney (in kidney yin vacuity).
3. **Ovulatory phase**. Transition from *yin* to *yang*. Blood and *qi* show a strong dynamic. Mid-cycle is ideal for solidifying the *ren mai* and *chong mai* and for supplementing the kidney. We can eliminate accumulations of dampness and phlegm and resolve heart and liver stagnation. The mucus should be plentiful and fertile.
4. **Luteal phase**. *Yang* phase. The fertile egg implants. The time before the onset of the period is well-suited for supplementing (kidney) *yang* and for moving liver *qi*.

If infertility—as is most commonly the case—is rooted in states of vacuity, treatment initially focuses on the kidney. In this context, recommendations vary slightly between the individual phases:

- On day 4–5 after the onset of the menstrual period (follicular development phase), supplement the kidney and nourish blood.
- During the intermenstrual phase (follicular maturation and ovulation), nourish and quicken the blood.

- In the luteal phase (development of the corpus luteum and secretion of progesterone), supplement the kidney, solidify *ren mai* and *chong mai*, and regulate the liver.
- During menstruation (atrophy of the corpus luteum), quicken the blood and regulate menstruation.[5]

■ Conception

On the physical level, a successful conception requires an adequate supply of blood and essence because the new life is formed from these. On the father's side, essence is passed on through the sperm; on the mother's side, it consists of the prenatal heavenly *gui* (see above) and postnatal *qi* in the form of blood. The mother's essence is her *yin* energy, but without her *yang* energy, namely the *ming men* fire, no conception can take place. This ministerial fire of water makes it possible for the spark of new life to ignite.

Ming Men—the Life Gate
Nan Jing 39, question on the life gate *ming men*: "The life gate refers to the place where the essences and spirits reside, where the semen is stored in the man, and where the uterus is suspended in the woman. Its *qi* is identical to that of the kidneys."[2]
The kidney is not only the source of water (kidney *yin*), but also of fire (kidney *yang*). In this context, we have to distinguish between the prenatal ministerial fire of the kidney and the imperial fire of the heart. The kidney fire from the *ming men* originates in the area between the two kidneys (CV-4) and is closely related to the *yuan qi* (original *qi*) and the *dong qi* (moving *qi*). The *ming men* is therefore not only the residence of water and fire, but also the root of *yuan qi*. It contributes to the nourishing effect of the *yin* in the viscera and assists in the development of their *yang*.

When the father's sperm-essence and the mother's blood unite, it is the uterus that forms the fetus out of these substances and nourishes and preserves it until birth. By transforming and preserving *jing* and blood, the uterus embodies the function of earth, from whose *qi* it originated.

Key Patterns of Female Infertility

We can find the following key patterns in female infertility:
- problems during ovulation or during the first half of the cycle
- problems during nidation or during the second half of the cycle

Problems During Ovulation or During the First Half of the Cycle

- kidney *yin* vacuity
- heart *qi* stagnation
- possibly complicated further by liver *qi* stagnation, dampness and phlegm, or blood stagnation

Problems During Nidation or During the Second Half of the Cycle

- kidney *yang* vacuity
- possibly complicated by liver *qi* stagnation, dampness and phlegm, or blood stagnation
- kidney *yang* vacuity that subsequently leads to spleen vacuity[4]

■ Pregnancy

Because of the absence of menstruation, pregnancy is a time of excess: on the one hand, an excess of *yin* because fluids collect; on the other hand, an excess of *yang* because the ministerial fire increases as well. Water and fire are inseparable inside the kidney. Hence, both increase as a result of the interrupted menses. This excess men-

strual blood, which is not just simply blood (see above), is transformed into essence during pregnancy to nourish the embryo and mother. As such, pregnancy depends not only on the mother's lifestyle during this time, but also especially on the existing state of kidney *qi*. For this reason, some women truly bloom during pregnancy while others feel exhausted instead.

Causes for a Miscarriage

Before Implantation of the Egg

- Due to *qi* stagnation or phlegm, the fallopian tubes are displaced.
- Due to kidney vacuity (*yin* and/or *yang*), blood vacuity or blood stagnation, the endometrium is of poor quality.

After Implantation of the Egg

- kidney vacuity
- *qi* and blood vacuity
- blood heat
- blood stagnation

■ The Pathology of Infertility from the TCM Perspective

Zhang Jiebin (ca. 1563–1640) summarizes the pathology of infertility in men and women in the *Jing Yue Quan Shu (Complete Knowledge of Medicine by Jing Yue [Zhang Jiebin])* as follows:

"Diseases of the Man
Disorders associated with conception are in the man located in the essence, in the woman in the blood. Without exception, they are conditions of vacuity. Vacuity conditions in the man manifest in nightly seminal emissions, clear essence, cold essence, and in failure of the penis to harden during foreplay; or [the essence] leaks out instead of shooting out; or there are repeated seminal emissions while dreaming; or the urine is impure and dribbles painfully; or [the man] abandons

himself to lust until his yin is vacuous; when yin is in a state of vacuity, the lumbus and kidney are painful and exhausted; or [the man] abandons himself to sexuality to the point where his yang has reached its utmost extreme; when yang has reached its extreme, it becomes violent and destroys yin or [the man] rubs it too strongly and persistently; when he has intercourse too strongly and persistently, the result is disharmony; or [the man] merely suffers from a hernia; when a hernia is present, the liver and kidney are displaced. This can be compounded by a yang vacuity; when yang is vacuous, there is too much cold; or it can be a yin vacuity; when a yin vacuity is present, there is too much heat. Conditions of this type are all diseases of the man. You cannot lay the blame [for infertility] completely on the woman. If you know the cause and a treatment is recommended, then carry out this treatment. When it is indicated to take measures against [the infertility], then take action. You must first try to find the responsibility in yourself and only afterwards turn to the woman. Then help is available in all cases.

Diseases of the Woman

The key factor in the woman is the blood. When blood and essence can come together, conception takes place. If you want to research her disorders, you will find all of them in the area of menstruation. If you want to cure her disorders, you will only be successful by regulating yin. Now, the menstrual period is blood and blood is yin. Yin corresponds to the moon. For this reason, the distance between periods is always one month. This is the normal state. When she is in a state of disease, we can find the following [manifestations]: Menstruation begins too early or too late, it comes twice in one month, it comes once in two months, it is interrupted because the blood is dried out, or it flows continuously without interruption; there is pain beforehand or there is pain afterwards; there are the colors pale red, black, or purple; there are blockages and therefore strings or pieces; if essence and blood are not replete, they transform into vaginal discharge; there is a state of vacuity and cold in the child's palace, as a result of which yang qi fails to form; there is heat in the blood, as a result of which yin qi fails to form; the menstrual water fails to discharge and the uterus fails to conceive as a result of blockages in the blood and qi. All these are disease states of the original yin. When the original yin is diseased, yin blood is insufficient and cannot develop a fetus. When yin qi is insufficient, [the uterus] cannot

hold the fetus. The strength for holding and developing lies entirely in the ming men (life gate). The life gate is precisely the sea of blood of the chong mai and ren mai, and the fetus depends essentially on the blood. Because blood does not form on its own, it is also substantially dependent on qi. These two are what we refer to as the 'original yin' (zhen yin). When you fill the ming men, you can say both in regards to blood and in regards to qi that you fill the yin; and the method of filling yin is precisely the way to strengthening the root and securing the foundation. This is what every person must not lack from adulthood on until old age. And if a person in addition gives up the foundation of the congenital and acquired source of life, how could they strive for descendants? For this reason, the only thing of importance for regulating menstruation and sowing seeds is to fill the ming men and to protect yang qi. Now, the storehouse of essence and blood is in the ming men, but the source of essence and blood lies in heart and spleen yang. The heart governs the blood. When you nourish the heart, blood is formed. The spleen and stomach govern nutrition. When you keep the spleen and stomach healthy, the qi [gained from food] is distributed, qi pulls, and the blood flows. Emotions, nutrition, and the above [-mentioned] channels [ren mai and chong mai] are all together without exception the sources for replenishing yin.

If you treat beginning and end indiscriminately, ignoring the proper order [of steps], this will not be sufficient to allow you to speak of the 'method for regulating menstruation and sowing seeds.'"[7]

■ Summary of Infertility in Tables

Tables **7.1** and **7.2** provide a summary of the most important patterns, symptoms, and diagnostic characteristics that arise in the context of infertility in men and women.

Table 7.1 Infertility in the man

Pattern	Symptoms	Tongue	Pulse
Kidney *jing* vacuity	Exhausted, forgetful, impaired vision and hearing, weakness and pain in the knees and LSC, shortened erection	Pale, limp	Deep, fine, weak
Kidney *yang* vacuity	Feeling of coldness, lack of libido, spermatorrhea, erection is often weak and only short, watery ejaculate (limited motility)	Pale, partly enlarged, with a thin white fur	Deep, weak, slow
Kidney *yin* vacuity	Feeling of heat, spermatorrhea, premature ejaculation, scant thick ejaculate, low sperm count	Red with scant fur	Thin, rapid
Blood stasis with *jing* vacuity	Chronic *qi* stagnation or trauma as prehistory; dry skin, varicose veins, pain in the lower abdomen	Purple, dark, possibly punctate hemorrhage	Deep, rough
Liver *qi* stagnation	Irritable, stressed, dizziness, tinnitus, weak erections, partly inability to ejaculate	Red margins, possibly congested SLV	Stringlike
Spleen *qi* vacuity and dampness	Increased phlegm, adiposity, edemas, feeling of fullness, soft stools, erectile dysfunctions	Large, inflated, with tooth marks, with a white sticky fur	Slippery
Damp-heat	Inflammations and obstructions in the genital area, spermatorrhea, premature ejaculation, possibly inability to achieve an erection, low sperm count, limited motility, possibly sperm antibodies, thick yellowish ejaculate	Red, with yellow slimy fur	Rapid, slippery
Qi and blood vacuity	Exhaustion, shortness of breath, paleness, dizziness, tinnitus, palpitations, weak erection	Pale, with thin white fur	Weak, vacuous

Note: LSC = lumbar spinal column, SLV = sublingual veins.

Table 7.2 Infertility in the woman

Pattern	Cycle	Blood	Symptoms	Tongue	Pulse
Kidney *jing* vacuity	Amenorrhea or irregular	Scant, bright	Exhausted, weakness and pain in the LSC and knees, tinnitus	Pale	Deep, weak
Blood vacuity	Delayed onset with mild pain in the lower abdomen	Scant, bright	Anemic, pale, listless, malnourished, constipated	Pale with scant fur	Weak, sometimes rough
Liver *qi* and blood stagnation	Amenorrhea or irregular	Dark red with clots	PMS, irritable and tense, feelings of pressure, pain, and tension, tension in the breasts.	Purple with blood macules	Deep, stringlike
"Cold uterus"	Normal or prolonged	Scant, dark with small clots	Feeling of coldness and cold pain in the lower abdomen, menstrual pain, frequent urination	Bright (vacuity), dark (repletion)	Deep, slow
"Hot uterus"	Normal or shortened	Strong bleeding	Feeling of heat, exhausted, dry mucous membranes (also endometrium!), scant stretchable ("fertile") cervical mucus	Red, with scant or no fur	Rapid, thin

Table 7.2 Continued

Pattern	Cycle	Blood	Symptoms	Tongue	Pulse
Spleen *qi* vacuity and dampness	Prolonged or amenorrhea, often with mid-cycle pain	Scant, bright	Excess phlegm, edemas, adiposity, vaginal discharge, soft stools	Inflated, with white slimy fur, tooth marks	Slippery
Damp-heat	Shortened	Scant, partly with phlegm mixed in	Edemas, tumors, inflammations in the small pelvis, yellowish discharge	Red, with slimy yellow fur	Slippery, rapid

Note: LSC = lumbar spinal column. PMS = premenstrual syndrome.

Bibliography

1. Focks C, Hillenbrand N (editors). *Leitfaden Chinesische Medizin*. Munich: Urban & Fischer; 2006.
2. Kubny M. *Qi—Lebenskraftkonzepte in China*. Heidelberg: Haug; 1995.
3. Lewis R. *The Infertility Cure*. Boston: Little, Brown and Company; 2004.
4. Lyttleton J. *Treatment of Infertility with Chinese Medicine*. London: Churchill Livingstone; 2004.
5. Maciocia G. *Die Gynäkologie in der Praxis der Chinesischen Medizin*. Kötzting: VGM Wühr; 2000.
6. Noll A. Sexuelle Störungen. In: Noll A, Kirschbaum B (editors). *Stresskrankheiten*. Munich: Urban & Fischer; 2006: 455–471.
7. Riegel A-M. *Das Streben nach dem Sohn. Fruchtbarkeit und Empfängnis in den Medizinischen Texten Chinas von der Hanzeit zur Mingzeit*. Munich: Herbert Utz; 1999.
8. Veith I, trans. The Yellow Emperor's Classic of Internal Medicine. University of California Press; 2002.

8 Worth a Thousand in Gold—The Quest for Perfect Children in Early China

Sabine Wilms

■ Introduction

What we refer to as infertility treatments in modern medicine was in early China included in the medical category of *qiu zi* (求子), literally "the quest for children." For cultural, social, and philosophical reasons, the significance of this topic in the historical Chinese context can hardly be overstated. It was therefore discussed not only in technical medical literature, but also in philosophical and cosmological texts, from both a Daoist and a Confucian angle.

On the one hand, what we traditionally identify as the Confucian perspective is a prescriptive set of ideas that is concerned with life in this world, in a socially meaningful and productive way that takes the cultivation of the self, the family, and the state as its goal. Harmony, balance, moderation, and order within and between these spheres of existence are necessary to ensure survival and continuity in the ever-changing cycle of life. In this context, women were recognized as essential participants for their role of producing and rearing male offspring, to guarantee the continuation of the family line from the past through the present into the future.

> Sons were of particular importance in the Chinese context because they were the only ones able to perform **ancestral sacrifices**.

In contrast to the social, moral, and political orientation of Confucianism, Daoist texts and authors focused on the natural world and the cosmic order as it was reflected not in the human realm but in the larger scheme of things. In that context, human reproduction was a mirror image, a metaphor, a window into the obscure processes of cosmogenesis and of birth, maturity, decay, and death that occurred in unceasing succession in all realms of the natural world.

Understanding this process of change was essential to the ultimate goal of Daoism, namely to exist in harmony with the *dao* (道 "way"), the way of the universe, which was expressed in the ideal of *wu wei* (無為 "non-action," but more accurately perhaps "not acting against the *dao*").

Considering the interpretation of reproduction in all early Chinese philosophical traditions, we understand why we find detailed references to the processes of conception, gestation, and childbirth in texts that we would otherwise classify as philosophical or cosmological. This multifaceted interest in the "quest for children" by male elite writers in early China should be kept in mind when we look at the information presented in the following paragraphs.

■ Sun Simiao and the *Bei Ji Qian Jin Yao Fang*

The following description of early medieval Chinese practices is drawn from a 7th-century text: the *Bei Ji Qian Jin Yao Fang* (備急千金要方), composed by Sun Simiao (孫思邈) around 652 CE. The title can be translated as *Essential 1000-Gold Formulary for Emergencies* and is in the following paragraphs abbreviated as *Qian Jin Fang*.

In this groundbreaking medical encyclopedia of over 5000 entries, the three volumes titled *Formulas for Women* form the first major section in the text, followed by pediatrics, general medicine, and, lastly, life-prolonging self-cultivation techniques. The information found in this text is of a clinical nature and was clearly intended for practical application. In addition to its intended use as medical knowledge on diagnosis, etiology, and therapy, it can also tell us indirectly about early Chinese culture, particularly in regard to views on gender.

The author of the *Qian Jin Fang*, Sun Simiao, is still venerated to this day in China as the "King of

Medicine" (*yao wang* 藥王), that is, one of the forefathers of Traditional Chinese Medicine in general. In addition to his medical fame, he is also known as an accomplished Daoist adept, alchemist, and pursuer of longevity, maintained close ties to the imperial court through much of his life, and was intimately familiar with Buddhist, Confucian, and Daoist philosophy. More relevant to the topic of this book, he is a key figure in the development of gynecology for being the first to stress the centrality of women's health for perpetuating the family lineage and to relate this to the individual practice of "nurturing life" (*yang sheng* 養生). He is also the first writer to explicitly state and justify the need for a literature of "separate formulas" (*bie fang* 別方) for women. His rationale is found in the famous often-cited introductory essay to the volumes on *Formulas for Women*. I am quoting it here at length because of its elegance and succinctness, the complexity of ideas raised, and its subsequent significance for the history of gynecology:

"The reason why women have special formulas is that they are different because of pregnancy, childbirth, and flooding damage (i. e., abnormal vaginal bleeding). Therefore, women's diseases are ten times more difficult to treat than men's. It is a classic saying that 'women are copious accumulations of yin *and are constantly inhabited by dampness.'*
From the age of fourteen on, [a woman's] yin qi *floats up and spills over, [causing] a hundred thoughts to pass through her heart. Internally, it damages the five viscera; externally, it injures the outward appearance. The discharge and retention of menstrual fluid is alternatingly early or delayed, stagnant blood lodges and congeals, and the central pathways are interrupted and cut off. It is impossible to discuss the entirety of damages and losses among these [conditions]. The raw and the cooked are deposited together [during digestion], vacuity and repletion intermingle with each other in confusion, malign blood leaks internally, and the* qi *in the vessels is injured and exhausted. [The woman's] intake of food and drink might have been intemperate, causing not just a single injury. Or she may have had sexual intercourse before [vaginal] sores have healed. Or she may have squatted over the privy without proper care, [allowing] wind to enter from below and thereby giving rise to the twelve intractable diseases. For these reasons, special formulas have been established for women. In cases where the nodal* qi *over the four seasons has caused illness and where vacuity or reple-*

tion of cold or heat have caused worry, then [women are treated] the same as men, the only exception being that if they fall ill while carrying a fetus in pregnancy, you must avoid toxic medicines!
In cases where their miscellaneous diseases are identical to men's, [the treatments] are dispersed throughout the various volumes and can be known from there. Nevertheless, women's predilections and desires exceed men's and they contract diseases at twice the rate of men. In addition, when they are affected by compassion and attachment, love and hatred, envy and jealousy, and worry and rancor, these become firmly lodged and deep-seated. Since they are unable to control their affects by themselves, the roots of their diseases are deep and it is difficult to obtain a cure in their treatment."

In these paragraphs, Sun Simiao constructs a multifaceted explanation for the medical need to recognize the female body as different. His discussion takes into consideration not only physiological factors, but also psychological and even cultural ones, all of which cause the diseases of women to be "ten times more difficult to treat than men's." This essay is a powerful appeal to physicians' humanitarian duty to heal female bodies, which are seen as particularly vulnerable for several reasons.

Because of the stresses of pregnancy, childbirth, and resulting hemorrhaging, they are prone to vacuity (*xu* 虛), which could lead to any number of physical and psychological problems. In addition, women's excess of *yin qi* associated with sexual maturation causes emotional instability, damage to the internal organs, menstrual disorders, and problems with the flow of blood and *qi* in the channels. When we read the essay above in conjunction with the individual formula entries that follow, the etiologies expressed by Sun Simiao reflect the notion that a vacuous female body, forced open in the process of childbirth, is liable to an invasion by cold and wind. Sneaking in through the vagina, these external pathogens can attack and block blood and *qi* in the channels and from there wreak havoc in any of the internal organs for years to come. Moreover, it turns out that the most dangerous pathology for women, in Sun's eyes, is the lingering presence of a substance called "malign dew" (*e lu* 惡露).

This evocative term refers to old blood left over in the uterus after childbirth, the most common symptom of which is blocked menstruation. It is considered extremely pathogenic and therefore has to be eliminated completely by means of numerous uterus-cleansing and blood-dispersing formulas. Associated with an endless list of symptoms not only inside the body for the rest of the woman's life, but also outside, "malign dew" is feared as highly offensive to the spirits.

To this day, a traditional Chinese woman's postpartum recovery is often covered by a host of taboos aimed at protecting her from premature contact with society and the natural environment. Postpartum taboos in the early gynecological literature express, on the one hand, the authors' paternalistic concern for the mother's extremely depleted and vulnerable physical state. On the other hand, though, the numerous references to magicoreligious etiologies and treatments reflect a simultaneous awareness of the pathogenic powers of the blood of childbirth and the risks of handling this substance.

To cite just one example, several centuries after the *Qian Jin Fang*, Chen Ziming (陳自明) (ca. 1190–1270 CE) compiled the *Fu Ren Da Quan Liang Fang (Comprehensive Good Formulas for Women* 婦人大全良方*)* in 1237. In particular, the section on childbirth contains a large percentage of religious treatments like invocations, talismans, astrological calculations, divinations, and various rituals to prevent offending the spirits during childbirth. Found in the lengthy discussion of postpartum taboos is even a strict warning that laundry that has been stained by the fluids of childbirth must not be dried in the sunlight, or one will risk injury by evil spirits.

To return to Sun Simiao's introductory essay, the effects of women's reproductive functions range from a general state of vacuity to specific conditions like emotional volatility during menstruation or the presence of rotting blood in the uterus for years after childbirth. This underlying and often invisible vulnerability can then lead to severe injuries from fairly harmless secondary causes like an immoderate diet, sexual intercourse during menstruation or too soon after childbirth, or an invasion of wind by an innocent visit to the outhouse.

After stressing that "women's cravings and desires exceed their husbands'…they contract illness at twice the rate of men and…because they are unable to control their emotions, the roots of their disorders are deep," the essay concludes by emphasizing the importance of childbearing for society at large. In the course of this argument, Sun first states that reproduction plays a central role in women's lives since "bearing children is the adult role in women's destiny and fate." Going further, he even advises that "specialists in the art of nurturing life (*yang sheng zhi jia* 養生之家) should particularly instruct their sons and daughters to study these three volumes of women's recipes until they comprehend them thoroughly" to prepare for any "harvests of unexpected surprises" and "to prevent premature and wrongful death." Even servants involved in childcare "cannot afford not to study them. Thus, they should routinely write out a copy and carry it on their person, clutched to their bosom, in order to guard against the unexpected."

In a subtle but highly significant twist, Sun Simiao hereby extends the elite practice of macrobiotic hygiene, that is, physical cultivation with the purpose of prolonging one's life, to cover not only the practitioner's individual body but to also include past and, most importantly, future generations. The importance of female bodies in this context becomes immediately obvious, a fact that the ancient sages had already recognized. Protecting and preserving women's health was therefore an essential task for any elite gentleman, since it could, if neglected or ignored, result in potentially grave consequences for society as a whole. This respect for the female body was doubtlessly further strengthened by Sun Simiao's personal and active involvement as a Daoist priest and practitioner of religious cultivation. In stark contrast with the negative association of the female body with impurity, transgression, and material desire in Buddhism, it was celebrated in Daoism for its identification with *yin* as complementary to *yang*, and with motherhood and the ability to give and nurture life.

■ Fertility Treatments in the *Qian Jin Fang*

With the essay described above, Sun Simiao laid the foundations from which to launch the first aspect of his *Formulas for Women*: a treatment program for "the quest for children." Containing six essays, 14 medicinal formulas, six moxibustion methods, and three "methods for converting a fe-male [fetus] into a male," it comprises about 6% of the *Formulas for Women*.

Before offering treatments though, Sun Simiao warns that even the best medicine is useless if the couple's basic destinies are mismatched (meaning that their birth signs do not follow the order of generation in the progression of the five phases) and the astrological constellations at the time of conceiving the fetus are inauspicious. If their birth signs are in harmony, however, they will still need to pay heed to Sun Simiao's medical advice and also guard against breaking taboos against sexual intercourse at inauspicious times, in order to en-sure their own and their offspring's future health and good fortune. Editors of the *Qian Jin Fang* from the Song period insert a reference here that meth-ods for determining the right time and day for "receiving a fetus" (*shou tai* 受胎) are found further back in the *Qian Jin Fang* in Volume 27 on "nurtur-ing life" (*yang sheng* 養生). It is interesting to note that these "methods for taboos and restrictions [on sexual intercourse]" are in a manuscript edi-tion of this text cited in the category for "the quest for children" and were therefore considered part of the *Formulas for Women*. This would suggest that methods of sexual intercourse aimed at safe-guarding and improving the result of conception (i. e., the fetus) were in early China sometimes con-sidered under the category of fertility treatments and sometimes under the category of longevity practices.

In other contemporaneous medical literature, such as the *Wai Tai Mi Yao (Arcane Essentials from the Imperial Library)* and *Ishimpo* (in Chinese, *Yi Xin Fang*), considerable space is devoted to these taboos and prognostications about the child's and parents' future in the section on "the quest for children." In a slight shift of emphasis, Sun Simiao offers a purely medical etiology of infertility in the next essay. Here, he states:

*"Whenever people are childless, it is caused by the fact that both husband and wife suffer from the **five taxa-tions** and **seven damages** and the **hundred illnesses of vacuity and emaciation**, with the disastrous result that the line of descendants is cut off."*

This seems in contrast to the popular notions of his time, most notably the *Zhu Bing Yuan Hou Lun (On the Origins and Symptoms of the Various Dis-eases* 諸病源候論*)*, which states:

"When women are without child, there are three rea-sons: First, that the tombs have not been worshipped; second, that the husband's and wife's yearly fate [a reference to their astrological constellations] are in a relationship of mutual conquest; and third, the hus-band or wife's illness. All these cause childlessness. If it is a case of tombs not having been worshipped or the yearly fates conquering each other, there are no medi-cines that can benefit."

Similar sentiments are expressed in the calendri-cal and astrological sections on childlessness in the *Wai Tai Mi Yao, Ishimpo*, and *Qian Jin Fang* cited above. Following this reference to non-med-ical causes of childlessness, Sun Simiao then pro-ceeds to discuss options for medical treatments. These are summarized here in a detailed case study to illustrate the treatment style and under-lying etiological reasoning found in Sun Simiao's *Formulas for Women*:

Case Study—An Interpretation of the First Section of *Qian Jin Fang*, "The Quest for Children"

In order to prevent or treat the medical cause of infertility, which Sun Simiao has previously iden-tified as the "**five taxations** and **seven damages** and the **hundred illnesses of vacuity and emacia-tion**," the author proposes a complex treatment plan:

First, the husband is treated for lack of offspring in conjunction with wind vacuity, clouded vision, and weakness and shortage of essential *qi*, by sup-plementing his insufficiencies with *Qi Zi San* (七子散 Seven Seeds Powder). The famous Yuan dynasty physician Zhu Zhenheng (朱震亨) (alternatively, Danxi 丹溪) later developed this formula into *Wu Zi Yan Zong Wan* (五子衍宗丸 Five Seeds Pills for Abundant Descendants), which is still used today as a treatment for infertility.

The wife is treated for lifelong inability to give birth with a "uterus-rinsing decoction," to be in-gested by the patient while she is wrapped in blankets. This preparation is supposed to induce sweating and cause the discharge of the illness in the form of accumulated blood, which will appear as cold red pus. Referred to as "this malign sub-stance" in the uterus, the root of the illness is identified as an accumulation of cold blood, which causes pain below the navel, irregular menstruation, and inability to receive the fetus. Sun Simiao stresses the importance of consuming an entire preparation of this medicine, if possible, because the illness might otherwise not be completely eliminated. On the next day, the woman should be treated with a suppository consisting of pulverized medicinals filled into a finger-sized silk bag and inserted into the vagina. This is to be applied repeatedly throughout the day while the patient is to remain in her chamber and rest until she has discharged a "cold malign substance" in the form of green-yellow cold liquid, which again represented the illness being expelled below.

The treatment should be concluded with *Zi Shi Men Dong Wan* (紫石門冬丸 Fluorite and Asparagus Pills), to be taken until the sensation of heat in the abdomen indicated a successful completion of the treatment.

Next, Sun Simiao lists a number of fairly complex medicinal formulas for the treatment of infertility in conjunction with symptoms such as heat above and cold below, inhibited menstruation, the 36 diseases of the lower burner, the myriad diseases of vaginal discharge, and the 12 abdominal conglomerations.

While the formulas differ based on the reason for infertility, such as the above-mentioned indications or a "blockage of the uterus that is preventing it from receiving the [man's] essence," they all share the goal of inducing a certain type of discharge below that indicates the expulsion of the illness, whether in the form of "long worms and green-yellow liquid," or "bean juice or snivel."

Thus, it appears that in Sun Simiao's eyes, infertility was caused by an accumulation of cold blood in the uterus that was treated by expelling it via the vagina, sometimes in combination with a "scrubbing" of the uterus or internal organs. In the midst of these formulas, we find two formulas with significantly less ingredients, said to be "used by the ancients," but fallen out of use in Sun Simiao's times. The first one treats the husband for insufficiency of *yang qi* and inability to cause transformation (i.e., in the woman's womb) or, if transformation did occur, failure to complete it. The second one seems like a rather standard treatment for women's infertility. Sun Simiao precedes these with the caveat that he has no personal experience using them, but has included them because of their popularity in ancient times. Throughout this section, Sun Simiao's choice of

medicinal ingredients reveals his underlying etiological ideas as well as treatment strategies.

The following discussion of medicinal actions is based on the understanding of a substance's efficacy during the early Tang period. Thus, I follow the descriptions in materia medica literature roughly contemporaneous to the date of composition of the *Qian Jin Fang*. For this purpose, I have relied on a critical edition of the *Shen Nong Ben Cao Jing* (神農本草經 *Divine Farmer's Classic of Materia Medica*), a Han period medicinal text that was edited and annotated by Tao Hongjing (陶弘景) in the early 6th century.

This text can therefore serve as an accurate reflection of materia medica knowledge slightly prior to the time when the *Qian Jin Fang* was composed. According to the descriptions of the actions of medicinals in this text, the formulas for treating infertility in the *Qian Jin Fang* contain medicinals like *po xiao* (impure mirabilite 朴消), *mu dan* (moutan 牡丹), and *tao ren* (peach kernel 桃仁) that eliminate evil *qi*, break up accumulations, and treat blood stagnation. These are combined with other medicinals: *xi xin* (asarum 细辛), *gan jiang* (dried ginger 干姜), *jie geng* (platycodon 桔梗), and *shu jiao* (zanthoxylum 蜀椒). These are warming, treat wind, dampness, cough, and counterflow *qi* ascent, and precipitate *qi*. They are also combined with medicinals like *tian men dong* (asparagus 天门冬), *niu xi* (achyranthes 牛膝), *wu wei zi* (schisandra 五味子), and *shan zhu yu* (cornus 山茱萸) that extend life and supplement insufficiencies, treat taxation damage and emaciation, nourish *yin*, and boost essence and *qi*, in addition to the above characteristics of warming, moving blood, or eliminating wind and dampness.

This choice of ingredients suggests a notion of infertility as caused by the inhibited movement of *qi* and blood due to vacuity, which in turn leads to cold stagnation and accumulations in the abdomen of a substance that Sun Simiao refers to as "this malign substance." The frequent use of medicinals like *fang feng* (asarum and saposhnikovia 防風) also indicates the notion that infertility might be caused by externally contracted wind-cold, which had to be dispersed and expelled by increasing the flow of blood and *qi* with supplementing, warming, and down-draining preparations.

In addition to medicinal formulas, the text lists several moxibustion techniques for treating women's infertility. The choice of moxibustion points is quite carefully differentiated by the particulars of the condition, such as:

- general infertility
- inability to have children because the mouth of the uterus is blocked
- inability to complete a pregnancy due to miscarriage with abdominal pain and leaking of red discharge
- blockage of the uterus so that she is unable to receive the [male] essence
- red and white leakage

Except for one use of *ran gu* (然谷 Blazing Valley), which is located on the ankle, the other points are all located in the area between the navel and the pubic bone: *guan yuan* (關元 Pass Head), *bao men* (胞門 Uterine Gate), *qi men* (气門 Qi Gate), and *quan men* (泉門 Spring Gate). These are for the most part still used today for the treatment of infertility.

Appended to the chapter on fertility is a short but significant section on manipulating the fetus's gender. As a brief introductory essay explains, the fetus is created by the interaction and mutual stimulation of *yin* and *yang*.

According to the standard medical notions of the time, the shape of the fetus was not settled until the end of the third month of pregnancy, and the mother's behavior and environment could therefore affect the fetus's physical and psychological characteristics. This was the basis for the popular practice of "fetal education" (*tai jiao* 胎教), discussed by Sun Simiao in the following chapter on pregnancy-related formulas. Regarding the fetus's gender, early medieval theories of conception and pregnancy are sometimes contradictory, suggesting either that the gender of the fetus was not yet fixed or that it could be transformed until the third month of pregnancy.

By the Song period, sexual differentiation had become identified with conception in medical literature, and instructions for changing the fetus's gender were therefore eliminated from elite doctors' gynecological texts. On the other hand, instructions for influencing the gender of the fetus during the act of intercourse, as, for example, by timing it in relationship to the woman's menstrual cycle, become more important. Being a formula text with only short essays, the *Qian Jin Fang* fails to provide a conclusive statement on this issue. Nevertheless, the formulas obviously reflect the belief that gender could be manipulated up to the third month of pregnancy, which, in most cases, meant converting a female fetus into a male.

Besides a complex formula of medicinals that mostly boost *yang, qi*, blood, and essence, Sun Simiao also lists several instructions of a decidedly magical flavor, such as the advice to "take a crossbow string, place it in a crimson bag, and have the pregnant woman carry it on her left arm" or to tie it around her waist below the belt. Another method calls for an ax to be hidden under the woman's bed. All of these actions needed to be performed secretly, a common feature in magical formulas. Interesting in this section is the curious combination of medical and magical thinking, but even the medicinal formulas include such ingredients as dog testicles and the head of a rooster from the top of the eastern gate.

■ Summary

1. The section on fertility treatments in the *Qian Jin Fang* includes formulas for treating male insufficiency of *yang qi*, as well as a reference to formulas in the section on "nurturing life" that is aimed at men. This shows that responsibility for the inability to procreate was not placed exclusively with the woman, but was shared between husband and wife. The creation of the fetus was seen as an act performed by two equal partners, with *yin* and *yang* intermingling and stimulating each other. As the essay states, "*Yin* and *yang* blend in harmony, the two *qi* respond to each other, and *yang* bestows and *yin* transforms." Jender Lee[5] has shown that in early medieval Chinese medicine, the treatment of infertility was shifted from sexual cultivation texts directed at men, called "texts of the bedchamber" (*fang zhong shu* 房中書), to medical formula literature on women's health. In this context, increasing attention was focused on ensuring the woman's reproductive health before and during pregnancy with medicinal formulas, rather than on the avoidance of calendrical taboos at the time of conception.

2. While the cause of male infertility was here simply diagnosed as insufficient *qi* (and treated in more detail in the section on "supplementing and boosting by sexual intercourse"), the

woman's condition was carefully differentiated depending on a sophisticated diagnosis that took into consideration the appearance of abdominal masses, sensation of cold, menstrual irregularities, white or red vaginal discharge, and the anatomical shape of her reproductive organs.

3. In all cases, treatment was directed at causing the discharge of cold blood, sometimes in connection with heat therapy, and the cleansing of the uterus, by using cold-expelling and precipitating medicinals. The stagnation and accumulation of pathogenic cold in the body's center was seen as caused by either the invasion of external wind-cold or a deep-lying insufficiency of *yin*, blood, and *qi*, which in any case predisposed the patient to the former.

4. The complexity of the medicinal formulas, requiring numerous non-household medicinal ingredients, suggests that this sphere of women's health care was not limited to the treatment by other female household members or local medicinal peddlers and midwives, but had also received the attention of concerned male literati like Sun Simiao.

5. In addition to medicinal formulas, Sun Simiao also included magical treatments as well as references, in the very first paragraph, to the superior power of astrology and fate, against which even the finest physician was helpless.

6. Thus, Sun Simiao recognized that, in this significant area of women's health, medicinal formulas did not exhaust his readers' need for different treatment modalities.

■ Pregnancy Treatments in the *Qian Jin Fang*

The second major category of the *Formulas for Women* volumes in the *Qian Jin Fang* covers pregnancy and comprises almost a quarter of the entire gynecological section. It is divided into three sections: "malign obstruction in pregnancy," "nurturing the fetus," and "the various diseases of pregnancy."

The comparatively short section on "malign obstruction in pregnancy" (*ren shen e zu* 妊娠惡阻) contains two long essays and four formulas. The

first essay describes a method for determining whether a woman is pregnant and for predicting the gender of the fetus and the time of birth, by diagnosing the pulse. Several important ideas about conception, pregnancy, and fetal development can be deduced from this advice:

- The fetus is created through the harmonious intermingling of blood and *qi*, *yin* and *yang*.
- Pregnancy is diagnosed by detecting increased movement and blood flow in the pulse of either the heart vessel, which governs the flow of blood, or of the kidney vessel, which governs reproduction.
- By the fourth month, the fetus's gender is fixed and can be diagnosed by the characteristics of the pulse (deep and replete for a boy, big and floating for a girl).

Sun Simiao also mentions several simpler methods for diagnosing the gender, such as:
- inducing the woman to spontaneously turn to the left (for a boy) or right (for a girl) or
- finding lumps in the right or left side of the husband's chest.

This section is reminiscent of folk advice given all over the world. It is significant that Sun Simiao chose to transmit this advice alongside and as equal to what we would consider more properly medical and sophisticated methods of pulse diagnosis, which were by necessity the domain of an educated physician with sufficient training and experience to distinguish such subtle differences.

The remainder of this chapter concerns the etiology and treatment of "malign obstruction" in pregnancy in strictly medical terms. It defines the condition as a combination of physical and psychological symptoms caused by the presence of wind-cold, a pathological accumulation of fluids below the heart, as well as a general stagnation of *qi* and blood. These are in turn ultimately due to the quintessentially feminine problems of vacuity and emaciation from taxation damage, insufficiency of *qi* and blood, and additional weakness of kidney *qi*, potentially aggravated by exposure to wind.

The next section on "nurturing the fetus" (*yang tai* 養胎) begins with an essay on "fetal education" (*tai jiao* 胎教). This practice is aimed at creating a model descendant who is "long-lived, loyal and filial, humane, righteous, intelligent, wise, and free of disease."

"Fetal education" prescribes the pregnant woman's ideal surroundings, activities (such as observing ritual performances, playing the zither, and reciting poetry), and composed mindset during the first 3 months of pregnancy, when the fetus "transforms in response to things, and its disposition and character are not yet fixed."

This information is standard and similar to advice cited in many other early texts. Following these instructions on fetal education, the *Qian Jin Fang* contains a varied list of prohibited foods, with the more mundane goal of preventing miscarriage, childbirth complications, or physical deformities.

Then, Sun Simiao quotes "Xu Zhicai's Month-by-month Formulas for Nurturing the Fetus," a text that is also cited in many other early medical texts: from the *Tai Chan Shu* (胎產書 *Book of the Generation of the Fetus)*, early Han period, to the *Zhu Bing Yuan Hou Lun (On the Origins and Symptoms of the Various Diseases)*, early seventh century, and the *Ishimpo (Formulas from the Heart of Medicine)*, tenth century, where it is identified as a quote from yet another text.

At times almost literally identical to the *Ishimpo* version, the quotation in the *Qian Jin Fang* describes the monthly progress in the fetus's gestation and notes the foods and acupuncture channels prohibited in each month. It also includes two decoction formulas for each month, one for the treatment of pathologies likely to occur during that month and the other for the treatment of damage to the fetus.

The last subsection of pregnancy treatments consists of "medicines for lubricating the fetus" (*hua tai yao* 滑胎藥). This is an important category of prescriptions, taken during the final stage of pregnancy to prepare the mother and fetus for childbirth and to ease labor, which is still used today. As a whole, this section stands out for the nuanced descriptions of symptoms and the specificity and complexity of the formulas. This suggests that prescribing medicinal decoctions for nurturing the fetus and in preparation for delivery were two areas of women's medical care that educated medical practitioners, whether professional or amateur, were actively engaged in during the time of the composition of the *Qian Jin Fang*.

The last chapter in this section, on the "various diseases of pregnancy" (*ren shen zhu bing* 妊娠諸病), presents a more diverse treatment style: it contains 10 sections on the conditions of stirring the fetus (*tai dong* 胎动) and repeated miscarriage;

leaking uterus; child vexation; heart, abdominal, and lumbar pain and intestinal fullness; cold damage; malaria; (vaginal) bleeding; urinary diseases; diarrhea; and water swelling: a total of 89 formulas and three moxibustion methods.

The treatments in this section run seamlessly from complex medicinal formulas, often with more than half a dozen ingredients, to simple home remedies such as drinking infant's urine or water in which the husband's leather boots have been washed. Ingesting pulverized cow manure, grease from a cart's linchpin, or charred fingernails and matted hair are recommended side-by-side with physical manipulations such as applying abdominal compresses of roasted buffalo manure mixed with vinegar, or burning moxa on *qi hai* (气海 Sea of *Qi*, CV-6), a point still used today for the treatment of abdominal pain, painful or irregular menstruation, and vaginal discharge. Much to our regret, it is impossible to determine yet whether these different treatment modes—as well as the etiologies they were based on—reflected the practices of different types of practitioners who were differentiated by gender, economic or social status, education, professionalization, family ties, or other factors.

All in all, though, the chapters on fertility and pregnancy in the *Qian Jin Fang* offer us a comprehensive glimpse into the sophistication, multiplicity, and variety of early Chinese notions regarding the causation as well as treatment of medical problems related to fertility, conception, and pregnancy. The level of attention and care, with which the woman was apparently treated throughout this process, shows yet again how high the *Qian Jin Fang* author Sun Simiao valued women's contribution in the efforts of the state, family, and individual to "nourish life" and safeguard the continuity between past, present, and future.

Bibliography

1. Li Jingrong et al. (editors). *Bei Ji Qian Jin Yao Fang Jiao Shi*. Beijing: Renmin weisheng chubanshe; 1996.
2. Ma Jixing (editor). *Sun Zhen Ren Qian Jin Fang*. Beijing: Renmin weisheng chubanshe; 1995.
3. Zhang Ruixian, Liu Gengsheng, et al. (editors). *Qian Jin Fang*, Part I. Beijing: Huaxia chubanshe; 1996.
4. Wilms S. Bei Ji Qian Jin Yao Fang, Essential Prescriptions Worth a Thousand in Gold for Every Emergency. 3 vols. on Gynecology. Portland: The Chinese Medicine Database; 2007.
5. Lee TD. Childbirth in early imperial China. Nan nü, Vol 7, No. 2, 2005: pp. 216–286.

Options and Methods in Fertility Treatment

4

Qi Gong and its Medical Applications

No discussion of the modes of treatment in Chinese medicine would be complete without mentioning *qi gong* as a therapeutic method. In spite of the fact that these techniques are used rather sparingly in clinic, *qi gong* offers an additional spectrum of treatment options. This method is still often neglected even in traditional Chinese hospitals. Just like acupuncture, *qi gong* has taken a long time to be acknowledged in the West. The two methods share certain characteristics, such as the treatment of the *qi* flow. Nevertheless, the practitioner works with needles in acupuncture, but with the bare hands in the diagnosis and treatment with *qi gong*. Often, the patient's body is not touched at all. As a consequence of the enthusiasm for and rediscovery of the old medical teachings, many hospitals and universities in China have carried out research projects and studies on *qi gong*. This has resulted in a growing acceptance, even beyond practicing patients and practitioners.

Because *qi gong* is also valued and demanded in China by Western practitioners who are studying there, simple methods are taught in the hospitals. Some physicians cultivate their own *qi* with a series of exercises from *qi gong*.

The Effects of *Qi Gong*

Qi gong is an old Chinese method for cultivating the body's own *qi*, the "vital energy." It requires regular practice times. *Gong* means "to work hard on something," "to apply real effort to acquire a skill."

Tsu Kuo Shih offers the following definition in his book *Qi Gong Therapy*:

"Qi gong *is the art of exercising* jing *(essence),* qi *(energy), and* shen *(spirit). The heart of* qi gong *is the training of* yi *(imagination) and* qi *(vital energy). The main goal of these exercises is to regulate the internal functions of the human body. We achieve this in* qi gong *by developing our power of imagination and breathing techniques, by guiding the inner* qi *towards realization, and by moving and strengthening the inner* qi*. The inner* qi *is the body's very own original* qi*. Therefore, we can achieve self-regulation and self-control of the internal organs by means of* qi gong*."*[5]

As a therapeutic principle, its effects are explained by the following factors:

- **Restoring vitality**. *Qi gong* restores vitality and replenishes exhausted energy reserves by means of calmness and rest. Deep relaxation affects the cerebral cortex. By remaining in a calm and relaxed state, we relieve the fatigue and overstimulation of the cerebral cortex and instead induce regeneration and invigoration. Targeted training calms hyperactive and overexcited sections in the system. After *qi gong* practice, the practitioner experiences a comfortable state of calmness and relaxation.
- **Conserving energy**. During *qi gong*, the body enters an "energy-conserving state," similar to that in deep relaxation or deep sleep (parasympathetic state). In this state, the metabolism and oxygen needs are reduced. Because the body hardly consumes any energy, excess *qi* can be collected.
- **The massaging effect on the abdominal organs**. Deep abdominal breathing and additional massage improve the functioning of the abdominal organs and therefore the supply of the entire organism.

The Three Treasures (*San Bao*)

In *qi gong* therapy, we invariably encounter the concept of the "three treasures"—*jing, qi,* and *shen.*

Jing

Jing—essence—refers to the foundation of vital activities, which is supplied by the kidney. We distinguish between:

- prenatal essence
- acquired essence

The term "essence" indicates that by transforming and refining an undifferentiated substance something precious has been created that must be cultivated and protected. The character *jing* can be translated as "something produced by distillation." The energy form *jing* is stored in the kidneys. Because of its "fluid" nature, it circulates throughout the entire body. Sperm and ovum are a form of this precious subtle essence. The man's *jing* can be squandered by excesses of any kind, but especially by sexual debauchery with repeated ejaculations. In women, frequent births, miscarriages, and intensive hormone therapy can lead to a loss of *jing*. In addition, the monthly build-up of the endometrium for the implantation of the ovum and the subsequent bleeding associated with the shedding of the endometrium consume *jing. Jing* is the basis for growth, reproduction, and development.

Qi

Qi—vital energy—includes all forms of energy, from the air that we breathe to the life-sustaining energy that animates our body. *Qi* is the life force that guarantees all emotional, mental, and bodily functions throughout our life. It goes hand in hand with breathing and finally leaves the body with our last breath. Health and illness depend on the strength and regular circulation of *qi*.

Shen

Shen—spirit—comprises a wealth of human characteristics such as charisma, consciousness, spirit, and personality. We can summarize *shen* as the spiritual, intellectual, mental, and especially communicative capacities of the person.

■ *Qi Gong* for Fertility Treatment in China

Master Li Jiacheng is a *qi gong* physician in Xi'an. He treats patients with *qi gong* and teaches them a *qi gong* method for self-practice. He recommends different exercises that can be utilized in infertility.

The Exercises

The main exercise aims at strengthening the lower *dan tian* (*dan tian qi gong*). In addition, specific exercises are taught for men (*nan dan gong*—men's *qi gong*) and for women (*nü dan gong*—women's *qi gong*) respectively. In kidney vacuity, a kidney-strengthening *qi gong* should be practiced. In addition, he also recommends a visualization technique for fertility through the "third eye" (see below).

Conserving *Jing*

The technique for "retaining *jing* (ejaculate)" is only recommended for men who have been practicing *qi gong* for a long time or are familiar with Daoist practices. Nevertheless, it is desirable to have more frequent sex with ejaculation during the time of ovulation and to be more reserved concerning ejaculation at other times. If an exercise program has been set up but pregnancy has still not occurred after 2 years, abstinence should be practiced for 3 months in order to prevent the loss of additional *jing*. If the general constitution is very weak, patients should always be given Chinese medicinals for supplementation as well.

Furthermore, a weakened constitution calls for a therapy according to the following treatment plan:

- rounds of treatments that last 7 days each with daily acupuncture, followed by breaks of 2–3 days or
- a series of three times 15 days of daily acupuncture with 3-day breaks in between

These recommendations should be modified for Western circumstances: daily acupuncture treatment is widely accepted in China, but would certainly be much less acceptable here.

Exercise and Therapy Plan

Concept 1—Easy Variation

Attend *qi gong* classes daily for 1 week, then consult the teacher once a month. In the meantime, practice daily.

Concept 2—Moderately Difficult Variation

Daily *qi gong* treatment and *qi gong* exercises for 1 week; then continue to practice *qi gong* exercises for 3 months. During this time, no sexual excess, be conservative with ejaculation (*jing*), and pay particular attention to the time of ovulation.

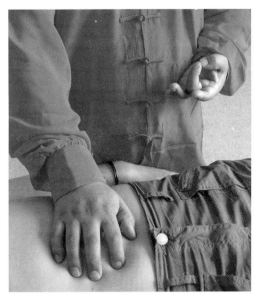

Fig. 9.1   *Qi gong* massage on the abdomen.

Concept 3—Difficult Variation

Daily *qi gong* treatment and practice for 1 month. Afterwards, continue with the exercises for 6 months and do not have sex during this time. Then return to the easier variation. Pay attention to the time of ovulation.

> In China, another recommendation is to take in somebody else's child. Most often, a child is adopted from an orphanage. The following notions are behind this: "a child attracts other children," and "if you do something good, something good will come back to you."

■ *Qi Gong* as Treatment by the Practitioner

One method of application is *qi gong* treatment (*wai qi* treatment) by a *qi gong* physician or *qi gong* practitioner. The practitioner uses concentrated *qi* to carry out a treatment through touch

(*qi gong* massage, *qi gong* acupressure) or without touch (*fa qi*—emitting energy) (**Fig. 9.1**).

This treatment is used primarily in the treatment of chronic disorders, for strengthening in conditions of weakness (also of individual organ systems) or for harmonizing the circulation of *qi* (e. g., in emotional imbalance). While the practice of *qi gong* is already widespread in the West, the method of external *qi gong* treatment by a physician or practitioner has still not received much attention. Working with external *qi* requires long practice, a good teacher, and a great feeling of responsibility.

In "external *qi gong* treatment" (*wai qi fa*), the practitioner first makes the diagnosis and establishes a treatment principle. The treatment of female and male patients is performed with the patient either sitting or lying. The physician or practitioner emits *qi* (*fa qi*). This occurs without touch, from a certain distance. As in the other treatment methods of TCM, the treatment stimulus can be determined discriminately. The two main treatment principles are *bu fa*—strengthening (supplementing/concentrating)—and *xie fa*—draining (discharging/dispersing)—in repletion states. The principle *bu fa* is applied in states of vacuity (exhaustion) and the principle *xie fa* in states of repletion (**Table 9.1**).

Table 9.1 The "eight treatment principles" in TCM

Principle	Action	Indication
Bu fa	Supplementing/concentrating	Filling *yin/yang*, in vacuity
Xie fa	Draining/dispersing	Sedating, distributing, dispersing, in repletion
He fa	Harmonizing	Soothing method
Wen fa	Warming	Treatment of cold disorders
Tong fa	Promoting flow	Removing blockages of *qi* and blood
Han fa	Promoting sweating	For invading pathogenic factors, also drafts
San fa	Resolving and dispersing	Eliminating pain and swelling
Qing fa	Clearing (heat)	Cooling, freeing in fever

Wai qi treatment is also used in the treatment of inoperable cancer conditions. In addition, it is commonly applied in emotional imbalance. A technique that is applied locally is *wai fa qi* with the sword finger (**Fig. 9.2**). It is applied on the forehead above the point *yin tang* to calm the spirit, or it can have a dispersing effect on compressed tissue.

Qi Gong as Self-treatment

The largest and most well-known aspect of *qi gong*, practiced by many people in and outside of China, consists of "methods for self-practice." This refers to mostly simple exercises that are demonstrated by a teacher and then again and again repeated by the student over a longer period of time. There are general exercises that are widely disseminated as *yang sheng* (method for cultivating health), such as the "eight brocades" or the "18 movements *tai ji qi gong*." Special exercises are often taught in clinics for certain disorders or symptoms, such as "lung *qi gong*" or "cancer *qi gong*." Such special exercises for the treatment of diseases are called **medical** *qi gong*. In all cases, it is important to practice continuously over an extended period of time to achieve the desired effect.

The *Dan Tian* Exercise

Master Li Jiacheng regards the practice of concentrating on the "lower *dan tian*" (*dan* "cinnabar,"

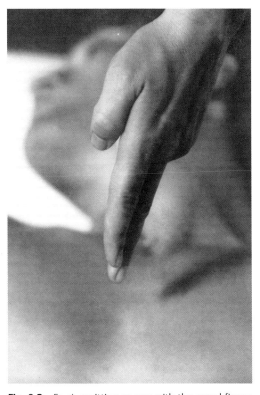

Fig. 9.2 *Fa qi*—emitting energy with the sword finger.

tian "field") as the most basic exercise for all *qi gong* methods. Before starting to practice other complicated *qi gong* exercises, practitioners should first be able to concentrate their *qi*.

A special characteristic of *dan tian qi gong* is the fact that it not only gathers *qi* and thereby strengthens the center and energy of the kidneys, it also has the effect of mentally harmonizing people who are too much "in their head."

Locating the *Dan Tian*

When you are instructed to "concentrate the mind on the *dan tian*," this normally refers to the lower *dan tian*. This is the area of the body that is closely related to the fundamental vital processes in the human body. In TCM theory and Daoist *qi gong* teachings, it is said that this is the place where the *ren mai* (conception vessel) and *du mai* (governing vessel) as well as the *chong mai* (thoroughfare vessel) start from. It is the pivot of the "true *qi*," the entire potential of the person and of its ascent and descent, opening and closing. It is the foundation for the creation of life, the basis of the five viscera and six bowels, the root of the 12 main channels, the meeting point of *yin* and *yang*, the gate of respiration, and "the land where fire and water flow together." It is the place where the man preserves his reproductive essence and where the woman can nourish the fetus. By concentrating on the *dan tian*, we can improve health and cure disease.

> The *dan tian* refers not to one precise point but to a region of the body. Different localizations for the *dan tian* are transmitted, the most popular of which is as follows: three fingers' breadths below the navel and, seen from the front, a third deep into the lower abdomen.

Specific Functions of the *Dan Tian*

- regulates *qi*
- strengthens prenatal *qi*
- invigorates the kidneys (with the result of strengthening *jing*)
- regulates the *qi* in the vessels and in the blood
- regulates *wei qi* (defense *qi*)
- regulates blood storage (*chong mai*, liver, uterus)
- warms the essence palace (gathering point of *jing*)

> The *dan tian* exercise:
> - helps to achieve inner calmness and composure
> - develops abdominal breathing
> - strengthens the spleen and stomach (correlated with the "earth phase" in the human

body) and hence also the functioning of all viscera and bowels
- supports kidney *yang*
- assists in making *qi* sink down from the upper body

"Dan Tian Qi Gong While Seated"—Sequence of the Exercise

First, the practitioner assumes a seated position in the lotus pose or cross-legged. The use of a meditation pillow is recommended. Gathering the legs and sitting on the ground facilitates the gathering of *qi* in the lower abdomen. But it is also possible to sit in a chair in a comfortable upright seated position. When sitting cross-legged, the right leg should be positioned on the inside and the left leg on the outside. This *yang bao yin* position (*yang* embraces *yin*) reinforces the gathering nature of this exercise. With the hands, we assume the *yin bao yang* position (*yin* embraces *yang*). The *yang* hand is placed directly on the *dan tian*. Here, *yang* lies underneath to support the warming process (**Fig. 9.3**).

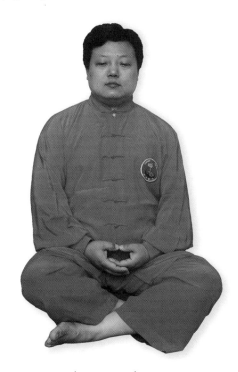

Fig. 9.3 Seated position in *dan tian qi gong*.

After assuming this position, quiet the mind and inhale and exhale calmly and naturally through the nose. Close the eyes gently or leave them cracked open. Rest the tongue on the palate. With your "inner vision," gaze at the tip of the nose, from there gaze down to the heart region, and then lastly all the way down to the *dan tian*. Remain here and "focus the mind on the *dan tian*." Gazing at the nose calms the breath, looking at the heart level calms the heart.

Patients with a cold lower abdomen can add a visualization of *tai yang*, the sun, during the *dan tian* concentration. This will lead to a faster concentration of *qi* and warmth. The most difficult part of this exercise is to calm the spirit. Experience suggests that you should start with a practice time of at least 20 minutes because an unskilled person will need at least 15 minutes to simply calm down. The duration of practice should then gradually be increased to 30 minutes, then to 45 minutes, and can finally be raised to 1 hour. The best time to practice is at night between 11 p.m. and 1 a.m., especially for men, and at noon between 11 a.m. and 1 p.m., especially for women. But you can also choose any other time of day.

To end this exercise, swallow the collected saliva in the mouth ("heavenly water") in three portions, in your imagination down to the *dan tian*. The hands are placed flat on the *dan tian*. Then stroke the abdomen in circles three times clockwise and three times counterclockwise. To conclude, lightly press the hands on the *dan tian* three times to close it.

Afterwards, clear the face by rubbing the hands and touching the face. For this, tap and stroke the legs. In the first few weeks, the legs may hurt, but this will stop with consistent practice. If the legs fall asleep, you can tap the points *zu san li* (ST-36) and *san yin jiao* (SP-6) to activate *qi* and blood.

Exercise "The Divine Visualization"

The foundation of this exercise comes from the method *kai tian mu* ("opening the third eye"). This is a traditional *qi gong* method with Daoist roots. It is believed to have originated many thousands of years ago and is related to the legendary figure of Er Long Shen, who is depicted in images with an open "third eye," as well as with the goddess Guanyin.

Master Li Jiacheng teaches this method and recommends using it in a modified form in the treatment of infertility. In place of the original medium, a red ball, use a divine visualization with the request for a child. For this purpose, you would in China pray to the Daoist god Lu Dong Bin, a deified monk. He is asked for help in disease. In the following paragraphs, we have reduced this exercise to two basic units:

1. Yu Bei She—*Preparatory Exercise while Standing*

- Stand with feet shoulder width apart, with knees relaxed.
- Look straight ahead.
- Let the gaze come back to about 30 cm in front of the face.
- There, visualize the image for 3–5 minutes in front of the third eye.
- The eyes are hereby opened only halfway.
- Practice for about 2 weeks.

Note. The third eye lies two finger breadths above the eyes in the center of the forehead. Visualization must be trained, up to twice a day. It is helpful to have a vivid image for the visualization. You can use a real image—for example, a statue of Guanyin—for a few days and afterwards work with this image in your imagination.

2. Gui Gong Shuang Shou—*Exercise with Knees in Folded Hands*

- Assume a kneeling position (the body is hereby straight; do not allow it to rest on the lower legs in the back!).
- Fold the hands loosely in front of the chest (prayer position, **Fig. 9.4**).
- The gaze is directed straight ahead into the distance.
- Make the gaze return slowly to 30 cm.
- Let the image appear (visualization, e.g., of Guanyin).
- The eyes are hereby half open, half closed.
- Remain in this position for 10–15 minutes.
- Slowly close the eyes.
- Now see the image through the third eye (in front of the body).
- Next, let the image enter the body through the third eye; slowly bring the image down to the lower *dan tian*.

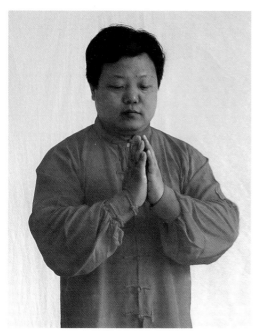

Fig. 9.4 Praying position during visualization.

focus on the *dan tian* ("cinnabar field"). All methods aim at improving the function of the female organism. Nevertheless, there is one exercise that should not be practiced in infertility. It effects the interruption of menstruation and is therefore obviously contraindicated in fertility therapy. Olvedi describes the exercise according to Master Li Zhi-Chang as "deer exercise for the woman."[4] This practice stimulates estrogen production and thereby prevents menstruation if practiced daily. This exercise is practiced by Daoist nuns in monasteries. By interrupting the menstrual bleeding, they conserve precious *jing* and can transform it into spiritual energy. After ending this practice, the menstrual period normally starts again.

The exercises of women's *qi gong* utilize a great number of self-massage techniques, especially for the breast and abdominal regions. The focus of these sets of exercises lies in **activating and regulating the "extraordinary vessels"** *ren mai, du mai, chong mai,* and *dai mai.* Hereby, diseases and disruptions can be influenced directly.

In the following, we describe three sets of exercises from the *nü zi qi gong* according to Liu Yafei. The exercises activate the *ren mai, dai mai,* and the female lower abdominal organs in the pelvis.

- Concentrate on the *dan tian* for 2–5 minutes.
- Then collect saliva and swallow it down to the *dan tian* three times.
- Let the hands slowly sink down to the *dan tian.*
- Circle the hands three times clockwise on the *dan tian,* then three times counterclockwise.
- Apply pressure with the hands on the *dan tian* three times.
- Slowly release the hands.
- Rub the hands and clear the face with them (see above).

Note. Practicing in a kneeling position is very difficult initially, but effects a strongly stimulating process.

Qi Gong for Women—*Nü Dan Gong* and *Nü Zi Qi Gong*

There are different sets of exercises for women's *qi gong.* Liu Yafei refers to them as *nü zi qi gong* ("*qi gong* for women and girls"). In addition to the word for woman (*nü*), Master Li includes in his term *nü dan gong* the word *dan*—to indicate the

Relieving the Chest and Massaging the Abdomen

- Press the point *shan zhong*:
  - Press *shan zhong* (CV-17) with the fingertips of both hands. Apply pressure during inhalations and release pressure during exhalations.
  - Repeat this exercise 9–18 times.
- Press *ren mai*:
  - Press *ren mai* from the jugular fossa (CV-22) to the upper margin of the pubic bone (CV-2) in nine steps from top to bottom. Apply pressure during inhalations, release pressure during exhalations.
  - Bring the hands back to the top.
  - Repeat this exercise three to nine times.
- Make *ren mai* porous:
  - While inhaling, guide the hands upward without touching. While exhaling, lower them on the central line down to the pubic bone.
  - Repeat the exercise six times.

- Massage the abdomen in both directions:
  - Both hands, placed on top of each other, describe circles over the entire abdomen (lower border: pubic bone, upper border: sternum).
  - First, circle nine times clockwise, then bring the hands to the lower *dan tian* and massage nine times in the opposite direction.
- Lift the *dan tian*:
  - Place the hands on top of each other. While inhaling, strongly lift the *dan tian* with the hands (balls of the little finger); while exhaling, lower it almost without touching it at all.
  - Repeat this exercise 9–18 times.
- Massage the *dan tian* diagonally:
  - From the iliac crest, massage diagonally downward in the direction of the groin and back upward. Apply equal pressure in both directions.
  - Repeat this exercise 9–18 times.
- Rub the *dan tian* in opposite directions:
  - Both hands describe contra-rotational circles on the abdomen.
  - Perform this exercise 9–18 times in one direction, then repeat in the opposite direction.
- Rub both flanks:
  - From the armpits, massage in six strokes from the outside in and from the top down. When bringing the hands back up, there is almost no outward movement; by raising the *qi*, the arms follow.
  - Repeat this exercise six to nine times.

Note. This set of exercises is particularly helpful for disorders in the breast: it resolves tension in the breasts in PMS and counteracts breast tumors. Furthermore, it has a supporting effect in blood vacuity and blood weakness. The contra-rotating massage strokes regulate the energy flow in the lower pelvis. Lastly, the abdominal massage results in strengthening the energy of the spleen.

Harmonizing the *Dai Mai*

- Rub the back with alternating hands:
  - The hands glide from the *dan tian* along the girdling vessel (*dai mai*) to the back.
  - Then stroke from the lumbar area (kidney region, BL-23) down to the coccyx (*wei lu*) with alternating hands. Simultaneously rotate the spinal column in spirals.
  - Repeat 9–18 times on each side.
- External harmonizing of the *dai mai*:
  - The pelvis describes external horizontal circles in a clockwise direction (like in hip circles).
  - The hands are hereby placed on the hips.
  - The legs are, of course, stretched, with the feet shoulder-width apart. The feet remain on the floor. The head is erect.
  - Circle 9–18 times in each direction.
- Internal harmonizing of the *dai mai*:
  - Rotate the pelvis in small horizontal circles. The movement is like a ball rolling in a basin.
  - While doing this, keep your attention constantly focused on the *dai mai*. The knees are now bent slightly. The abdomen is kept soft. The exercise is carried out "internally."
  - Perform the exercise in both directions, 9–18 times per side.
  - To conclude, bring the hands to the kidney region and rub 18 times downward from the hips to the sacrum.

Note. This set of exercises stimulates the circulation of *qi* and blood in the pelvis. It regulates the girdling vessel, strengthens kidney *yang*, and holds the organs in a natural position.

Moving the *Dan Tian* in Circles

- Move it in circles forward and backward:
  - For this purpose, connect the areas *hui yin* (CV-1) with *ming men* (GV-4) and *dan tian* in your imagination. The hands can accompany this vertical circular movement of the pelvis.
  - After 9–18 times, change direction: now connect *hui yin, dan tian*, and *ming men*. Perform the exercise in this direction 9–18 times as well.
- Circle the *dan tian* sideways:
  - The pelvis makes sideways circular movements. First clockwise, so that the left *dai mai* is connected with the right *dai mai* and then with *hui yin*. The *dan tian* is the center around which the pelvis circles.

– Repeat the exercise 9–18 times. Then connect the right *dai mai* with the left *dai mai* and then with *hui yin*.

Note. In this set of exercises, a "web of *qi*" is constructed around the *dan tian*. The *yuan qi* is improved, and stagnations of blood and phlegm can be resolved. These exercises are particularly helpful for menstrual complaints, but also in infertility and frigidity.

Qi Gong for Men—*Nan Dan Gong*

For men as well, there are special *qi gong* exercises. These aim primarily at strengthening sexual and kidney strength. One example is the following exercise *tie dan gong*.

Tie Dan Gong—Exercise for Strengthening the Lower Body

The exercise *tie dan gong* is recommended for men —an exercise for strengthening the lower body and the genitals. In this practice, self-massage also plays a key role. The stroking massage of the abdomen is regarded as particularly important. In addition, the testicles are kneaded and lifted and the spermatic cords and testicles are turned. The kneading massage, turning, and lifting of the testicles have a supporting effect on sperm production and the secretion of male sex hormones. Another characteristic is the stretching of the penis and testicles. This practice is said to enrich the pubic area with *qi* and blood. The improved circulation leads to improved function.

Conserving *jing*, in this case ejaculate, plays an important role in Chinese culture. Thus, we can read in the classic text *Su Nü Jing* (*Classic of the Plain Maiden*) from the 3 rd century CE:

"If a man loves once without surrendering his semen, it will strengthen his body. If he loves twice without surrendering it, his eyes and ears will function better. After the third time, all diseases disappear. After the fourth time, he will find peace in his soul. After the fifth time, the heart and blood circulation are revitalized. After the sixth time, his loins are envigorated. After the seventh time, his buttocks and thighs are strengthened. After the eighth time, his skin becomes delicate. After the

ninth time, he will achieve longevity. After the tenth time, he will become like an immortal."[4]

These words express the effects that a loss of essence can have when it is squandered wastefully. "Excessive sexual activity" can lead to severe overspending of *jing*. The above-mentioned classic also gives age-specific recommendations. Accordingly, a man between 30 and 40 years of age should only ejaculate once a day if he is of excellent health, otherwise only on every second day. There are also other statements that recommend ejaculation every 3 days at the most. The advice given above (see p. 103) applies to infertility problems.

Exercises for the Areas *Ming Men, Hui Yin*, and the Kidneys

In addition to the *dan tian* exercises, further exercises focus on *ming men, hui yin*, and the kidneys. The following paragraphs describe the significance of these areas.

Ming Men—Life Gate

The point *ming men* lies on the *du mai*, below the spinous process of the second lumbar vertebra, between the *shen shu* (kidney transport points), on the backside of the navel as it were. It is therefore also referred to as the rear *dan tian*. *Ming men* lies exactly between the kidneys and is connected to them. It promotes communication between the kidneys, the navel, the heart, the lungs, and the brain. *Ming men* is seen as the source of vitality, as the ruler over the ministerial fire, and as the essence palace.

Ming men is called the "sea of *jing* and blood", in comparison to the spleen and stomach, which are regarded as the "sea of water and food." Both seas together—as manifestation of the correlative phases earth and fire in the human body—serve as foundation for the five viscera; the *yin qi* and *yang qi* of the five viscera can only be produced and developed through them. While *ming men* is attributed to fire, the kidneys correspond to the water element.

Among the two phases fire and water, fire warms and moves water, while water as the foundation of life is also the origin of fire. Fire and water must support each other. They are dependent on each other and cannot separate. Kidney water and *ming men* fire are known as prenatal *yin* and *yang*.

Hui Yin—Meeting of *Yin*

The area *hui yin* (CV-1) is located on the perineum, between anus and urethra. It is the starting point of the *ren mai, chong mai,* and *du mai*. In the old times, Chinese physicians referred to it as the origin of the sea or else as the lower *dan tian*. It was also said to be the source of procreative *jing*. This region is linked to sexuality in both sexes. The old texts state that 1.3 *cun* in front of the *hui yin* point is where the *jing* (male sperm) is stored and where the female uterus is located. In recent years, physicians and *qi gong* practitioners have been regarding the two kidneys, *ming men*, the lower *dan tian*, and *hui yin* as a center for regulating human energy. Most recently, it has been clinically proven that stimulating the region of the lower *dan tian*, *hui yin*, and *ming men* has the effect of increasing the secretory activity of the hypophysis and adrenal gland.

Shen—The Kidneys

The kidneys store the essence *jing*. The *jing qi* of the five viscera and six bowels is stored in the two kidneys and flows together in the lower *dan tian*. As regulator of the body's vital activity, the kidneys are closely related to growth, development, reproduction, and the aging process. They influence the functions of the brain and of the endocrine system, including the sex hormones.

Bibliography

1. Lewis R. *The Infertility Cure*. London: Little Brown; 2004.
2. Lie, FT. *Wissenswertes vom Qigong*. Hamburg: Kolibri; 1993.
3. Maciocia G. *Die Grundlagen der Chinesischen Medizin*. Kötzting: VGM Wühr; 1994.
4. Olvedi U. *Das Stille Qigong*. Munich: Heyne; 1994.
5. Shih TK. *Qi Gong Therapy*. Barrytown: Station Hill; 1994.
6. Wenzel, G. *Qigong im Westen*. Schwarzach: Eigenverlag; 1990.
7. Yafei L. *Frauen-Qigong*. Lehrfilm DVD. Roge: AV Recording; 2005.
8. Yuanping W, Zi D. *Medizinisches Qigong*. Kötzting: VGM Wühr; 1996.

Procedure on the Back of the Body
- *Gun fa* Roll to open the surface.
- *Rou fa* Knead the back *shu* points to supplement the *qi* of the viscera and bowels.
- *Di an fa* Press the points BL-13, BL-15, BL-43, BL-20, BL-21, BL-23, and GV-4 to supplement *qi*.
- *Rou fa* Knead the sacrum.

Procedure on the Front of the Body
- *Mo fa fu* Stroke the abdomen in circles.
- *Di an fa* Press ST-36, SP-3, SP-6, CV-12, and CV-6 to supplement *qi*.
- *Tui fa* Push the spleen channel in the direction of its course.

Treating Liver *Qi* Stagnation with *Tui Na*

Symptoms
- increased eye pressure
- grinding the teeth
- tense chewing muscles
- neck and shoulder tension
- upper abdominal pain
- heart palpitations
- stomach stress
- digestive disorders
- menstrual complaints
- general tension
- irascibility
- quickly getting annoyed
- tense pulses

Treatment Principle
Harmonize liver *qi*.

Point Selection
GB-34, LR-3, LR-13, LR-14, TB-6, PC-6, BL-18, GB-21, GB-30

Procedure on the Back of the Body
- Place hands on the patient's back, calm the patient, make contact.
- *Gun fa* Roll lightly to open the surface.
- *Nie fa* Pinch skin folds, loosen connective tissue.
- *Zhuo fa* Knock (bird head pecking), stimulate the points (**Fig. 10.1**).
- *Di an fa* Acupressure on the back bladder points, harmonize.

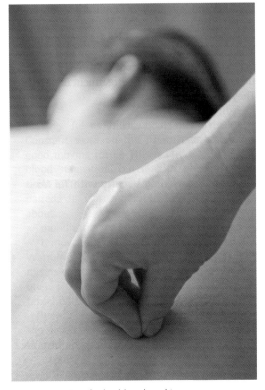

Fig. 10.1 *Zhuo fa*—bird head pecking.

- *Mo fa* Stroking the three lines.
- *Rou fa* Knead the back stretchers.
- *Tui fa/rou fa* Push and knead the neck and shoulder muscles.
- *Na fa* Grasp the shoulder muscles (**Fig. 10.2**).
- *Rou fa* Knead the sacrum (in pelvic blockages).
- *Rou fa* Make circles on GB-30, opening.
- *Tui fa* Push the back.
- *Chui fa* Knock lightly.
- *Tui fa* Push, establish a connection to the legs.

Procedure on the Front of the Body
- *Na fa* Grasp, loosen the neck.
- *Fen tui fa* Dividing strokes, clear the forehead.
- *Rou fa* Knead, loosen the chewing muscles.
- *Zhuo fa* Knock CV-17 to stimulate breathing.

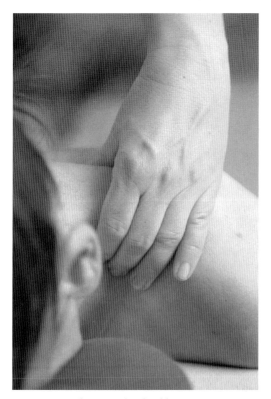

Fig. 10.2 *Na fa*—grasp the shoulder area.

- *An fa*   Press the shoulders down.
- *Tui fa*   Push, release the upper abdominal region.
- *Tui fa*   Push with the finger tips, comb between the ribs.
- Rou fa   Describe circles, release the *mu* points of the liver (LR-14), gallbladder (GB-24), and spleen (LR-13)
- *Mo fa*   Stroke *ren mai*, connect above and below, relieve the stomach.
- *mo fa fu*   Stroke the abdomen.
- *An fa*   Press the iliac wing.
- *Dou fa*   Shake, loosen the arms and legs.
- Rou fa   Describe circles, release LR-3 and GB-34.
- *Tui fa*   Push, relax hands and feet.
- *Di an fa*   Press PC-6.

■ Description of a *Tui Na* Technique and its Effect

In this section, we describe a representative technique of *tui na* therapy and explain its effect. Any *tui na* technique can generally be categorized into a characteristic quality. As such, we speak on the one hand of **yang techniques**, which are executed with strength and intensity and are therefore used for the method of *xie fa* (dispersal). A more gentle execution, on the other hand, can be described as a **yin technique**, which is used accordingly in the method of *bu fa* (supplementation). One example of a *yang* technique is a short heavy blow (*pai fa*) on a certain area of the ribs, such as to release a muscle cramp. A typical *yin* technique would be slow stroking in the abdominal area (*mo fa*).

Most often, the areas of the body where a technique is applied correspond to the technique itself: Thus, the *yin* side of the body, such as the abdomen, is primarily treated with *yin* techniques. Exceptions are severe repletion states in this area like stomach cramps. On the body's *yang* side, such as the back, it is more common to apply *yang* techniques. Likewise, we primarily use *yang* techniques on the *yang* channels and *yin* techniques on the *yin* channels.

Each individual technique can, of course, be applied strongly or gently. It is possible, for example, to apply the *pai fa* technique (hitting with cupped hands) also in mild succession for the purpose of stimulation. On the other hand, we can apply a *mo fa* technique (circling strokes) also in repletion cases like constipation if it is intensified and executed in the appropriate direction.

The Technique of Pressing—*An Fa*

The Chinese term *an*, from the phrase *an mo*, is translated into English as "pressing." In its classical application, the quality of *an fa* is more commonly described as a *yang* technique (*fa* "method, technique"). *An* ("pressing") with the finger corresponds to classic acupressure, or *di an fa* ("point pressing") in Chinese.

In *an fa*, we apply pressure with the thumb, middle finger, index finger, bent fingertips, but also the wrist, whole hand, both hands (on top of each other or side by side), tip of the elbow, lower arm, or even the foot, tip of the foot, or heel.

In classic finger pressing, selected points are fixated and pressed with the tip of the finger or thumb. Hereby avoid injuring the skin or losing the point. It is possible to work with both hands and to hold two points simultaneously. Indications for finger pressing (*an fa*) are typically *a shi* points (pain points; *a shi* "ouch").

However, *an fa* can also have a gentle quality. In that case, the practitioner presses and holds only gently. Any pressing of a point such as the kidney *shu* points (BL-23) in kidney *yang* vacuity with nausea, when executed too strongly, would harm the patient. Points on the body with an energetic vacuity must therefore only be held (**Fig. 10.3**). The technique of holding delivers a concentration of energy to this location and corresponds to the method of *bu fa* (supplementing).

As such, these points have more of a *yin* character. They are empty and soft; a deep hollow opens up in which finger pressure is applied to stimulate energy. When you find such a point, the patient has the feeling of "comfortable, I want to be held here!" This point attracts the finger pressure like a magnet; in vacuous exhausted states, the sensation is like a battery getting recharged.

An Fa Technique in Infertility

In the context of fertility treatment, the following section describes the *an fa* technique for supplementation at the point CV-4. Supplementing on this point is often neglected in other descriptions; hence, we explain it here in more detail.

CV-4 is a point on the abdomen and we therefore choose mild pressure with the finger. The middle finger is used for this purpose (**Fig. 10.4**). It is best because it has the perfect length for sink-

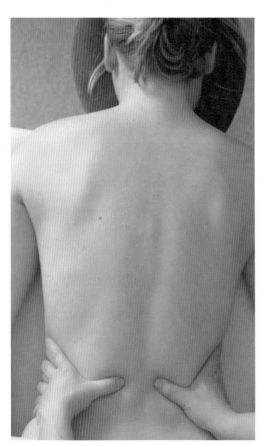

Fig. 10.3 Gentle *an fa*—finger pressure on BL-23 (kidney *shu* point).

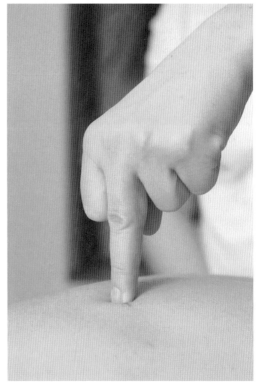

Fig. 10.4 *An fa*—finger pressure with the middle finger.

ing into the soft belly. The thumb is a finger that is utilized more for draining techniques because it is the strongest finger. The index finger is here regarded—in a vacuity state—as too penetrating in its application. At a point like CV-4, it is important in vacuity states to sink down carefully, to rule out any energetic injury. Because there is no obvious *de qi* sensation at a vacuous point, you must pay great attention to really arriving at and being in contact with the point. This occurs while you slowly sink down from the surface of the skin to the point. Then the point is held.

It is important that the therapist has neither cold fingers nor long fingernails. Hold gentle pressure here for at least 1 minute. The breathing should, of course, be flowing gently. The therapist's shoulders must be relaxed, the feet well grounded. Cover the surrounding areas of the patient's body because the patient easily cools down in quiet phases of a *tui na* treatment. After the treatment time on this point is over, release pressure gently; move the middle finger back to the surface of the skin and then leave skin contact. This treatment is carried out with special concentration.

■ Self-massage in Infertility

Patients often come with the question: "What else can I do on my own?" Here, self-massage—*zi shen an mo*—offers an effective complementary therapy. At the same time, it closes the gaps between professional treatments, which in the West generally take place once or twice a week while patients in China are most commonly treated on a daily basis. Self-massage can be applied every day.

Exercise—Strengthening Kidney *Yang* and Warming the Lower Abdomen

In this application, the hands should be warm. Begin therefore by rapidly rubbing the surfaces of the hands against each other until you generate warmth. Another method is to shake the wrists rapidly, ideally while standing, for 3–5 minutes. This not only generates heat in the hands but creates a comfortable warm feeling throughout the whole body. A necessary precondition is, though, that the knees and shoulder joints are relaxed:

- **Rub the *dan tian*.** Here, we mean the lower *dan tian* (see Chapter 9). Because prolonged standing weakens the kidneys, rubbing the *dan tian* should be done while seated or lying down. The patient can thereby concentrate fully on the application:
  - Place the hands on top of each other on the lower abdomen, women with the right hand underneath and men with the left hand underneath.
  - Now circle the hands on the *dan tian*, first clockwise then in the opposite direction. The pressure should be gentle, but still maintaining contact with the body.
  - The circling can be applied on top of the clothing and should be carried out at least 36 times in each direction.
  - To finish, rest the hands calmly on the *dan tian* for a while.
  - During the entire exercise, breathe deeply into the abdomen so that you raise and lower it.
  - Instead of counting a specific number of circles, you can also just take 5 minutes for each direction, followed by 5 minutes to rest on the *dan tian*.
  - At the end, exert light pressure on the *dan tian* three times to close it.
- **Warm the loins and lower back.** This exercise can be performed standing or sitting:
  - After warming the hands by rubbing, place them backwards on the kidneys.
  - The hands can remain for 2–3 minutes before you begin circling them on the kidneys (*rou fa shen*).
  - The circling movement should be carried out with an emphasis on the inward movement. This has a supplementing effect, and the rubbing furthermore is warming and feels very comfortable. Anybody with a healthy shoulder region can perform this exercise.
  - A time frame of 5 minutes or a count of 100 circles is appropriate.
  - Following this, place the hands on top of each other on the lumbar spinal column. With light pressure, push the hands downward onto the sacrum (*tui fa*). This also generates comfortable warmth. Do this at least 20 times.
  - To finish, rest the hands on the sacrum for a short while.

- **Stimulate the kidneys by knocking.** Knocking (*chui fa*) has a very stimulating and, if applied more strongly, penetrating and releasing effect. While standard *tui na* technique avoids knocking techniques in the kidney region or at least does not apply strong knocking and hitting techniques here, we can apply at least knocking techniques with great efficacy in self-massage. They have a good effect on weakened, insufficient kidneys. They can support kidney *yang* and *yin*. At the same time, the swinging movements have a loosening effect on the lower back:
  - First, form the hands into loosely balled fists.
  - Now knock loosely and lightly on the kidney region with the dorsal part of the hand.
  - This technique can be carried out 200–300 times.
- **Knock on the sacrum.** Light knocking on the sacrum strengthens kidney *yang* in particular. At the same time, the vibrations reach the organs in the lower abdomen. They can cause mild tingling and warmth. In patients with stagnations in the lower abdomen, they stimulate movement and flow:
  - This exercise is most easily carried out with loosely balled fists that hit with the "eye of the fist" (the thumb side).
  - Continue knocking for 2–3 minutes.
- **Rub the soles of the feet:**
  - First, you can apply sharp rubbing (*ca fa*) with the edge of the hand in the area of the arch to warm the foot. By means of rapid frequency, you can achieve a warming effect as if with a small saw.
  - You can also take the foot in both hands and warm it by rubbing.
  - Then circle the ankles. This opens the channels and improves the energy flow.
  - Now treat the point *yong quan* (KI-1). Hereby, it is best to apply the rubbing technique (*rou fa*).
  - Place the thumb very flatly and broadly with the surface of the highest joint down.

- With light pressure, describe slow circles on the point. The rubbing warmth creates a supplementing effect on the kidneys.
- Sustain this rubbing for at least 1 minute; it must be done on both feet.
- **Knock the sole of the foot.** This is also an old technique, for lifting kidney *yang*:
  - For this purpose, take small wooden clappers and take turns beating the sole. This must, however, be done by another person.
  - On your own, you can also knock the soles with the knuckles of the balled fist.
  - Continue knocking for 5–10 minutes.
  - This technique can also be combined with the previous ones.
- **Knock like a pendulum.** This stimulates the *qi* in the lower abdominal region. In addition, you generate mild warmth that radiates in the treated areas:
  - This position is performed standing, with the feet shoulder-width apart.
  - The hands are formed into loosely balled fists.
  - At the same time, hit the lower abdomen with one hand and the sacrum with the other.
  - Alternate the fists continuously from front to back and back to front like a pendulum.
  - Repeat this knocking 6–18 times.
- **Rub the ears.** The ears are the sense organs associated with the kidneys. In kidney vacuity, we can always find cold ears. Warming the ears by rubbing and massaging also has an effect on the kidneys. This method is excellent for self-massage; you can do this more frequently throughout the day for 1–2 minutes each.

Bibliography

1. Lie FT, Skopek H. *Chinesische Heilmassage, Tuina-Therapie, Akupressur. Band IV: Praxis und Theorie der Neuen Chinesischen Akupunktur*. Vienna: Maudrich; 1992.
2. Zhang E. *Chinese Tuina*. University of TCM: Publishing House of Shanghai; 2002.

11 Moxibustion

Annette Jonas

■ General Effect

Moxa therapy or **moxibustion** is a form of treatment in TCM. Like acupuncture, it treats the points of the body. The two treatment methods are often applied simultaneously, which is why the term *zhen jiu*, "needling and burning," is common in China. The Western term moxibustion is derived from the Japanese word *mogusa*, which also means something like "burning."

The herb moxa is used for burning; it is the foliage of wormwood, Artemisiae argyi folium (*ai ye*). This herb contains essential oils, including cineol and thuja oil, as well as choline, resins, and tannin, the vitamins A, B, C, and D, potassium chloride, iron, and magnesium. These active ingredients are released during burning, and heat is generated. From the TCM perspective, moxa therapy—when applied in certain locations—can set processes in motion and expel states of cold in particular.

> Moxibustion releases a substance in the skin's sweat glands that stimulates the nerve endings in the skin. This stimulation affects the pituitary and adrenal glands, causing the secretion of hormones. The warmth improves circulation and stimulates the metabolism. The body's immune system is supported as well by the warmth.

In fact, **disease prevention** plays an eminent role in moxa therapy. There is an expression that you should not go on a far trip without first having stimulated the *qi* with moxa.

Forms of Moxibustion

Moxa Cigar

A moxa cigar is a piece of rolled-up moxa medicinal, ca. 20 cm long and wrapped in thin paper that also burns off during moxibustion. The length and thickness roughly correspond to those of a large Havana cigar. The end is lit and the glowing part is held over the appropriate area. In an indirect procedure, you can also cut off a piece of cigar and stick it on an acupuncture needle (fire needle, **Fig. 11.1**). Moxa cigars are an excellent tool in fertility treatment, especially since patients can also take them home to use (**Fig. 11.2**).

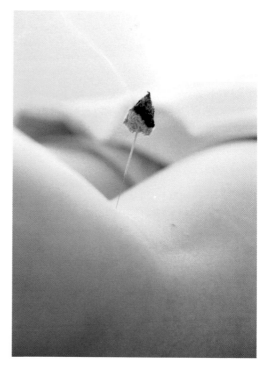

Fig. 11.1 Treatment with the fire needle—indirect moxa technique.

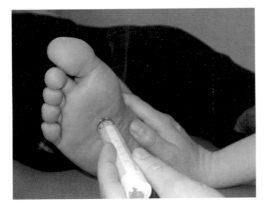

Fig. 11.2 Treatment with the moxa cigar on the foot.

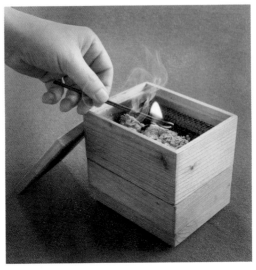

Fig. 11.3 Moxa box

Moxa Cone

In this technique, moxa wool is shaped into small cones that are placed directly on the skin or on a medium (salt, a slice of ginger, garlic). Also available are industrially pre-manufactured moxa cones with a sticky bottom, which are placed directly on the skin. Because this procedure requires some skill, it is better to apply moxa cones in the clinic or hospital than at home.

Moxa Rice Grains

Moxa rice grains are also shaped by hand from moxa wool. After burning off, they must be quickly removed from the skin with tweezers.

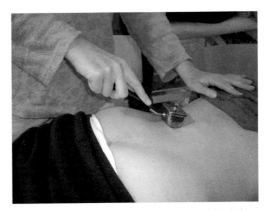

Fig. 11.4 A moxa stove in the treatment of the kidney area.

Moxa Box

The moxa box is a small wooden box with a grate and a vent, in which you burn the moxa (**Fig. 11.3**).

Moxa Stove

A moxa stove usually has a small handle by which you hold it over the treatment area (**Fig. 11.4**).

Moxa Plasters

Moxa plasters are plasters with moxa that you stick on the skin. A newer product is small packages ("herbal heatpack") that are attached with an adhesive bandage and contain iron filings in addition to the moxa. The iron oxidizes when the package is opened. This generates heat, and the moxa can unfold its effect.

Range of Applications for Moxibustion

The main areas of application cover numerous symptoms, including:
- infertility in the man
- menstrual disorders in the woman
- weakness of the bladder and kidney

Moxibustion is particularly suited for use in the treatment of *yang* vacuity states with cold symptoms. Nevertheless, we can also successfully supplement *yin* vacuity patterns. Particularly worth mentioning is its use in **disturbances in the hormonal area**:
- impotence of the man
- frigidity or lack of libido
- involuntary or premature seminal emission
- weak erections
- feeling of cold in the back

Treatment Principles of Moxibustion

In the application of the "eight treatment principles," the most commonly used methods are *xie fa* (dispersal/draining) and *bu fa* (supplementation/concentration). These two main methods can be applied in moxibustion as well. With regard to fertility treatment, we fall back on the method of *bu fa* by means of moxibustion and use *wen fa* (warming) as an additional method (see **Table 9.1**, p. 105). *Xie fa* and *bu fa* differ in the strength of stimulation. While we use a strong stimulation in xie fa, bu fa consists of a gentle stimulation.

The **indication** for *bu fa*, the supplementing technique, is a state of insufficiency or vacuity. This application should always include a clear intention of filling and stimulating. Indications for *wen fa*, the warming technique, are cold disorders and patterns of *yang* vacuity.

Moxibustion should have the effect of gradual warming or stimulating. **Criteria for evaluating** the successful effect of the technique are the patient's reactions:
- The warmth is experienced as comfortable.
- Pressure and massage are experienced as comfortable (combinations are possible).
- The moxa smell is experienced as comfortable.
- Gentle activation and movement improve the condition.

The **key factor** in the application of this method is to have sufficient time at your disposal. Generally speaking, moxibustion is not a short therapy. Nevertheless, a daily treatment time of 10–20 minutes should be sufficient. If you add further points, the duration can, however, certainly increase to 30–45 minutes.

Easiest in **application** is moxibustion with the **cigar**, whether in clinic or at home. The use of **moxa cones** is somewhat more complicated, but on the other hand extremely effective when applied directly. The **moxa box** is also very good for its dispersing effect, but has the disadvantage of making the room very smoky. The **moxa stove** is slightly less smoky; you must be careful, however, not to burn yourself on the metal body.

Necessary supplies for working with moxa cigars are:
- the moxa cigar
- a lighter
- an ashtray
- a moxa extinguisher

For application at home, it is very important to extinguish the cigar completely to avoid fire damage. Moxa cigars cannot be stubbed out like tobacco cigars; instead, the embers must be smothered. The glowing end must be placed in a container filled with sand or uncooked rice if no moxa extinguisher is available.

■ The Use of Moxibustion in Fertility Treatment

Because the effect of moxa is strongly warming and *yang*-stimulating, states of *yang* vacuity constitute the main indication for moxibustion. Nevertheless, it is also possible to use moxa to supplement *yin* or blood.

Patterns in fertility treatment that can be treated with moxa are:
- kidney *yang* vacuity
- *qi* and blood vacuity
- cold stagnating in the lower abdomen

Kidney *Yang* Vacuity ("Weakness of the Lumbus") in Men and Women

Symptoms
- impotence
- aversion to sex
- cold (especially in the lower back, knees, and feet)
- frequent or night-time urination
- weak back
- insufficiently straightened posture
- lower back pain
- weak motivation
- weak erections
- pale tongue
- deep weak pulse

Treatment Principle
Supplement kidney *yang* and warm *yang*.

Point Selection
- ventral: CV-4, CV-6, KI-3, KI-7, KI-1
- dorsal: BL-23, BL-52, *jing gong* assistant point, GV-4, *ba liao*

Medium
In former times, practitioners treated this condition with aconite moxibustion. They ground aconite into a fine powder, mixed it with a little alcohol, and shaped it into a base on which they burned moxa cones; especially effective in impotence and premature seminal emission. Aconite, however, is toxic and no longer available in pharmacies. Instead, you can use ginger, for example.

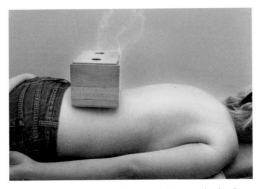

Fig. 11.5 Treatment with a moxa box on the back.

Application
- With a **moxa cigar**, treat each point individually or draw a line.
- Set the **moxa cones** on each of the selected points. Three to five or five to seven moxa cones are recommended for KI-7.
- Position the **moxa box** sideways across the lower back (*shen shu/ming men*). Make sure that the heat does not become too strong. The height of the box can be adjusted accordingly (**Fig. 11.5**).
- Treat the individual points for 5–10 minutes. Leave the moxa box in place for 10–15 minutes.

Qi and Blood Vacuity ("Weak Earth") in Women

Symptoms
- weakness
- fatigue
- lack of appetite
- weak extremities
- paleness
- blood deficiency
- amenorrhea
- rather pale tongue
- vacuous pulse

Treatment Principle
Supplement spleen *qi* and strengthen the blood.

Point Selection
CV-6, CV-8, ST-36, SP-6, BL-43, BL-20, BL-21, CV-12, KI-3, BL-23

Application
- With a **moxa cigar**, treat each point individually.
- Set the **moxa cones** on each of the selected points. Three to five moxa cones per point are recommended.
- Position the **moxa box** on CV-12.

Cold Stagnating in the Lower Abdomen ("Cold Lower Abdomen") in Women

Symptoms
- cold lower abdomen
- aversion to cold
- dysmenorrhea
- paleness
- livid tongue
- slow and tense pulse

Treatment Principle
Expel the cold and warm the body.

Point Selection
CV-4, GV-4, BL-23, BL-52, *ba liao*

Medium
Ginger

Application
- Apply the **moxa cigar** or **moxa cone** on each point.
- Position the **moxa box** on top of the lower back at the level of BL-23 or the sacrum.

General Treatment Recommendation in Fertility Treatment

On the basis of a weakness and vacuity of *yang* energy, the main treatment principle is **supplementing** (*bu fa*) and **warming** (*wen fa*) kidney *yang*:
- every day, 10 minutes of moxibustion with a moxa cigar on the **lower abdomen** in the area of CV-4
- every day, 10 minutes of moxibustion with a moxa cigar on the **lower back** in the area of GV-4/BL-23

For domestic use, we recommend moxibustion on the lower abdomen. Patients can carry out this treatment on their own.

■ Localization and Application

For **point-specific application**, the use of the moxa cigar is ideal, but you can also apply moxa cones or self-adhesive moxa. For **linear application**, an imaginary line is drawn between points that are interrelated or lie on one channel. For this purpose, it is most common to use the moxa cigar. For **regional application**, you can position a moxa box or roll on a moxa plaster.

The Most Important Points in the Treatment of Infertility

Points on *Ren Mai*

CV-4, CV-6, CV-8, and CV-12. These points can be treated individually, but you can also draw an imaginary line from CV-8 to CV-4. Move the moxa cigar back and forth on this line:
- CV-4, *guan yuan*: strengthens original *qi* and the kidneys, nourishes *yin* and blood
- CV-6, *qi hai*: supplements *qi* and *yang*
- CV-8, *shen que*: supplements original *qi* and also the blood; direct and indirect (with medium underneath) moxibustion is possible
- CV-12, *zhong wan*: supplements the center, expels dampness; use of moxa box is possible

Points on *Du Mai*

GV-4 and GV-20:
- GV-4, *ming men*: strengthens kidney *yang*, longer treatment (ca. 10 minutes)
- GV-20, *bai hui*: lifts *yang qi*

Points on the Bladder Channel

BL-17, BL-18, BL-19, BL-20, BL-21, BL-23, BL-52:
- BL-17, *ge shu*: strengthens *qi* and blood; treat individually or together with BL-18 and BL-19
- BL-20, *pi shu*: has a *qi*-supplementing effect, direct moxa
- BL-21, *wei shu*
- BL-52, BL-23, GV-4: you can draw a line from BL-52 through BL-23 and GV-4

123

- BL-23, *shen shu*: strengthens the kidneys
- BL-52, *zhi shi*: strengthens the kidneys, in conjunction with BL-23

Points on the Spleen and Stomach Channels

ST-36, SP-6:
- ST-36, *zu san li*: supplements *qi*; frequent moxibustion is possible
- SP-6, *san yin jiao*: supplements *qi* and *yin*

Points on the Kidney Channel

KI-1, KI-2, KI-3, KI-6, and KI-7:
- KI-1, *yong quan*: supplements the kidneys; do not use in vacuity heat; for best effect, alternate moxibustion with rubbing
- KI-2, *ran gu*: supplements the kidneys; do not use in vacuity heat
- KI-3, *tai xi*: supplements the kidneys; *yin* and *yang* aspect
- KI-6, *zhao hai*: supplements the kidneys
- KI-7, *fu liu*: supplements kidney *yang*; longer treatment (five to seven moxa cones)

■ Problems in the Application of Moxa Therapy

Moxa therapy is a treatment that is frequently neglected in clinical practice. There are various reasons why the whole range of this excellent old therapeutic method is not employed to its fullest extent. The greatest problem lies in the **regular application**. Because it is impossible in Western clinical practice to carry out moxa treatment on a daily basis, the patient must be instructed on how to repeat treatment according to directions at home, daily or possibly every other day.

Application in the Hospital or Clinic

The application requires time. Unlike with acupuncture, the practitioner must remain actively involved during the entire treatment. The applica-
tion can only take place in an enclosed room because the **moxa smell** would otherwise bother other patients. After treatment, the room must be aired out thoroughly and is not useable for additional treatments for a while. The moxa smell remains in the air for a long time. The clothing of both the practitioner and the patient continues to smell of moxa for a while.

Application at Home

For domestic application, we primarily recommend the moxa cigar because its use is comparatively simple and does not cause as much smoke as, for example, the moxa box. Nevertheless, the same problems arise as in clinical practice, with the difference that the application takes place directly at home and could cause problems for other family members. This is the main reason why application at home is not more common. The recommendation of "smokeless moxa" (moxa coals) is not always accepted either. Also, moxa coals are less effective and quickly develop strong heat. The desired effect, however, can only occur with regular correct application.

Dangers

In addition, the patient must be alerted to the following dangers:
- **Danger of burns.** The application of moxa must be carried out with the necessary distance and movement. A static application with insufficient distance can easily cause burns on the skin.
- **Danger of soiling and damage.** After a certain time of smoldering, the moxa ashes of the cigar must be tapped off. If ashes fall on any clothing or furniture, this can quickly lead to burns or soiling. It is especially important that you do not stub out the moxa cigar after use. This action destroys the structure of the cigar tip, parts break off, and ashes can fall onto the skin or clothing when you relight the cigar.
- **Danger of continued glowing.** Moxa cigars must be extinguished correctly. If you do not have a moxa extinguisher at home, the embers should be smothered in a container full of sand. When

trying to stub out a cigar, there is the risk that it will continue to glow and cause a fire.

The following quote comes from Chen Yanzhi, a famous physician from the Jin dynasty (265–316 CE):

"To be able to practice acupuncture, you must be well-trained. Moxa, on the other hand, can be applied by anybody."[2]

Bibliography

1. Brodde A. *Brennen mit Moxa-Kraut.* Schorndorf: WBV; 1981.
2. Hölting H. *Die Moxa-Therapie.* Vol. 2. Munich: Ehrenwirth; 1995.
3. Maciocia G. *Die Grundlagen der Chinesischen Medizin.* Kötzting: VGM Wühr; 1994.
4. Wühr E. *Quintessenz der Chinesischen Akupunktur und Moxibustion.* Kötzting: VGM Wühr; 1988.

12   Acupuncture

Andreas A. Noll

From the perspective of TCM, the numerous functional—and, in the course of time, occasionally also substantial—disorders of reproductivity and sexuality are disturbances in the area of circulation and the production of *qi* and blood. After a decisive diagnosis especially of the affected channels (also in the sense of main, *luo*, muscle, and extraordinary channels), we can then regulate the distribution of *qi* by means of the channel system.

We commonly use acupuncture points that experience has shown to be very effective, such as:
- SP-6, SP-7, SP-8, SP-9, and SP-10
- ST-36 and ST-40
- CV-4 and CV-6
- LR-3 and LI-4
- LR-5
- KI-3, KI-6, and KI-7
- GV-4
- BL-23 and BL-32

These are so-called "*qi* holes" that have proven extremely effective in the treatment of many andrological and gynecological problems with acupuncture and moxibustion.

This chapter deals with unusual, less familiar options in acupuncture and moxibustion therapy. Especially in the lower abdomen and on the liver channel below the lumbar area, there are quite a few points that have an outstanding effect in fertility disorders. This effect depends on the specific combination with other points on the same or a connected channel. The focus of this chapter lies in the description of the effects found in classical Chinese sources of acupuncture. In this context, we discuss points that are less familiar in standard clinical practice (**Fig. 12.1**).

The following points are located on top of or next to the center line (i. e., the median line that runs from the navel to the center of the symphysis), and then 1 to several *cun* each below the navel (**Table 12.1**).

■ Points on the Pubic Line 5 *Cun* below the Navel

The points on the pubic line 5 *cun* below the navel include the following (**Table 12.1**):
- CV-2
- KI-11
- ST-30
- SP-12

CV-2: *Qu Gu*—Curved Bone

Here, the liver channel crosses the *ren mai*. As the sea of *yin*, this point is particularly important for the reconstruction of *yin* (and blood) in the first part of the menstrual cycle. We use this point especially when we find a stagnation of fluid (e. g., cysts, discharge, gummed-up fallopian tubes). In addition, the *ren mai* functions as the reservoir for essence. Thus, when states of exhaustion arise after pregnancy, miscarriage, or hormone therapy, treating this point can help by strengthening essence and *qi*.

Indications from the *Zhen Jiu Da Cheng* (针灸大成 *Great Compendium of Acupuncture and Moxibustion)*[12]

- seminal emissions
- weakness and vacuity in the five viscera
- extreme cold and fatigue due to vacuity
- feeling of fullness in the lower abdomen
- difficult urination with dribbling urine
- ulcers and hernias
- pain in the lower abdomen
- bloody vaginal discharge

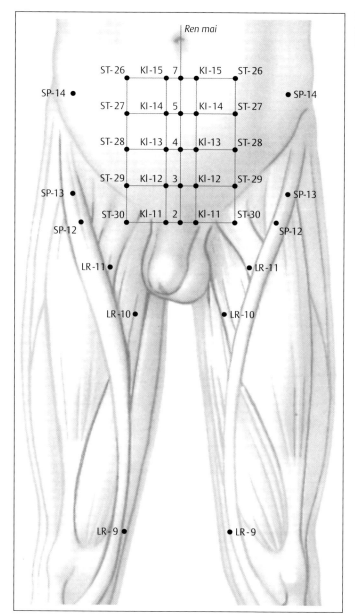

Fig. 12.1 Survey of acupuncture points on the lower abdomen that are important in fertility treatment.

Ren mai

ST-26 KI-15 7 KI-15 ST-26
SP-14
ST-27 KI-14 5 KI-14 ST-27
ST-28 KI-13 4 KI-13 ST-28
ST-29 KI-12 3 KI-12 ST-29
SP-13
ST-30 KI-11 2 KI-11 ST-30
SP-12

SP-14

SP-13
SP-12

LR-11

LR-11

LR-10

LR-10

LR-9

LR-9

Combinations

Suitable combinations are, for example, with:
- LU-7, *lie que*: for opening the *ren mai* in patients with general *qi* vacuity
- SP-6, *san yin jiao*: for cysts
- SP-9, *yin ling quan*: for vaginal discharge

KI-11: *Heng Gu*—Transverse Bone

The kidney channel and *chong mai* meet at this point; hence we find these key indications: general exhaustion after having spent all essence—this can be refilled to a certain extent by opening the *chong mai*—and impaired kidney and bladder functions.

Table 12.1 Points on the lower abdomen between navel and symphysis that are important in fertility treatment, and their indications and effects

Locali-zation	Center Line[a]		0.5 Cun from the Center Line		2 Cun from the Center Line		3.5 Cun from the Center Line	
1 cun below navel	CV-7	Accumulations of yin and blood	KI-15	Vacuity and stagnation of qi	ST-26	Balances out cold and vacuity	SP-14	Qi ascent
2 cun below navel	CV-5	Regulates and strengthens qi and yang	KI-14	Accumulations of yin	ST-27	Affects yin and qi	–	–
3 cun below navel	CV-4	Original qi and yin stagnation	KI-13	Qi vacuity	ST-28	Moves fluids	–	–
4 cun below navel	CV-3	Yang vacuity	KI-12	Insufficiency of kidney qi and kidney essence	ST-29	Upbears and downbears qi	SP-13	Qi repletion and ascent
5 cun below navel	CV-2	Kidney qi vacuity, dampness	KI-11	Dampness, general vacuity	ST-30	Resolves blockages	SP-12	Repletion, cold

[a] Center line from the navel to the center of the symphysis.

Indications from the *Zhen Jiu Da Cheng*

- frequent painful and urgent involuntary urination
- urinary dribbling
- pain and tautness in the penis
- feeling of fullness in the lower abdomen
- painful and red eyes
- general vacuity of the five viscera
- loss of essence

Combinations

Suitable combinations are, for example, with:
- KI-3, *tai xi*: for general exhaustion, for example, after intensive hormone therapy
- KI-6, *zhao hai*: for rising heat and states of disquietude
- KI-10, *yin gu*: for accumulations of dampness like prostatitis and vaginal discharge

ST-30: *Qi Chong—Qi* Thoroughfare

At this point, the *chong mai* ("sea of blood") joins the stomach channel; this is therefore an excellent point for influencing blood, *jing*, and, via the stomach channel, also postnatal *qi*. Furthermore, because the *chong mai* is the "sea of the 12 channels," we can resolve obstructions and blockages in the entire abdomen here.

Indications from the *Zhen Jiu Da Cheng*

- fullness in the abdomen
- inability to lie on the stomach
- hernia
- heat in the large intestine
- abdominal pain with fever
- pain in the testicles and penis with atrophy of the genitals
- *qi* ascending from the lower abdomen and attacking the heart
- fullness and tension in the abdomen with strong pain, obstructed breathing
- back pain with stiffness in the lower back

- feeling of heat in the stomach in cold damage disorders
- female infertility
- pain in the small intestine
- menstrual irregularities
- ascent of fetal *qi* during pregnancy (i. e., nausea and vomiting in the mother)
- retained placenta
- difficulties during delivery

Combinations

Suitable combinations are, for example, with:
- SP-4, *gong sun*: when you want to open the *chong mai* as the sea of blood, especially in the second half of the menstrual cycle
- ST-36, *zu san li*: when *qi* rises too much in this phase
- SP-10, *xue hai*: for premenstrual pain, but also for pain during ovulation

SP-12: *Chong Men*—Thoroughfare Gate[*]

The "thoroughfare" mentioned in the point name here is also the *chong mai*, which can be reached at the adjoining point *qi chong* (ST-30). Since the liver channel and spleen channel intersect here as well, we can effectively resolve all kinds of stagnation with this point. Hence, it guarantees access to the thoroughfare of blood (*chong mai*).

Indications from the *Zhen Jiu Da Cheng*

- cold in the abdomen with *qi* repletion
- painful formation of tumors in the abdomen
- *shan* (mounting) pain

- impaired milk production during breastfeeding
- the fetus pushes upward and encroaches on the heart region, as a result of which breathing is impaired

Combinations

Suitable combinations are, for example, with:
- SP-10, *xue hai*: for myomas and painful menstruation
- LR-1, *da dun*: for intense pain in the lower abdomen (penis, vagina), also after surgery
- LR-5, *li kou*: for swelling/pain/itching in the external genitals

◼ Points on the Line 4 *Cun* below the Navel

The points on the line 4 *cun* below the navel include the following (**Table 12.2**):
- CV-3
- KI-12
- ST-29
- SP-13

CV-3: *Zhong Ji*—Central Pole

CV-3 is an extremely important point since all *yin* channels of the leg intersect here with *ren mai*, which is known as the "sea of *yin*." Hence, its range of indications includes any energetic state that is characterized by the accumulation of *yin* (especially cold and fluids). *Yang* is vacuous; the lower abdomen feels cold and swollen. Especially

Table 12.2 Points on the line 4 *cun* below the navel

Localiza-tion	Center Line[a]		0.5 *Cun* from the Center Line		2 *Cun* from the Center Line		3.5 *Cun* from the Center Line	
4 *cun* below the navel	CV-3	*Yang vacuity*	KI-12	Insufficiency of kidney *qi* and kidney essence	ST-29	Upbears and downbears *qi*	SP-13	Repletion and *qi* ascent

[a] Center line from the navel to the center of the symphysis.

[*] This point is also translated as "Surging Gate" in English.

129

in women with *yang* vacuity and infertility, applying moxibustion on this point can help.

Indications from the *Zhen Jiu Da Cheng*

- accumulations of cold *qi*, which occasionally stretch into the breasts
- sensation of heat in the abdomen
- formation of masses below the navel
- *ben tun* (running piglet) disease
- excessive sweating in the genital area
- swelling of the vagina
- *yang* vacuity
- frequent urination
- infertility in women and involuntary seminal emissions in men
- persistent vaginal discharge after childbirth
- retained placenta
- irregular menstruation
- formation of masses due to blood stasis
- swelling and pain in the pubic area
- cold in the lower abdomen
- heat and itching in the genital area
- hunger with no desire to eat
- corpse-like loss of consciousness
- the menses arrive and the couple enters the bedroom (i.e., they have sexual intercourse)
- the bladder is full but there is no discharge of urine
- in women's infertility: use this point four times and the woman will become pregnant![4]

Combinations

Suitable combinations are, for example, with:
- SP-6, *san yin jiao*: for stagnation in the lower abdomen
- GV-4, *ming men*: for aversion to sex and feeling cold, especially in the feet
- ST-36, *zu san li*: for general cold and weakness

KI-12: *Da He*—Great Manifestation

Here we are obviously dealing with a point that is so important that the early Chinese masters of acupuncture felt compelled to capture this in its name! This is where the kidney channel meets with *chong mai*—hence, we can strengthen essence and its mobilization through this point: indications are impotence and tendency to miscarriages.

Indications from the *Zhen Jiu Da Cheng*

- seminal emissions with general exhaustion
- contraction of the penis
- pain in the penis
- red and painful eyes, beginning in the inner corner of the eye
- bloody vaginal discharge

Indications from the *Qian Jin Yi Fang* (千金翼方 *Supplemental Prescriptions Worth a Thousand in Gold)*[11]

- red and turbid vaginal discharge in women
- seminal emissions and great exhaustion in men
- shrinking of the penis
- pain in the penis

Combinations

Suitable combinations are, for example, with:
- KI-3, *tai xi*: for simultaneous fear, lumbar pain, and weakness in the lumbus
- LR-3, *tai chong*: for simultaneous impotence and emotional blockages

ST-29: *Gui Lai*—Return!

This passionate exclamation is directed at the failure of *qi* and *yang*, which can lead to sagging of the uterus and inability to raise the penis, but also to failed descent of the testicles from the abdomen. Cold and weakness impede *qi*, especially in the first phase of the menstrual cycle. It is therefore preferable to treat this point with moxibustion.

Indications from the *Zhen Jiu Da Cheng*

- *qi* ascent
- undescended testicles with pain in the penis
- hernias
- accumulation of cold in women

Combinations

Suitable combinations are, for example, with:
- SP-6, *san yin jiao*: for prolapse of the uterus or bladder

- LR-3, *tai chong*: for simultaneous impotence and emotional blockages
- LR-8, *qu quan*: for swelling and itching in the genitals

SP-13: *Fu She*—Bowel Abode

This point is characterized by its usefulness in states of repletion with simultaneous *qi* ascent. As the *jiao hui* (intersection) point of the spleen, liver, and *yin* linking channels, it resolves blockages, as a result of which the *qi* that is ascending counterflow is able to reach the lower burner. The term "abode" in the name of the point furthermore indicates that we can resolve accumulations here; not only material ones but also mental "accumulations"—when the carousel of thoughts will not stop or when you are unable —for example, during sexual intercourse—to pay attention to other people because you are too preoccupied with yourself.

Indications from the *Zhen Jiu Da Cheng*

- hernia that can be pushed back or not
- pain around the hernia with *bi* (impediment) syndrome, in which the pain rises upward to the heart
- feeling of swelling in the abdomen
- feeling of cold in the extremities, especially in the tips of the fingers and toes—apply moxa five times

Combinations

Suitable combinations are, for example, with:
- ST-40, *feng long*: for constipation and flatulence
- PC-6, *nei guan*: for simultaneous nausea
- ST-44, *nei ting*: for blocked ability to absorb

■ Points on the Line 3 *Cun* below the Navel

The points on the line 3 *cun* below the navel include the following (**Table 12.3**):
- CV-4
- KI-13
- ST-28

CV-4: *Guan Yuan*—Pass Head

Hardly any other point has as many different names as this extremely essential point, which lies a hand's width below the navel. Its names range from "Child Palace" to "Birth Gate" and "Bodily Sluggishness." Through this point, we can effectively stimulate original *qi*, the active component of essence, and thereby also the person's *yang*. It is preferable to use moxibustion, especially for signs of stagnating *yin* in the lower burner and excessive *yang* in the upper burner.

Indications from the *Zhen Jiu Da Cheng*

- extreme cold
- weakness and exhaustion
- colic-like pain below the navel that radiates to the genitals
- pain through the navel that radiates to the genitals
- pain due to formation of masses or cold in the abdomen
- seminal emissions
- turbid vaginal discharge
- blood stasis and hernias
- headache due to wind

Table 12.3 Points on the line 3 cun below the navel

Localization	Center Line[a]		0.5 *Cun* from the Center Line		2 *Cun* from the Center Line		3.5 *Cun* from the Center Line	
3 *cun* below the navel	CV-4	Stagnation of original *qi* and of *yin*	KI-13	*Qi* vacuity	ST-28	Moves fluids	–	–

Note: [a]Center line from the navel to the center of the symphysis.

131

- concentrated dark urine that is discharged only with difficulty
- hot white vaginal discharge
- *lin* (strangury) disorders
- retention of urine due to stones in the urinary tracts
- diarrhea
- *ben tun* (running piglet) disorders radiating to the heart
- menstrual problems
- being cut off from pregnancy
- loss of essence
- exhaustion and heat
- the gate to the uterus is blocked and cold
- bleeding during pregnancy
- vile discharge after childbirth that will not stop

Combinations

Suitable combinations are, for example, with:
- KI-2, *ran gu*: for extremely cold feet
- GV-4, *ming men*: for aversion to sex and feelings of cold
- KI-1, *yong quan*: for simultaneous states of unrest and insomnia

KI-13: *Qi Xue—Qi* Point

Just like the point *guan yuan* (CV-4), which lies right next to it, this point has an effect on original *qi*. But in addition, we can also use this point to influence the *qi* that has its source in the lung but is collected by the kidney and is essential for reproduction and all other basic functions of the human organism. Additional names for this point are "Child Gate" and "Gate of the Uterus."

Indications from the *Zhen Jiu Da Cheng*

- *qi* sensations that rise from the lower abdomen into the chest and throat
- persistent diarrhea
- lumbar pain
- menstrual disorders
- redness and pain in the eye, radiating from the inner corner of the eye

Combinations

Suitable combinations are, for example, with:
- KI-27, *shu fu*: for inability to breathe deeply
- KI-7, *fu liu*: for other symptoms of *qi* vacuity in the kidney
- KI-6, *zhao hai*: for rising heat sensations

ST-28: *Shui Dao*—Waterway

The name says it all—water, in whatever form, finds it way when we treat this point. Accumulations of fluid include urine as well as blood and the fluids in the intestine.

Indications from the *Zhen Jiu Da Cheng*

- stiffness and spasms in the lower back
- cold in the bladder
- accumulations of heat in the triple burner
- tension in the lower abdomen in women
- pain radiating from the external genitals
- tumor in the uterus
- cold in the vagina
- retention of urine and stool

Combinations

Suitable combinations are, for example, with:
- SP-5, *shang qiu*: for edemas
- SP-9, *yin ling quan*: for urine retention
- SP-10, *xue hai*: for menstrual pain

■ Points on the Line 2 *Cun* below the Navel

The points on the line 2 *cun* below the navel include the following (**Table 12.4**):
- CV-5
- KI-14
- ST-27

Table 12.4 Points on the line 2 *cun* below the navel

Localization	Center Line[a]		0.5 *Cun* from the Center Line		2 *Cun* from the Center Line		3.5 *Cun* from the Center Line
2 *cun* below the navel	CV-5	Regulates and strengthens *qi* and *yang*	KI-14	Accumula-tions of *yin*	ST-27	Effect on *yin* and *qi*	–	–

[a] Center line from the navel to the center of the symphysis.

CV-5: *Shi Men*—Stone Gate

The name of the point refers to its use in fertility problems—since a woman who is unable to bear children is known as a "stone woman" in China. Because of its contraceptive effect, this point has traditionally been forbidden for treatment with acupuncture, while moxibustion was recommended. Nevertheless, the name also refers to accumulations in general, that is, obstructions, blockages, and swelling in the lower abdomen.

Indications from the *Zhen Jiu Jia Yi Jing* (针灸甲乙经 *Systematized Classic of Acupuncture and Moxibustion*)[13]

- strong pain in the chest and abdomen with severe sweating
- fullness in the abdomen and edemas
- *shan* (mounting) disorders in the lower abdomen
- pain around the navel
- urine retention due to *qi* stagnation
- yellow urine
- *qi* repletion
- loss of urine due to weakness
- fullness in the abdomen
- *ben tun* (running piglet) disorders with *qi* ascent
- alternating heat and cold
- vomiting
- difficult urination
- abdominal pain coming in waves
- encumbered speech due to a stiff tongue
- swollen penis
- pain in the lower back, stretching into the lower abdomen
- strong pain in the lumbus and abdomen that stretches to the genitals, with difficult urination
- the testicles are shrunken and painful

- the evil collects in the abdomen and causes hernias
- persistent discharge of breast milk
- infertility
- itching in the pubic area[4]

Combinations

Suitable combinations are, for example, with:
- SP-10, *xue hai*: for severe menstrual pain and myomas
- LR-5, *li kou*: for vaginismus

KI-14: *Si Man*—Fourfold Fullness

Similar indications as its neighbor, CV-5: accumulations in the lower abdomen. This point has a *qi*- and blood-moving effect as well, which it could in the present context unfold particularly for the purpose of triggering ovulation.

Indications from the *Zhen Jiu Da Cheng*

- all binding and accumulations
- diarrhea
- accumulation of water in the large intestine
- severe pain in the lower abdomen
- strong aversion to cold
- redness and pain in the eyes
- menstrual disorders
- infertility
- *qi* sensations that rise from the lower abdomen into the chest and throat

Combinations

Suitable combinations are, for example, with:
  KI-1, *yong quan*: for severe painful blockages in the lower abdomen
  BL-57, *cheng shan*: for painful constipation

133

ST-27: *Da Ju*—Great Gigantic

In this case, the "gigantic" that the point name refers to is the abdomen in which all *qi* and *yin* can collect; there is not much left over for supplying the periphery, or for the production and distribution of blood and *qi*. As obstacles for a pregnancy, we here find sluggishness, problems with dampness (e. g., cysts), and perhaps blood vacuity.

Indications from the *Zhen Jiu Da Cheng*

- fullness and tension in the lower abdomen
- restlessness and thirst
- difficult urination
- hernias
- hemilateral paralysis
- atrophy of the muscles in the extremities
- insomnia
- fright palpitations

Combinations

Suitable combinations are, for example, with:
- SP-6, *san yin jiao*: for abdominal pain and erectile dysfunctions
- TB-6, *shi gou*: for diarrhea
- SP-9, *yin ling quan*: for vaginal discharge and turbid urine

■ Points on the Line 1 *Cun* below the Navel

The points on the line 1 *cun* below the navel include the following (**Table 12.5**):
- CV-7
- KI-15
- ST-26
- SP-14

CV-7: *Yin Jiao*—Yin Intersection

Here, *yin* gathers in the form of *chong mai, ren mai*, and the kidney channel. By treating this point with moxibustion, we can resolve accumulations of *yin* and blood—characterized by severe stabbing pain.

Indications from the *Zhen Jiu Da Cheng*

- strong pain as if someone were plunging a knife into the abdomen
- feeling of fullness in the upper abdomen with pain that radiates to the genitals
- hernia pain
- dampness
- sweating and itching in the pubic area
- muscle spasms in the lumbus and knee
- heat under the navel
- nosebleed
- bleeding from the uterus
- turbid vaginal discharge
- persistent lochia
- cold pain around the navel
- infertility
- collapsed chest in children

Combinations

Suitable combinations are, for example, with:
SP-10, *xue hai*: for stagnating bleeding
LR-8, *qu quan*: for varicocele

KI-15: *Zhong Zhu*—Central Flow

The name expresses the moving power of this point. While the neighboring point CV-5 is able to treat pain from stagnation of *yin* and *xue*, this point has more of a quickening effect on anything that is too sluggish in the lower abdomen: menstruation, defecation, and urination.

Table 12.5 Points on the line 1 *cun* below the navel

Localization	Center Line[a]		0.5 *Cun* from the Center Line		2 *Cun* from the Center Line		3.5 *Cun* from the Center Line	
1 *cun* below the navel	CV-7	Accumulations of *yin* and blood	KI-15	Vacuity and stagnation of *qi*	ST-26	Balances out cold and vacuity	SP-14	*Qi* ascent

[a] Center line from the navel to the center of the symphysis.

Indications from the *Zhen Jiu Da Cheng*

- heat in the lower abdomen
- hard stools and constipation
- diarrhea
- lumbar pain
- redness and pain in the inner corner of the eye
- irregular menstruation

Combinations

Suitable combinations are, for example, with:
- SP-3, *tai bai*: for constipation
- KI-4, *da zhong*: for simultaneous kidney vacuity and fright

ST-26: *Wai Ling—Outer Mound*

This point has a pronounced effect on *yang*. Besides using it for strengthening *qi* in general (of the lung as well!), we can use this point also in cases with cold and *yang* vacuity in the lower abdomen.

Indications from the *Zhen Jiu Da Cheng*

- pain in the abdomen
- feeling of emptiness in the chest
- pain around the navel

Combinations

Suitable combinations are, for example, with:
- PC-6, *nei guan*: for feeling of emptiness in the chest
- SP-4, *gong sun*: for cold pain in the abdomen

SP-14: *Fu Jie—Abdominal Bind*

"Abdominal binds" are large masses of substrate that can cause severe abdominal swelling. In addition, though, we can also resolve feelings that are pent up in the belly—such as when you are unable to really "speak straight from the gut."

Indications from the *Zhen Jiu Da Cheng*

- severe *qi* counterflow with violent coughing
- pain around the navel
- feeling of cold in the abdomen
- diarrhea
- *qi* ascending and attacking the heart

Combinations

Suitable combinations are, for example, with:
- ST-37, *shang ju xu*: for acute diarrhea
- LR-3, *tai chong*: for rage in the gut
- LR-2, *xing jian*: for concurrent heart attack

■ Important Points on the Liver Channel

The following points on the liver channel from the lumbar area down to the knee are used only very rarely in conventional acupuncture practice (**Table 12.6**). Nevertheless, they show a remarkable effect in the treatment of reproductive and sexual disorders. Like almost all points on the liver channel, they are able to resolve blockages in the flow of *qi* and blood. Because the liver channel, as well as its *luo* network vessels and muscle channel, runs to the lower abdomen and genitals and this is furthermore a place where pathogenic heat, cold, and dampness can lodge and block sexuality and reproduction, the therapeutic application of these points can offer substantial benefits.

LR-9: *Yin Bao—Yin* Bladder

The name of the point indicates its efficacy in disorders of the bladder and uterus. It can be needled especially in cases with painful disorders of the genitals but also for cramping before or during menstruation that is caused by *qi* stagnation.

Table 12.6 Points on the liver channel that are important in fertility treatment

Point	Point Name	Localization	Indication/Effect	Technique
LR-9	*Yin bao—Yin Bladder*	4 *cun* above the medial epicondyle of the femur	Pain, blockages of *qi*	Needling
LR-10	*Zhu wu li—Leg Five Li*	3 *cun* directly below ST-30, a pulse is palpable here	Blockages, itching in the genitals; for strengthening	Supplementing needling, moxa
LR-11	*Yin lian—Yin Corner*	2 *cun* directly below ST-30, 1 *cun* above LR-10	Infertility	Preferably moxa!
LR-12	*Ji mai—Urgent Pulse*	1 *cun* below the pubic crest, 2.5 *cun* from the center line, pulse	Blockages of *qi* and blood	Caution: needling—preferably moxa!

Localization

On the inside of the thigh, 4 *cun* above the medial epicondyle of the femur, in a depression between two muscles.

Indications from the *Zhen Jiu Da Cheng*

* pain in the lumbar area, radiating into the lower abdomen
* difficult urination
* enuresis
* irregular menstruation

Combinations

Suitable combinations are, for example, with:
* LR-5: for irregular menstruation
* CV-3, ST-28, SP-9: for urinary disorders

LR-10: *Zhu Wu Li—Leg Five Li*

The number "five" in the point name indicates the extraordinary strengthening effect of this point, which develops its fortifying and harmonizing effect from the middle, the center, outward. Accordingly, this point should only be used for supplementing treatment (moxa), that is, especially for vacuity states with simultaneous blockages. In addition, though, the point is also particularly effective for itching in the genital area.

Localization

Three *cun* directly below ST-30 where you can detect a pulse.

Indications from the *Zhen Jiu Da Cheng*

* feeling of tension in the abdomen
* blockage with feeling of heat
* desire to lie down

Lei Jing Tu Yi (類經圖翼 **The Illustrated Wings of the Classified Canon)**[14]

Wind heat in the intestines, inability to urinate, wind exhaustion, desire only to lie down, inability to lift the four limbs.

Combinations

Suitable combinations are, for example, with:
* LR-5, SP-10: for itching in the genitals
* TB-8, TB-10, ST-45, LI-3: for desire to sleep and no desire to move

LR-11: *Yin Lian—Yin Corner*

This point unfolds its effect in *yin*, that is, it strengthens the blood and kidney energy and promotes the flow of *qi* and blood, especially in the context of fertility problems.

Localization

Two *cun* directly below ST-30, 1 *cun* above LR-10.

Indications from the *Zhen Jiu Da Cheng*

* infertility in women: three moxa cones on this point, and she will bear a son immediately

Combinations

Suitable combinations are, for example, with:
* CV-4, ST-29, SP-6: for irregular menstruation

LR-12: *Ji Mai*—Urgent Pulse

An urgent, tense, and stringlike pulse at this location indicates that the *qi* in this area is blocked by cold or emotional factors like anger and tension.

Localization

One *cun* below the pubic crest, 2.5 *cun* from the center line, in the middle between ST-30 and LR-11, slightly to the outside, where a pulse can be detected. Be careful during needling and moxa because of the femoral artery!

Indications from the *Huang Di Nei Jing, Ling Shu* (黄帝内经灵枢 *The Yellow Emperor's Inner Classic, Magic Pivot)*[10]

* cold in the center burner, with pain radiating into the lower abdomen and testicles

* pain on the inside of the thigh—here, it is better to treat with moxa than with needles!

Combinations

Suitable combinations are, for example, with:
* LR-1, CV-4: for inflammation of the testicles, edemas of the scrotum, and pain in the penis
* LR-5: for itching in the genitals
* LR-3: for erectile dysfunctions

Bibliography

1. Geng J. *Selecting the Right Acupoints*. Beijing: New World Press; 1995.
2. Kirschbaum B. *Die 8 Außerordentlichen Gefäße in der Traditionellen Chinesischen Medizin*. Uelzen: ML; 2000.
3. Litschauer J. *Zhenjiu-Akupunktur und Moxibustion*. Munich: Pflaum; 1975.
4. Lorenzen U. *Mikrokosmische Landschaften*. Munich: Müller & Steinicke; 2006.
5. Lorenzen U, Noll A. *Die Wandlungsphasen der Traditionellen Chinesischen Medizin*. Vols. 1–5. Munich: Müller & Steinicke; 1992–2002.
6. Morant GS. *Chinese Acupuncture*. Massachusetts: Paradigm; 1972.
7. Porkert M, Hempen CH. *Systematische Akupunktur*. Munich: Urban & Schwarzenberg; 1985.
8. Youbang Ch, Liangyue D, Kai Z. *Essentials of Contemporary Chinese Acupuncturists' Clinical Experiences*. Beijing: Foreign Languages Press; 1989.
9. Zeitler H. *Akupunkturtherapie mit Kardinalpunkten*. Heidelberg: Haug; 1981.
10. *Huang Di Nei Jing Ling Shu* [Yellow Emperor's Inner Classic, Magic Pivot], 1st century CE, 黄帝内经灵枢
11. *Qian Jin Yi Fang* [Supplemental Prescriptions Worth a Thousand in Gold], 7th century CE, 千金翼方
12. *Zhen Jiu Da Cheng* [Great Compendium of Acupuncture and Moxibustion], 1601, 针灸大成
13. *Zhen Jiu Jia Yi Jing* [Systematized Classic of Acupuncture and Moxibustion], 3rd century CE, 针灸甲乙经
14. *Lei Jing Tu Yi* [The Illustrated Wings of the Classified Canon], dated to 1624, 類經圖翼

13 Chinese Dietetics

Beatrice Trebuth

When friends and family members all around are having babies, couples with an unfulfilled desire for children have a hard time. Expectations and pressures are great; the feeling of having failed in something intended by nature burdens them. A wish that of itself is nothing but pure love of life becomes an act of planning and precautionary measures.

It is easy to say that things happen more easily when they are carried out straight from the gut, rather than when desired and controlled by the mind. The contraceptive pill may have turned all of biology upside down, but it has proven to be of great help in terms of family planning and compatibility with a professional life. Furthermore, we live in a world that is more and more shaped by life on the outside, in which the perfectly organized person has become the trendsetter, dominating the inner world of the self. Reflecting back onto ourselves and our way of life becomes necessary.

To understand eating as cultivation of life, to rethink and change our personal dietary habits means to throw an anchor into the fast-flowing river of life and to take time off for mental and physical "nurturing." In addition to providing joy in life, pleasure, leisure, and satiation, as well as the material substances for blood and the fluids, food also supplies our bodies with *qi* and with the fire that mobilizes precious essences and warms the kidneys, which gives us vital warmth and the strength to conceive. In many meditation practices and health-related exercises in Asia, mentally focusing on the area of the lower abdomen, the lower *dan tian*, serves to strengthen kidney energy and essence (*jing*). This is where the transformation both of food and of vital energy takes place, this is where all power gathers and from where it is distributed—a place of quiet.

■ Food Culture and Dietetics

Our culture-specific knowledge of food and eating has developed from an originally holistic understanding, such as we find in Hildegard von Bingen (1098–1179), Paracelsus (1493–1541), or later, Rudolf Steiner (1861–1925), to an isolating, analytical way of thinking and acting. In high-tech laboratories, biochemists create new, clever convenience foods and assemble nutrients, flavorings, and preservatives in an attempt to imitate nature and match consumer preferences.

When we turn to the public for answers to the question of what a healthy diet is, we find great confusion. We are eating products whose origin, history, and manufacturing conditions we know little about. They are foreign to us, even though we consume them. Our need and ability to prepare meals is decreasing. A majority of our food is already prepared; it must merely be heated up or can even be eaten immediately. As a result, important everyday practices are becoming obsolete. Eating is no longer the comprehensive process of shopping, preparing, consuming, and digesting; rather, eating is focused more and more on nothing but the intake of food. Eating thus is slipping out of our consciousness, becoming something that we determine or own only partially. Reflecting back for a moment, we know that there can be no true knowledge of proper eating without the ability to prepare our own meals. Only that knowledge allows us to confidently deal with potential risks, helps in the evaluation of dishes and products, and at the same time opens our eyes to the pleasures of eating—to the fulfillment found in a successful meal that concretely connects the needs of body and soul.

Chinese dietetics provides answers to the following questions. What dishes and products are good for the body? What does the body truly need? How do we evaluate them? And how can each person actively participate in his or her own healing process?

The energetic effect of food on the organism lies at the center of Chinese dietetics, from the Greek *diaita* ("cultivation of life"). We absorb *qi* from food and thereby directly supply the body. Hence, food is gentle medicine by means of which our life force is strengthened to the point where the organism can maintain its equilibrium or be lead back to it.

▪ To Preserve and Protect *Jing*

Human *qi* is supplied by three sources:
- the inborn potential, kidney *jing*
- respiration
- food

The **kidney** as the reservoir of *jing* (essence) directs the harmonious course of the biological vital processes in all stages of life. Birth, childhood, adolescence, and old age are all directed by *jing*, the source of life in our deepest origin. At the same time, *jing* is a substance or energy that we inherit from our parents. A precious limited "bundle" that must be protected because once squandered it is difficult to renew. Healthy kidney *jing* is not only decisive for our constitution, but is also connected directly to our ability to have children. The spleen has the function of absorbing *qi* from food and from spiritual and emotional dimensions and of transforming this into the body's own essences. The essences gathered by the spleen supplement the *jing* of the kidney and prevent excessive losses. Attention to diet can protect *jing* from rapid consumption and replenish it on a daily basis.

In addition, *qi* is absorbed via the lung from the cosmos and universe, to accumulate in the chest space and mix with the other forms of *qi*. It stands for rhythmics in the body and is responsible for **respiration** and all other rhythmic movements in the body. Hence, a fine interplay exists between the different forms of *qi* that move, warm, transform, hold, and protect the body. It is therefore

important to always keep in mind that deep breathing and movement in fresh air have a great influence on our *qi*.

Across generations, people in ancient China were conscious of preserving their energy reserves. To strive for harmony and be attentive to maintaining health—this allowed them to come closer to their goal of longevity. It meant that they had to guard their *jing*, to cultivate it, and use it sensibly. What a contrast to Western cultures, where we have adopted an exhausting and hedonistic philosophy of life for many centuries. Herein, thoughts of how long we may live play no role. To scale down the pace of life, to rest—this does not fit into a script of life with success at all costs. Nevertheless, men and women must pay with their *jing* and *qi* when years go by that exhaust the energy reserves. Creating balance in life helps to preserve *jing*. To live with constant stimulations and challenges requires nothing less than to periodically turn inwards, calm the spirit, and create a quiet environment. Meditation, *tai chi, qi gong*, and a balanced diet high in **nutrition** create this balance.

Jing is consumed naturally by life in and of itself in different ways. There are tragic events, accidents, life crises, and also in women every pregnancy, all of which wear greatly on our vital reserves. In addition, though, influences that appear unspectacular from the outside also affect *jing* and the constitution.

In the pursuit of thinness, women have for years been consuming tropical fruits or juice for breakfast, eating raw foods and salads, yogurt or soft cheese, and drinking mineral water to fight hunger—with the firm belief that this was healthy. There is hardly a woman who has not tried any diets, and many have experienced long periods of time with exhausting attempts to lose weight. Excessive fasting with a one-sided diet of cold foods harms the metabolism and the enrichment of kidney *jing* by the transformation process in the spleen. The function of the spleen in turn depends on the necessary heat supplied by our diet. The weight gain that tends to occur after diets results from this weakening of the digestive fire and of spleen *qi*.

In Chinese dietetics, fasting and purification diets are adapted to the individual constitution. Fasting does not mean completely abstaining from

139

eating but eliminating toxins and accumulations from the body by taking the individual's constitution into consideration.

In order to fulfill their wish for children, parents must have *qi* and *jing*, which can be strengthened in a period of preparation for a potential pregnancy. A conscious lifestyle with a strengthening diet supports a positive end result. In the event of a pregnancy, the child profits. When parents are able to give their child strong *qi* and *jing* at the beginning of life, the child will start and live his or her life with strength and good *jing*. Parental *jing* as well as the nutrition received during pregnancy, after birth, and in childhood shape constitution and health in adulthood—an eternal cycle!

Jing and Diet

To supplement *jing* by means of healthy eating, we need foods that are able to support the growth and development of body and soul. At the same time, we need foods that direct their energy straight to the kidneys, to thereby support it in its function of storing essence. In Chinese dietetics, black soybeans, cooked with a small amount of seaweed and some sea salt, are a traditional recipe for this purpose. Because *jing* is closely related to blood, some of the fortifying foods listed below are not only *jing* tonics but also excellent foods for strengthening blood, such as meat and seaweed.

In order to transform food into substances produced by the body and to mobilize essence or *jing*, we require warmth. Processes of transformation all the way to the blood are based on a strong digestive fire in the spleen and stomach, the organs of the center, which in turn warm the ministerial fire in the kidney. Hence, even the best *jing* tonics can only develop their effect fully when our diet is strengthening the *qi* of the center, as a result of which targeted supplements can then be digested and assimilated effectively.

Nature has provided us with certain substances that accelerate the development of life in the animal and plant realms and can therefore strengthen our energies, including the *jing*, on a variety of levels:

- **Royal jelly**, the food of the queen bee, is produced from the pollen and secretions of the worker bees. It provides the queen with valuable energy—and *jing*-strengthening food for astonishingly rapid growth, fertility, and a long life. Not as strong as royal jelly but still a powerful support for *jing* is **pollen**, the food of young bees. It contains almost all nutrients required by humans as well.
- **Chicken** or **duck eggs** are *jing* on their own, extremely concentrated in their protein content, and probably one of the most common and simplest supplements.
- Similarly useful and strengthening are **fish eggs** (roe). **Caviar** is valuable not only because of its price and rarity; rather, it is an excellent *jing* tonic. **Oysters** are *jing* food as well; they are considered an aphrodisiac and influence the cells that produce the sperm.
- **Milk** is regarded as transformed blood and in the form of **breast milk** contains everything that the baby needs to grow. In Chinese dietetics, untreated cow's, goat's, and mare's milk complement the diet to supplement in states of insufficiency or weakness—of course, always whilst taking the condition of the digestive fire into account: milk is recommended in patterns with *yin* and blood vacuity, but not in phlegm-dampness patterns.
- **Seeds** and **nuts**, such as sesame and almonds, contain not only the fertilized germ cells, but also the nutrients for a new potential plant. For this reason, they are an appropriate source for strengthening *jing*.
- In addition, **oats, ghee** (clarified butter), **artichoke leaves**, and **nettles** also have a special effect on *jing*.
- Good *jing*-strengthening soups are cooked fresh from **marrow bones**, eaten for several days, and after a break for a few more days.

Note: it is important to know that to build strength, **time** is the key factor that brings success. All tonics only make sense when taken consistently over a longer period of time!

- Even small amounts of **meat, fish**, and internal organs like **liver** and **kidney**, when pure in quality, are already sufficient to have their nutrients and energetic potential transformed into blood and tissue.

Additional important plant-based products that nourish *jing* and blood are **seaweed** and **microalgae**. They contain trace elements that are important for many bodily processes, as well as for the production of the gametes and hormones that control their development. Seaweed can be cooked in soups, broths, or with legumes, or prepared as a vegetable. Because it is very high in iodine, though, we must first rule out diseases of the thyroid gland.

Microalgae like spirulina and chlorella are very ancient plants that are priceless in their significance for humans. Due to their high content of chlorophyll, protein, and nucleic acids, they can support the production of blood and renew cell structures. While both of them strengthen the body in general, spirulina, which is colder by nature than chlorella, is stronger at nourishing blood, fluids, and *yin*. Both are indicated in states of cold and phlegm-dampness in the lower burner. Start with low dosages because their cold quality and cleansing effect can potentially cause problems. Spirulina in powder form is mixed into juice or grain water. It is more digestible and absorbable in this form. The powder dissolves more easily with a dash of lemon juice and also becomes more palatable. Chlorella is taken in tablet form.

■ Certified Organic Food and its Preparation

The quality of *qi*, blood, and tissue is determined by the substances that we provide for the body. Toxins and artificial substances in our food and environment affect the *jing* that is necessary for strong and healthy gametes. The quality of the woman's ovum and the man's sperm can be influenced positively by the purity of food. To eat food that is fresh but not organically produced is therefore not enough. Biologically speaking, organic production means that plants were able to grow or animals were raised without being exposed to chemical fertilizers, pesticides, antibiotics, or hormones. Shopping at natural food stores or organic vegetable stands at the market furthermore motivates us to buy vegetables in season, which at the same time strengthens the body in any given season. Nature must be prepared well before it is able

to produce the body's own substances—*qi* and blood, but also warmth. The following **cooking methods** support the process of transformation. As **yin-increasing** methods of preparation, use the following:

- cooking vegetables in their own juices
- steaming
- blanching
- boiling in water

As **yang-increasing** methods of preparation, use the following:
- grilling
- roasting
- baking
- prolonged braising

Food is processed to increase its digestibility. Ways to prepare food before cooking it are:
- cutting
- grating
- chopping
- slicing
- pureeing
- marinating

By contrast, the following are methods that add important enzymes to food without heating it:
- sprouting
- lactic acid fermentation
- any other fermentation

Assuming that a person is healthy, the **distribution of food groups** can look like this:
- 30% cooked grains (e.g., rice, millet, polenta, spelt or wheat grits, quinoa, bulgur, rye, rolled oats)
- 35% vegetables and fruit in cooked form, as well as seaweed, lettuce, and sprouts from seeds
- 10% legumes (e.g., lentils, peas, beans, sprouts, miso, tofu, and other soy products)
- 10% meat, fish, broths, eggs, and milk products
- 15% raw fruits and vegetables, nuts and seeds, and fats

Overemphasizing any one of these groups invariably causes an imbalance. Too many animal products can cause dampness and phlegm. Excessive amounts of grain in the form of bread, pasta, and whole grains lead to dampness and *qi* stagnation. An excess of raw foods damages *yang*. Too little protein leads to insufficiency of blood. The goal is the right balance!

■ Chinese Dietetics

Thermal Nature

The particular thermal nature of individual foods determines the selection and balance in the composition of any diet. In this context, we differentiate between:

- hot
- warm
- neutral
- cool
- cold

In patients with insufficiency of blood and fluids, we emphasize cool foods. If we are more concerned with boosting active energies and warmth, on the other hand, neutral and warm foods are stressed. Cool foods harmonize and build *qi*, warm foods strengthen *qi* as well as *yang*.

We can witness a rapid therapeutic effect in foods with a cold or hot nature. Thus, cold foods can quickly lower *yang* in internal heat, while hot foods heat up the body and expel cold in cases of *yang* vacuity and internal cold.

The **thermal nature** of foods is also related to the channels; in this context:

- Hot and warm foods influence more the *yang* **aspects**, that is, kidney, liver, heart, and spleen *yang*.
- Neutral to warm foods have a very strong effect on the **center**.
- Cool to cold foods effect the *yin* **aspects**, such as lung, kidney, liver, and stomach *yin*.

In addition to the thermal nature, the **flavor** and its effect are also significant for classifying a certain food. Through the nourishing aspect and its energetic potential, each of the five flavors develops a typical effect in correspondence to the associated phase. The energy movements show the effect of a particular food:

- **Sourness** draws energy inward and downward and can thereby preserve the fluids. A strategy that must be used with care in liver *qi* stagnation!
- **Bitterness** directs energy downward, drains, and can dry dampness. It is important that we distinguish natural bitter compounds, as they are present in plants, from artificial ones. In patients with insufficiency of fluids, for example, coffee, cocoa, coffee substitute, black tea, and red wine are counterproductive.
- **Sweetness** spreads in all directions; it is the most important flavor for boosting *qi*, it provides fluids, and it balances. In accumulations of dampness and phlegm, though, all sweet fruits and sweeteners must be given up.
- **Acridity** directs energy outward, enlivens blood, and resolves stagnation. Nevertheless, inherent in this dynamic force is the danger that too much acridity disperses *qi* and *yin* and causes dryness.
- **Saltiness** descends, moistens dryness, and softens solidifications.

■ *Yang*, Warmth, and Food

Yang has the following functions:
- moving
- nourishing
- warming and activating (the processes in the body)
- protecting (the body)
- holding (the organs in their place in the body)

Yang vacuity hence results in a lack of warmth and therefore in feeling cold. Kidney *yang* vacuity can also mean an insufficiency of *jing*, in which case it concerns more the *yang* aspect of *jing*, corresponding to the ministerial fire or the gate of life (*ming men*). This is the driving force for all transformations in the body and provides the dynamic activity for ovulation at the point of transition from *yin* to *yang*. The *yin* and *yang* aspects of the essence must be in perfect harmony, because *yin* in the form of water, essence, and blood needs the warming action of *yang* as ministerial fire in the kidney. Kidney *yang* vacuity generally coincides with vacuity of spleen *qi* and *yang*, as a result of which transformation and movement of fluids and food are impaired and accumulations of dampness and cold arise. In cases of general vacuity of *qi* and blood that has arisen as a result of spleen *yang* vacuity, we see not only cold sensations in the lumbus and knees but also digestive problems with loose stools, lack of appetite, and fatigue. Kidney *yang* vacuity also affects the man with regard to fertility and can be the cause of impotence, low sperm count, and reduced sperm motility.

In dietetics, **strengthening the spleen** is obviously of primary importance, so that it can fulfill its function of transforming food and drink into blood, fluids, and *qi*. Otherwise, the kidney is unable to store enough postnatal *jing* and fails to receive the necessary warmth that in turn warms the spleen in its activity.

Icecream and cold drinks, raw foods, tropical fruits, dairy products, and frozen foods should be avoided. Stay away from denatured sweeteners like refined sugar, but also avoid excessive consumption of wholesome sweeteners like honey, maple syrup, or whole cane sugar, which are extreme representatives of the sweet flavor; in small amounts they have a strengthening effect on spleen *qi*, but too much leads to dampness and phlegm.

The best way of boosting the spleen and kidney is with broths that have been cooked for a long time. But beware in cases of vacuity or repletion heat in the liver and heart or in pronounced liver *qi* stagnation! In such cases, we can balance the warm nature of broths with a shorter cooking time and cooling types of vegetables and grains as added ingredients.

Recommended Diet for Boosting Kidney *Yang*

Postnatal kidney *yang* depends on food energy, which is produced in the center burner. To boost *yang* and *qi*, we recommend the following:

- warm, cooked dishes, a substantial warm breakfast (e. g., broth, rice congee, legumes, vegetables with toasted grains)
- depending on the severity of the *yang* vacuity, use more warming foods and spices
- two to three hot meals per day
- periodic proteins in the form of lean meat and fish
- easily digestible grains, simply prepared meals (only two to three ingredients per dish)
- *yang*-increasing cooking methods

Table 13.1 gives an overview of foods that boost kidney *yang* and spleen *qi*. Because *qi* and warmth are the foundation of all vital processes, you may want to adopt these recommendations as standard diet and modify them depending on the energetic diagnosis.

Table 13.1 Foods for boosting kidney *yang* and spleen *qi*

Food Group	Examples
Grains	Toasted short-grain rice, long-grain rice, basmati rice, oats, buckwheat, quinoa, sweet rice, toasted millet, amaranth
Vegetables	Leeks, green onions, kale, savoy cabbage, carrots, pumpkins, sweet potatoes, yam roots, Brussels sprouts, onions, sweet chestnuts, fennel, corn on the cob, parsnips, turnips
Spices	Cloves, garlic, fennel seed, aniseed, black pepper, fresh ginger, fenugreek, cinnamon bark, rosemary, star anise, nutmeg, oregano, thyme, basil, juniper berries, cardamom, coriander, turmeric, caraway, vanilla, horseradish
Legumes	Black beans, peas, lentils, garbanzo beans
Fruits	Sweet apples, apricots, plums, peaches, coconuts, lychees, figs, sweet cherries, raspberries (grated, dried, or stewed with spices)
Leaf lettuces and herbs	Corn salad, radicchio, endives, lollo rosso, batavia; chives, parsley, basil
Meat and fish	Beef broth, lamb, chicken, deer, sheep and goat; salmon, trout, prawns, mussels, carp
Dairy products	Sheep's and goat's milk
Fats and oils	Olive oil, sesame oil, walnut oil, flaxseed oil, butter, ghee (clarified butter)
Nuts and seeds	Walnuts, pistachios, hazelnuts, peanuts; sesame
Drinks	Fennel tea, star anise tea, liquorice root tea, hot water, apple or grape juice with hot water
Other	Barley malt, rice malt, palm sugar, molasses, maple syrup, honey, whole cane sugar

The following cooking methods are recommended:

- baking in the oven
- boiling with red wine or sake
- cooking vegetables in their own juices: the vegetables can still be slightly crunchy inside
- blanching of sprouts and lettuces

Tips for meals: roasted walnuts with leeks; leeks with prawns; black bean soup with warming spices and seaweed; stew; rice congee (100 g rice in 1 L water, simmered for 4 hours); chicken or beef bouillon, fish soup.

Yin, Blood, Fluids, and Food

Yin energy in the body is the inner, quiet, preserving, and moistening force that balances the outwardly-directed, active, stimulating, and warming yang energy. In its origin, yin is an internal and quiet energy. A lifestyle that for years demands more than a person can handle damages the yin in the kidneys, which are the origin and foundation of yin and yang and of water and fire within the body. Kidney yin vacuity, heat, and dryness, as well as unhealthy loss of essence jing causes an imbalance between yin and yang and over an extended period of time also an exhaustion of kidney yang.

Professional **women** often live with a double burden: in addition to the constant household chores, they perform their job, often many hours under taxing conditions like sitting in front of a computer screen for a long time; they are surrounded by technology and sit in air-conditioned offices with stale air. Regular breaks for regeneration, sufficient sleep, and a diet that builds qi, blood, and fluids would here be necessary to balance the yin-taxing living and working conditions. It is only natural that yin furthermore decreases with age and lessens fertility in women past the age of 30 who want to have children. The production and amount of fluids and secretions, the build-up of the endometrium, the production of fertile vaginal mucus, and the maturation of the follicles are all based on strong yin energy.

Similarly, **men** cannot simply ignore a yin-consuming lifestyle either. Internal heat as a result of yin vacuity affects sperm development and growth.

Building up yin requires time and poses a special challenge for a lifestyle that emphasizes yang. It makes sense to adopt measures that can build strength and health long before any pregnancy. To make time for regeneration in the workday, to change one's lifestyle in small steps including sufficient sleep and physical exercise that is enjoyable, to compensate for one-sided activity, and to decide on a strengthening balanced diet—all these can replenish energy resources.

Blood is an important yin substance that is primarily built by a good spleen function but also by a good kidney function. Disturbing influences on the spleen, kidney, and liver over a longer period of time cause blood vacuity. Excessive work during the night prevents the liver from storing and regenerating blood at night. Many hours of work on the computer weaken liver blood, but can be compensated well with a blood-building diet.

To build blood and yin, we need foods that nourish the body's own substances and stimulate and increase fluid production in the body. A yin-nourishing diet follows the same principles as one for building blood: include sufficient greens and other vegetables, plant- and animal-based proteins, and moistening grains like wheat. The nutritious oils in seeds and beans moisten and produce fluids. Because excessive consumption of meat, eggs, and cheese causes heat and accumulations of phlegm, it is best to combine plant and animal proteins with soy products, legumes, meat, and small amounts of dairy products.

Cooked, mild, juicy dishes instead of raw foods, fruits, dairy products, bread, and cheese support the spleen in the production of blood.

Coffee, cocoa, red wine, black and green tea, alcohol, and hot spices like curry, pepper, ginger, garlic, or cinnamon dry the blood and fluids and should therefore be avoided. A diet that overemphasizes these foods over a longer period of time, just like an internal imbalance, can lead to the development of blood heat. If this blood heat manifests as strong menstrual bleeding or skin irritations, these spicy, warm or hot, and bitter drying foods must be avoided at all cost.

Recommended Diet for Boosting Kidney Yin

To absorb fluids and vital substances from food, we must boost the center. Building yin requires time

Table 13.2 Foods for boosting kidney *yin*

Food Group	Examples
Grains	Millet, barley, short-grain rice, wheat, spelt
Vegetables	Carrots, Chinese cabbage, bamboo shoots, champignon and shiitake mushrooms, cucumbers, potatoes, pumpkins, white radishes, beets, celeriac, asparagus, tomatoes, white cabbage, green beans, yam roots, zucchinis
Legumes	Black soybeans, mung beans, kidney beans, lentils, peas, mung bean sprouts, soybean sprouts, lentil sprouts
Spices	–
Fruits	Watermelon, honeydew melon, pears, apples, apricots, blackberries, raspberries, mulberries, blueberries, mangoes, lychees, bananas, pineapples, plums, sweet cherries, red grapes, raisins, longan, red dates, figs, avocados
Leaf lettuces and herbs	Alfalfa sprouts, chickweed
Meat and fish	Pork, duck, chicken, cow's and pig's kidney, rabbit, goose; squid, carp, sardines, fish soup, shrimp, shellfish (e. g., clams, oysters)
Dairy products	Yogurt, cheese in small amounts, cow's, sheep's, and goat's milk
Fats and oils	Butter, olive oil, raw sesame oil, flaxseed oil
Nuts and seeds	Peanuts, walnuts; sunflower seeds, black sesame
Drinks	Horsetail tea, chickweed tea, pear juice with warm water, rose hip tea, flaxseed tea
Other	Kudzu or agar agar, eggs, coconut milk, wheat germ, wheat tea (in the evening), sea vegetables, sea salt, tofu, tempeh, miso, soy sauce, spirulina, aloe vera, small amounts of sweetener (e. g., molasses, grain syrup)

and continuity in the implementation of dietary recommendations (at least 3 months). To strengthen kidney *yin*, we recommend the following:
- highly nutritious proteins (legumes, meat, and dairy products)
- nuts and seeds
- steamed vegetables with a cool nature
- stewed fruit
- smaller meals throughout the day
- light, *yin*-nourishing meals in the evening (e. g., pureed vegetable soup, semolina porridge with stewed fruit)
- soups, broths, grain soups
- small amounts of dairy products

Table 13.2 gives an overview of foods that boost kidney *yin*.

The following cooking methods are recommended:
- cooking vegetables in their own juices
- steaming
- blanching
- pureeing
- boiling in lots of water

Tips for meals: black beans with seaweed; pureed vegetable soup; stew; congee; stewed fruit thickened with agar agar or kudzu.

Recommended Diet for Building Blood

To produce blood, we need special nutrients. The proportion of proteins gained from consuming meat and legumes is higher. To successfully build blood, a longer period of time is necessary (at least 3 months), just as in building *yin*. During this time, you must select blood-supporting foods from **Table 13.3** on a daily basis and create tasty meals with them. Particularly significant are:
- plenty of dark green plants high in chlorophyll (e. g., green vegetables, fresh herbs, or salads)
- grains, meat, legumes, sea vegetables, sea food
- high-energy foods that strengthen spleen *qi* because it serves as the foundation of blood

Table 13.3 Foods for building blood

Food Group	Examples
Grains	Spelt, wheat, oat, amaranth, short-grain rice, sweet rice, mochi
Vegetables	Carrots, Swiss chard, spinach, broccoli, beets, curly kale, mushrooms, sweet potatoes, green beans, eggplants, celery, nettles
Spices	Parsley root, artemisia
Legumes	Black soybeans, kidney beans
Fruits	Figs, dates, apricots, grapes (especially red), lychees, sweet cherries, apples, longan, mulberries, coconuts, berries (e. g., blueberries, raspberries, blackberries), avocados
Leaf lettuces and herbs	Green lettuces, corn salad; parsley, watercress, alfalfa sprouts
Meat and fish	Beef, chicken, bone marrow, cow's, chicken's, or duck's liver; squid, perch, eel, oysters, mussels
Dairy products	Cream, soft cheese
Fats and oils	Butter, olive oil, sesame oil, flaxseed oil
Nuts and seeds	Hazelnuts, pine nuts; yellow and black sesame, sunflower seeds
Drinks	Red juices (e. g., from red grapes, beets, sweet cherries), rosehip tea, nettle tea, raspberry leaf tea
Other	Seaweed, spirulina, chlorella, wheat grass, eggs, molasses

The following cooking methods are recommended:

- cooking vegetables in their own juices
- steaming
- blanching

Tips for meals: red fruit pudding; chicken soup; spinach with egg and sesame; corn salad with fried chicken liver.

■ Dampness, Phlegm, and Food

Accumulations of phlegm and dampness in the body are most commonly the result of other pathologies, such as kidney *yang* vacuity, liver *qi* stagnation, or blood stasis. In TCM, they are described as complex events in which fluids congeal in certain locations or systems and consequently impede their functions. In infertility, we find these disturbances in the ovaries, fallopian tubes, and uterus, potentially manifesting as ovarian cysts, endometriosis, or blocked fallopian tubes. In men, accumulations of fluids can lead to impotence, prostatitis, and congealed sperm, and can lower sperm quality.

Accumulations of phlegm and dampness in the body are directly related to dietary habits. They are the result of unhealthy one-sided eating habits with a preference for rich and sweet foods. Moistening foods must first be transformed by the body before they can be utilized. The spleen performs the function of transformation, also moving the transformed fluids and liquids to supply the skin and tissues. If the spleen is weak, dampness is not transformed but deposited in the tissues where it can congeal into phlegm. Excess weight or a tendency to gain weight usually follow. Bad eating habits or an impaired digestive function can also lead to accumulations of fluid and phlegm. We can prevent this with a diet that contains only small amounts of rich greasy foods and incorporates foods that can help to support the transformation of fluids and to resolve stagnation. A bitter herbal digestif after a heavy meal, for example, prevents the accumulation of fluids. Nevertheless, if signs of an internal collection of fluids and phlegm are already present, fatty foods such as duck, goose, pork and sausage, dairy products, desserts and sweets like chocolate and ice cream, white flour products, bread, noodles, and deep-fried foods must be limited or avoided. Milk, yogurt, and cheese form the largest and most popular part of our diet, but are at the same time the greatest evildoers in our Western culture. Several studies show a relationship between the inability to digest dairy products or excessive consumption of dairy products and weakened ovarian function. Another study found that fertility in women between 30 and 40 years of age was lower in populations with high milk consumption, and that the age-related decline in fertility was higher.[2]

In infertility in conjunction with dampness and phlegm in the lower burner, easily digestible, simple, fully cooked foods form the basis for rebuilding spleen *qi*.

The proportion of vegetables should be higher than that of grains because grains in excess can be too sweet and too heavy in patients with accumulations of fluids. Foods with bitter cool, bitter cold, and slightly acrid flavors are those that support the body in the transformation of dampness and phlegm. In cold patterns, you can also add warming spices such as fennel seed, fenugreek, or ginger to support kidney *yang*. If heat is present, acrid warming spices like garlic, cinnamon, nutmeg, and pepper, and vegetables with a warming nature like the onion family and leeks must be avoided. Cooling and phlegm-resolving foods like seaweed, barley porridge, and aduki and mung beans are an excellent choice here.

Recommended Diet for Transforming Dampness and Phlegm

The following general dietary recommendations are promising when applied consistently over a longer period of time (at least 3 months):
- simple composition of meals
- aromatic spices for the spleen
- a high proportion of vegetables
- easily digestible grains
- no late-night dinners
- a nutritious cooked breakfast
- no or very little meat, no dairy or white flour products
- in phlegm heat: seaweed

Table 13.4 gives an overview of foods that support the transformation of phlegm and dampness.

The following cooking methods are recommended:
- stir-frying in the wok
- cooking vegetables in their own juices
- roasting

Table 13.4 Foods for transforming dampness and phlegm

Food Group	Examples
Grains	Whole-grain basmati rice, toasted buckwheat, toasted barley, polenta, toasted oats, toasted millet, long-grain rice, amaranth, quinoa, rye
Vegetables	Carrots, kohlrabi with leaves, pumpkins, leeks, corn on the cob, radishes, rutabaga, onions, celery, horseradish, shallots, pakchoi
Spices	Fresh ginger, garlic, coriander, cardamom, nutmeg, cloves, oregano, lovage, marjoram, white pepper, rosemary, dried orange and grapefruit peel, juniper berries
Legumes	Aduki beans, black soybeans, kidney beans, lentils, garbanzo beans, fava beans, soybean sprouts
Fruits	Papayas, pears, dates
Leaf lettuces and herbs	Watercress, lettuce, alfalfa sprouts, dandelion leaves; cilantro leaves, chives, parsley, thyme, basil, dill
Meat and fish	Small amounts of turkey and chicken, quail; clams, anchovies, carp
Dairy products	Goat's milk, goat's cheese
Fats and oils	Olive oil
Nuts and seeds	Unsalted pistachios; pumpkin seeds, flaxseeds
Drinks	Boiled water, small amounts of: green tea, red tea (*pu erh* and *tuo cha*), bancha tea, lapacho tea, chai tea, grain coffee, jasmine tea, buckwheat tea
Other	Seaweed (kombu, hijiki, wakame, nori), small amounts of soy milk

Tips for meals: aduki beans cooked with a slice of fresh ginger, a piece of wakame, a twig of thyme, and dried orange peel, served with basmati rice; barley porridge: cook 50 g toasted barley in 1 L water until done and press through a strainer, sweeten with a little barley malt if desired; basmati rice with spices.

◼ *Qi* Stagnation and Food

Qi facilitates the communication between the organ systems and between the internal and external parts of the body. When *qi* can move freely and smoothly in the entire person, body and spirit are in harmony. In the menstrual cycle, it is the free flow of *qi* that moves the egg during the time of ovulation in the fallopian tube to the uterus. But *qi* is also the important driving force that discharges the blood during menstruation. Ovulation and menstruation are two central moments that depend on liver *qi* and its unimpeded movement.

Similarly, the heart also affects these processes; as emotional center of the entire body, it houses the spirit *shen* and depends on the free flow of *qi* and the supply of energy from the liver. The heart is directly connected to the uterus via the *bao mai*, one of the extraordinary channels. Emotional and mental stress therefore affects the free flow of *qi* and the supply of blood to the uterus. When life is experienced or lived as stressful, and when problems with becoming pregnant understandably cause additional feelings of anxiety, fear, pressure, and frustration, the probability that *qi* will stagnate becomes very high. To prevent this, the easiest and most effective but most difficult exercise is certainly meditation: If you succeed in completely freeing the spirit from all the muddled voices in the head and in allowing body and mind to be completely unwavering, *qi* and blood will find no place where they could stagnate. Physical exercise is another practical strategy for moving *qi* and freeing the mind. A regular rhythm in life with breaks for relaxation, consistent meal times, and sufficient sleep lessens the effects of stress and *qi* stagnation.

While the emotions have the greatest influence on the unimpeded movement of *qi*, a balanced diet also supports the energetic state of the liver by promoting the production of *qi*, blood, and fluids. The dietary principles for boosting spleen *qi* as well as building blood are important because the *qi* flow of the heart and liver depend on blood.

Rich and fatty foods in particular, as well as eating too much all at once overtax the liver, as a result of which *qi* stagnates and the liver is unable to perform its function of distribution. Eating less is therefore the first step that we can take to lessen stagnation. This is followed by limiting saturated fats like red meat, bacon, cream, cheese, and eggs, and bad fats like in margarine and refined oils, and especially highly processed foods with chemical additives.

We can also address stagnation with an appropriate combination of foods. Instead of combining fruit or sweets with grain, fruit on its own is certainly an appropriate light snack. Similarly, meat and dairy products in a meal can promote stagnation. Instead, combine rich foods with lighter ones that are easier to digest, for example, meat with green vegetables low in starch instead of with potatoes or grains.

The moderately acrid flavor in foods, spices, and herbs has a stimulating effect on liver *qi*. Too much of the acrid warm flavor, though, would promote the heat that can easily arise from stagnation. To counteract this, foods with a bitter cool and slightly sour flavor are an appropriate addition.

Recommended Diet for Liver *Qi* Stagnation

The following general changes in diet and lifestyle will help to maintain the free flow of *qi* and resolve stagnations:
• Easily digestible meals, main meal in the morning.
• Lots of vegetables, less grains, eating less especially in the evening.
• Sprouts and salads are important.
• Mildly acrid foods move *qi*.
• A little sweetness relaxes.
• In liver *qi* stagnation with heat: no horseradish, pepper, prawns, or crayfish.
• Movement and relaxation: *qi gong, tai chi*, relaxation through self-hypnosis, yoga.

Table 13.5 Foods for liver *qi* stagnation

Food Group	Examples
Grains	Barley, millet, rye, basmati rice, sweet rice
Vegetables	Celery, leeks (especially Chinese leeks), artichokes, carrots, radishes, kohlrabi, cauliflower, broccoli, asparagus, white cabbage, spinach, turnips, beets, onions
Spices	Rosemary, bay leaf, cardamom, coriander, marjoram, cumin, turmeric, dill, pepper, lovage, horseradish, fresh ginger
Legumes	Aduki beans
Fruits	Kumquats, lychees, tangerines, peaches, plums, melons, grapefruits
Leaf lettuces and herbs	Dandelion, alfalfa sprouts and any other sprouts, radishes and their leaves, green leaf lettuces, bitter lettuces: endives, arugula, chicory, cress, watercress; mint, chives, basil, fresh bay leaf, dill, or rosemary
Meat and fish	Crabs, prawns, crayfish
Dairy products	Soft cheese
Fats and oils	Small amounts of butter or ghee (clarified butter), olive oil, untoasted sesame oil
Nuts and seeds	Pine nuts, black sesame
Drinks	Orange blossom tea, lemon balm tea, rose petal tea, jasmine flower tea, passionflower tea, chamomile tea, peppermint tea, toasted rice tea, barley water
Other	Small amounts of barley malt, rice and date syrup, sugar-cane juice, honey; dry fruits, peel of lemons, oranges, and grapefruits

Table 13.5 gives an overview of foods that are recommended in liver *qi* stagnation. The energetic pattern in liver *qi* stagnation is closely linked to the emotional state. The recommended ingredients, when incorporated into daily meals and taken consistently for at least 3 weeks, can thereby support the process of promoting free flow.

The following cooking methods are recommended:
- stir-frying in the wok
- steaming
- cooking vegetables in their own juices

Tips for meals: freshly squeezed celery juice; one tablespoon apple cider vinegar in one glass of water, sweetened with honey; sweet rice with pine nuts; leek soup; daily fresh basil.

■ Blood Stasis and Food

Blood stasis is the result of congested *qi*. Prolonged cold symptoms, dampness and phlegm, or damp-heat can lead to stagnation in the woman's reproductive organs. This affects the *chong mai* as the "sea of blood" and the heart as the ruler of the blood; both regulate the smooth filling and discharge of blood and control blood circulation. Here, a well-aimed diet can only be a small part of the therapy; nevertheless, it makes sense not to amplify an existing blood stasis with the wrong diet, but instead to assist in resolving it with proper foods. Depending on the cause at the root of the blood stasis, the therapist composes an appropriate diet plan. The selected foods that can easily move blood are incorporated into the meal plan on a regular basis, together with foods recommended for liver *qi* stagnation. The same foods and meal combinations are to be avoided as in liver *qi* stagnation. Cold raw foods and drinks that constrict the circulation of *qi* and blood must be avoided at all costs. Particularly recommended, on the other hand, in blood stasis are **eggplants**, which promote particularly the circula-

Table 13.6 Foods for blood stasis

Food Group	Examples
Grains	Barley, Chinese pearl barley ("Job's tears")
Vegetables	Eggplants, kohlrabi, leeks, parsnips, shallots, pakchoi, onions, chestnuts, taro roots, black mushrooms ("wood ears")
Spices	Turmeric, nutmeg, oregano, rosemary, cayenne pepper, white pepper, ginger, garlic
Legumes	Black soybeans, kidney beans, aduki beans
Fruits	–
Leaf lettuces and herbs	Chives, basil
Meat and fish	Shrimp
Dairy products	–
Fats and oils	–
Nuts and seeds	–
Drinks	–
Other	Kombu, vinegar, small amounts of red wine

tion in the uterus and help relieve menstrual disorders caused by blood stasis.

Recommended Diet for Blood Stasis

Foods that disperse stagnant blood tend to be acrid and/or warm or hot. Nevertheless, use cayenne pepper, ginger, garlic, and alcohol only with caution in patterns with heat or *yin* vacuity symptoms. In *qi* and *yang* vacuity as well, an excess of these ingredients would disperse *qi* too strongly and exacerbate the vacuity.

In blood stasis, we recommend supplementing the diet daily with the foods listed in **Table 13.6** for a longer period of time.

Tips for meals: sliced eggplant, baked in the oven with a little oil; pureed eggplant with spices; aduki beans cooked with konbu and seasoned with a little red wine and spices.

Bibliography

1. Bensky D, Gamble A. *Chinese Herbal Medicine—Materia Medica*. Seattle: Eastland; 1993.
2. Cramer DW, Xu H, Sahi T. Adult Hypolactasia, Milk Consumption, and Age-specific Fertility. *Amer J Epidemiology*.1994;139:282–289.
3. Engelhardt U, Hempen CH. *Chinesische Diätetik*. 3rd ed. Munich: Urban & Fischer; 2006.
4. Flaws B. *Das Yin und Yang der Ernährung*. Munich: Heyne; 1997.
5. Heider de Jahnsen M. *Das Große Handbuch der Chinesischen Ernährungslehre*. Aitrang: Windpferd; 2006.
6. Holmes P. *The Energetics of Western Herbs*. Artemesis: Snow Lotus; 1998.
7. Leggett D. *Selbstheilung durch Ernährung*. Munich: Goldmann Arkana; 2004.
8. Lu HC. *Chinese System of Food Cures*. New York: Sterling; 1986.
9. Lyttleton J. *Treatment of Infertility with Chinese Medicine*. London: Churchill Livingstone; 2004.
10. Noll A, Kirschbaum B. *Stresskrankheiten*. Munich: Urban & Fischer; 2006.
11. Pitchford P. *Healing with Whole Foods*. Berkeley: North Atlantic; 1993.
12. Schneider C. *Kraftsuppen nach der Chinesischen Heilkunde*. Sulzberg: Joy; 1999.
13. Temelie B, Trebuth B. *Das Fünf Elemente Kochbuch*. Sulzberg: Joy; 1999.
14. Yeoh A. *The Tao of Eating and Healing*. Singapore: Times Books International; 1992.

14 Chinese Medicinal Therapy in Threatened or Recurrent Miscarriage and in Pregnancy

Walter Geiger, Karin Rudzki

■ Miscarriage and Recurrent Pregnancy Loss from the Perspective of Western Medicine

Let us first explain the different types of miscarriage because considerable differences exist depending on whether we want to save the pregnancy or whether we can no longer do so:

Definitions

By definition, we speak of a **miscarriage** up to the 20th week of pregnancy or with a lost fetus weighing less than 500 g. Beyond this limit, we speak of a **premature birth** or **stillbirth**. During the first trimester, we speak of an **early pregnancy loss**, afterwards of a **clinical spontaneous abortion (miscarriage)**.

Over 50% of all incidents of bleeding in early pregnancy (i. e., in the first 12 weeks of pregnancy or the first trimester) are a matter of abnormal pregnancies. The risk of miscarriage drops with increasing length of pregnancy. Ninety percent of all miscarriages fall in the time up to the 12th week of pregnancy.

In the majority of miscarriages in the first trimester, we find chromosomal changes and also deformations like neural tube defects or lip-jaw-palate clefts. Metabolic disorders of the pregnant woman (e. g., diabetes mellitus, hypo- or hyperthyroidism) or infections can trigger a miscarriage as well. Lastly, malformation of the uterus and myomas can lead to miscarriage, but only after the 12th week of pregnancy due to the fetus's increasing need for space.

Threatened Abortion

Threatened abortion refers to bleeding in early pregnancy, possibly accompanied by labor-like pain in the lower abdomen; in this case, the possibility of an intact pregnancy still exists. We see scant bleeding, sometimes—not always—accompanied also by mild abdominal pain, but with an intact pregnancy under ultrasound. If a local infection is found in the vagina or cervix, the patient receives antibiotic treatment. There is no specific therapy for this form of miscarriage, except for rest or even bedrest if necessary. Nevertheless, the risk of a miscarriage later on in the pregnancy is higher than in pregnancies without any bleeding.

Missed Abortion

The embryo shows no heartbeat in the ultrasound, and sometimes we see brown spotting. If there is no evidence of any embryonic tissue in the amniotic sac, we can speak of a "wind egg." Biomedicine responds swiftly with surgical evacuation, to avoid severe bleeding and a rising infection, as well as by giving anti-D immunoglobulin to rhesus-negative women to avoid rhesus incompatibility in subsequent pregnancies.

Incomplete Abortion

Spontaneous miscarriage is most common between the eighth and 12th week of pregnancy, but also often occurs only after the 12th week. Parts of the placenta remain in the uterus, as a result of which a follow-up curettage and possibly anti-D injection are necessary. Most often, the underlying reason is a developmental disorder in the child.

Incipient Abortion

This refers to an impending miscarriage with bleeding, contractions, and cervical dilation. This will be treated in the same way as an incomplete abortion.

Septic Abortion

This is the most critical form of miscarriage, requiring both surgery and high doses of antibiotics.

Habitual Abortion

In a patient with a history of three or more miscarriages, biomedicine speaks of habitual abortion. Two percent of all couples are affected by this. In up to 50% of these couples, it is impossible to furnish evidence of the specific cause of miscarriage.

Causes of habitual abortion include:
- Chromosomal changes in one parent in the form of numerical changes in the chromosome set or a rearrangement of genes within chromosome pairs (translocation).
- Polycystic ovary syndrome, often combined with overweight and insulin resistance, which also represent risk factors for recurrent miscarriage.
- Thyroid disorders, especially hypothyroidism and autoimmune thyroid diseases.
- Diabetes mellitus with impaired metabolism.
- Uterine deformities and, related to this, failure to nourish the implanted egg sufficiently (in 50–60% of habitual abortions).
- Myomas or polyps can present a mechanical obstacle.
- Infections: especially chronic endometrial infections from chlamydia, mycoplasma, and ureaplasma urealyticum (rising cervical infections are more likely to cause spontaneous abortion).
- Coagulation factors: factor V Leiden mutation, protein C, protein S, or protein Z deficiency,

defects in the antithrombin system, prothrombin mutations, hyperhomocysteinemia. In all these cases, hypercoagulability of the blood is present. In addition to a higher risk of miscarriage, we also see a higher risk of thrombosis, as well as in the more advanced stages of the pregnancy a higher risk of retarded intrauterine growth and HELLP syndrome. The formation of microthrombi leads to impaired vascularization in the area of implantation and in the later stages to impaired supply. Treat with heparin injections; but if bleeding occurs, heparin must be stopped immediately!
- Immunological factors: at the site of implantation, the body reacts with both rejection and assistance. In this reaction, the rejection involves primarily natural killer cells while the assistance involves primarily cytokines and growth factors that are produced and secreted by immunocompetitive cells. Implantation can be disturbed by both an excessive rejection or an insufficient presence of cytokines and growth factors, but also by the production of irregular autoantibodies in the context of a false activation of the immune system.
- In women with habitual miscarriages, irregular autoantibodies that can also cause **thrombophilia** are much more common than in normal women. Thrombophilia causes the formation of local blood clots in the area of nidation; the result is faulty implantation, which ultimately causes the death of the embryo. In terms of therapy, we can consider giving small doses of heparin in combination with small doses of acetylsalicylic acid (ASS).
- Environmental toxins: continuous exposure can cause habitual miscarriages, but not a single contact. Most noteworthy are especially lead, copper, mercury, vinyl chloride, pesticides, sulfur dioxide, cadmium, and organic solvents. Some substances can also affect male fertility.
- Psychological factors: here we find two groups of women: those who originally reject motherhood, and those who do not feel adequate to the responsibility.
- Male sub- or infertility is of lesser significance.

◼ Miscarriage and Recurrent Pregnancy Loss from the TCM Perspective

Threatened Abortion

From the TCM perspective, the four key signs for a threatened miscarriage are:
- disquieted fetus with a downward-pulling, sinking feeling
- back pain
- lower abdominal pain
- vaginal bleeding

The key treatment strategy in threatened abortion is to avoid the miscarriage by swift treatment with Chinese medicinals.

We distinguish between vaginal bleeding in pregnancy and disquieted fetus, which manifests with abdominal and back pain and a downward-pulling feeling in addition to bleeding. Back pain is one of the key symptoms in threatened abortion, in which case there is a relationship between the intensity of the pain and the severity of the imminent miscarriage.

In the *Jing Yue Quan Shu (Complete Works of Jing Yue)* published in 1624, we read:

In women, the kidney is connected to the uterus but it also controls the back. In severe back pain during pregnancy, unpreventable miscarriage is imminent."[12]

Pathology

The pathology of threatened abortion basically consists of a disharmony of the *ren mai* and *chong mai* (conception and thorough fare vessels), as a result of which nourishment of the fetus with *qi* and blood is insufficient. This disharmony of the *ren mai* and *chong mai* is very often compounded by weakness in the kidneys. Additional disease patterns are blood deficiency, *qi* deficiency, and sinking *qi*, as well as blood heat and blood stasis.

Causes and Disease Development

Possible causes for threatened abortion are a weak constitution, overwork, excessive physical and psychological strain, chronic illness, and traumas.

As a result, kidney *qi* is not secure and cannot hold the fetus. In this context, heavy lifting damages kidney *yang*; chronic diseases exhaust *qi*, blood, and essence. Anger, rage, and frustration can lead to liver *qi* constraint, which transforms into liver fire and produces heat in the blood. Falls and other traumas can injure the *ren mai* and *chong mai*.

Treatment Principle

The most important treatment principle in threatened miscarriage is to quiet the fetus and to supplement the *ren mai* and *chong mai*, thereby also strengthening kidney *qi*. Additional important treatment principles are:
- nourish the blood
- supplement and upbear *qi*
- cool the blood
- stanch bleeding.

Medicinal Therapy

In TCM, **quieting the fetus** means the use of medicinals that are known to prevent miscarriage. These medicinals can be deployed in accordance with the predominant disease pattern! The most commonly used medicinals include:[4]

For Kidney Vacuity
- *du zhong* (Eucommiae cortex)
- *tu si zi* (Cuscutae semen)
- *sang ji sheng* (Loranthi seu visci ramus = Taxilli herba)
- *xu duan* (Dipsaci radix)

For Blood Deficiency
- *e jiao* (Corii asini colla)
- *bai shao yao* (Paeoniae radix alba)
- *shu di huang* (Rehmanniae radix praeparata)
- *sang ji sheng* (Taxilli herba)
- *he shou wu* (Polygoni multiflori radix)

For *Qi* Vacuity
- *bai zhu* (Atractylodis macrocephalae radix)
- *huang qi* (Astragali radix)
- *ren shen* (Ginseng radix)
- *shan yao* (Dioscoreae rhizoma)

For *Qi* Stagnation
- *sha ren* (Amomi fructus)
- *zi su geng* (Perillae caulis)

For Heat
- *huang qin* (Scutellariae radix)

For Bleeding
- *ai ye* (Artemisiae argyi folium)
- *e jiao* (Corii asini colla)
- *di yu* (Sanguisorbae radix)
- *duan long gu* (Mastodi ossis fossilia calcinata)
- *duan mu li* (Ostreae concha calcinata)
- *sang ye* (Mori folium)

To Warm the Uterus
- *ai ye* (Artemisiae argyi folium)
- *bu gu zhi* (Psoraleae fructus)

To Astringe, Secure, and Strengthen Kidney Essence
- *fu pen zi* (Rubi fructus)
- *wu wei zi* (Schisandrae fructus)
- *jin ying zi* (Rosae laevigatae fructus)
- *lian zi* (Nelumbinis fructus)
- *ma huang gen* (Ephedrae radix)

It is very important to stanch the bleeding. You should also always supplement kidney *yang* to strengthen the upbearing effect of *du mai*, because a threatened miscarriage is characterized by a descending movement of a *yin* nature. Dr. Cong Chun-Yu, a famous physician, swears by *tu si zi* for this purpose and likes to use it in daily doses of as much as 150 g.[12] *Tu si zi* supplements kidney *yang*, increases *yin*, and secures essence, stops diarrhea, and improves the vision.[2]

Many other physicians also see *tu si zi* as a key medicinal for threatened abortion. Lyttleton concurs with this opinion as well, but warns against prescribing this herb for threatened abortion in doses of more than 30 g per day, because she believes that it can otherwise even trigger a miscarriage itself.[10] A similar rule applies to *dang gui* (Angelicae sinensis radix): on the one hand, it is used for threatened miscarriage in the popular formula *Dang Gui Shao Yao San* (Chinese Angelica and Peony Powder) from the classic *Jin Gui Yao Lüe* (*Essential Prescriptions of the Golden Coffer*). On the other hand, though, some authors suspect that *dang gui* can trigger uterine contractions because of its sharp blood-moving nature. Please note that you should avoid excessively hot and spicy medicinals when supplementing, and excessively bitter and cold medicinals when eliminating heat. Hence Giovanni Maciocia also recommends caution in the selection of medicinals:

"In addition, there are three treatment methods that should not be used during pregnancy, especially in threatened abortion. First, you should not promote sweating since this can lead to yang collapse. You should also not move downward (i. e., promote bowel movements) because this can cause yin collapse. And lastly, you should not stimulate urination, such as with medicinals that eliminate dampness like yi yi ren (Coicis semen), because the bodily fluids could be damaged as a result."[12]

Disease Patterns

The most important disease patterns in threatened abortion include:
- kidney *qi* vacuity
- spleen and kidney *qi* vacuity
- blood deficiency
- blood heat
- blood stasis

Kidney *Qi* Vacuity

Symptoms
Threatened abortion, most commonly in early pregnancy; with back pain, a feeling of collapse in the lower abdomen, minor vaginal bleeding, exhaustion, weak legs, frequent urination, a pale tongue, and a deep weak pulse.

Causes and Disease Development
Vacuity of the kidneys and insecure *ren mai* and *chong mai* cause insufficient nourishment of the fetus and "disquieted fetus."[1]

Treatment Principle
Supplement kidney *yin* and kidney *yang* and quiet the fetus.

Medicinal Therapy
The main formula is *Shou Tai Wan* (Fetal Longevity Pill), which supplements kidney *qi* and secures and holds the fetus. We achieve this effect with the medicinals *tu si zi*, *sang ji sheng*, *xu duan*, and *e jiao*; many current modifications additionally contain *du zhong* to increase the effect of the formula. All in all, this is an excellent formula for consolidating the kidneys and stabilizing the pregnancy. By means of supplementing the kidneys, kidney *qi* can hold the fetus, and fetal *qi* can itself become strong.

In the gynecological wards of Chinese hospitals, a drop in the basal temperature during pregnancy is interpreted as a sign of weak kidney *yang*. This is treated accordingly with kidney *yang* and *qi* tonics, as well as with medicinals that keep the uterus warm.[10]

Spleen and Kidney *Qi* Vacuity

Symptoms
Threatened abortion, especially towards the end of the first trimester; with back pain, downward-pulling pain in the lower abdomen, a dull pale face, fatigue, lack of appetite, heart palpitations, thin and pale red blood, increased bleeding after physical exertion, a pale tongue, and a deep weak pulse.

Causes and Disease Development
Persistent chronic illness as well as inadequate nutrition can lead to *qi* and blood vacuity, as a result of which the woman is unable to provide enough nourishment for the fetus, and a miscarriage threatens.

Treatment Principle
Supplement and upbear *qi*, strengthen the spleen, nourish the blood, and quiet the fetus.

Medicinal Therapy
The most commonly used main formula is *Tai Shan Pan Shi San* (Rock of Taishan Fetus-Quieting Powder). It is composed of the key medicinals for strengthening and upbearing *qi*, for example, *huang qi*, *dang shen* (Codonopsis pilosulae radix), and *bai zhu*, in combination with blood supplements like *e jiao, bai shao yao*, and *shu di huang*, supported by kidney tonics like *tu si zi* or *xu duan*. In cases with sinking spleen *qi*, we frequently recommend modifications of *Bu Zhong Yi Qi Tang* (Center-Supplementing *Qi*-boosting decoction) in combination with kidney *yang* supplements. Medicinals for quieting the fetus are employed in accordance with the predominant disease pattern (see p. 153).

Conception is closely related to the *chong mai* and *ren mai* and the kidneys as the prenatal source of life; the postnatal source is the spleen. The development of the fetus is dependent on the transformation and production of *qi* and blood by the spleen and stomach. The fetus relies on the mother's blood and essence for nourishment, but also on her *qi*, which holds the fetus in the uterus. The food essences fill the *ren mai* and *chong mai*. When the fetus's nourishment is insufficient, the holding power of the *dai mai* is weakened and a miscarriage becomes possible. The famous Chinese physician Ye Tianshi wrote on this topic:

"Conception is completely dependent on nourishment by the food essences of the blood and on protection by qi."[6]

In cases where essence and *qi* are damaged, Lyttleton also uses *huang qi, bai zhu*, and *dang shen*, in combination with the formula *Shou Tai Wan*, that is, *qi*-supplementing, stabilizing medicinals that astringe and upbear *qi* and secure the fetus.[10]

Blood Deficiency

Symptoms
The future mother develops anemia with symptoms like fatigue, heart palpitations, and paleness.

Causes and Disease Development
Blood deficiency is rarely the direct cause of a threatened miscarriage, but can contribute to delayed fetal development.

Treatment Principle
Nourish the blood.

Medicinal Therapy
Some authors recommend *Dang Gui Shao Yao San* to treat lower abdominal pain during pregnancy. This formula should be used in the initial stage of a threatened miscarriage with lower abdominal pain and vaginal bleeding. It relaxes the muscles, relieves pain, regulates the liver, nourishes the blood, and stabilizes the fetus.

Lyttleton recommends removing *chuan xiong* (Ligustici chuanxiong rhizoma) from the original formula because the combination with *dang gui* can cause uterine contractions. *Dan shen* (Salviae miltiorrhizae radix)—also from the category of blood-moving medicinals—on the other hand, supposedly improves blood circulation in the endometrium and in the placenta.[10]

The physician Li Wenguang believes with regards to *dang gui* that those oils that are not very volatile stimulate the uterus, while its highly volatile oils do not have this effect. *Dang gui* should therefore be added to the formula only at the end of the decocting process and be boiled for a shorter time. We can thus see a need for further discussion with regards to the safety of medicinals like *dang gui*. Bensky comments:

"Angelica sinensis rad. [dang gui] is very well-known as the number one herb in gynecology, harmonically warming without drying, tonifying without congesting, and always gently enlivening the blood. During pregnancy, however, it should be used with great caution and only when the therapist has a good understanding of its applications in this clinical situation."[2]

Chen, by contrast, states:

"Dang gui is a blood tonic that is commonly prescribed in pregnancy for building blood... Nevertheless, you should always exercise great caution in the treatment of pregnant women and only employ medicinal substances when the advantages outweigh the risks."[3]

In *dang gui*, we attribute a supplementing effect to the "head" of the root (*dang gui tou*) and a blood-moving effect to the "tail" (*dang gui wei*); the entire body of the root (*dang gui shen*), which is most commonly used today, is "slightly more supplementing than moving."[2]

Other authors recommend to treat blood deficiency with modifications of the formula *Si Wu Tang* (Four Agents Decoction) with *shu di huang, dang gui, bai shao yao*, and *chuan xiong*, or with the formula *Ba Zhen Wan* (Eight Gem Pill) and other blood-building medicinals like *he shou wu, sang ji sheng* or *gou qi zi* (Lycii fructus).

Blood Heat

Symptoms
Threatened miscarriage with back and abdominal pain, vaginal bleeding with bright red blood, heat sensations, thirst, disquietude and disturbed sleep, a red tongue with yellow fur, and a replete rapid pulse.

Causes and Disease Development
This pattern tends to develop out of *yin* vacuity, which favors the formation of heat in the blood. The heat pushes the blood out of the uterine vessels. Additional causes of blood heat are anger,

liver fire, or the consumption of excessively spicy foods and coffee and alcohol abuse.

As soon as the heat reaches the heart, the risk of miscarriage is high because the connection from the heart to the uterus via the *bao mai* (the uterine vessel) is disturbed. Lyttleton comments on this pattern:

"Heart qi controls the opening of the uterus. When a factor like liver fire agitates heart qi, this can result in opening the uterus. The discerning physician therefore always checks the connection between the heart and kidneys at the beginning of pregnancy... He or she secures the fetus with spirit-soothing acupuncture, herbal medicine, and counseling, whenever the woman is highly agitated and frightened."[10]

Treatment Principle
Quiet the fetus, cool the blood, and discharge heat.

Medicinal Therapy
To discharge heat from the heart and liver, Xia Guicheng, a famous gynecologist from the Jiangsu Provincial Hospital in Nanjing, recommends *gou teng* (Uncariae ramulus cum uncis), *chao huang lian* (Coptidis rhizoma frictum) and *lian zi xin* (Nelumbinis plumula). In cases of disquieted sleep or insomnia, she recommends *chao suan zao ren* (Ziziphi spinosi semen frictum), *wu wei zi, he huan pi* (Albizziae cortex), *fu shen* (Poria cum pini radice), *bai zi ren* (Platycladi semen), *long chi, mu li* (Mastodi dentis fossilia calcinata), and *gui ban* (Testudinis plastrum), to restore communication between the heart and the kidneys.

We can also use modifications of *Gu Jing Wan* (menses-securing pill) with medicinals like *gui ban, bai shao yao, huang qin, huang bai* (Phellodendri cortex), or *di gu pi* (Lycii cortex).

Blood Stasis

Symptoms
The main symptom is abdominal pain, but we also find scant vaginal bleeding. The tongue and pulse are inconspicuous.

Causes and Disease Development
Blood stasis is often triggered by trauma to the uterus, for example, as the result of a fall; but it can also arise from medical interventions during in vitro fertilization.

Treatment Principle
Move the blood, quiet the fetus, supplement and upbear *qi*.

Medicinal Therapy
Possible choices are *Tao Hong Si Wu Tang* (Peach Kernel and Carthamus Four Agents Decoction) or *Shao Fu Zhu Yu Tang* (Lesser Abdomen Stasis-Expelling Decoction).

There are certainly authors who warn against neglecting moving blood as a treatment option during pregnancy. Li Guangrong, for example, believes that:

"[T]he uterus can only develop when the blood circulates freely, and therefore the problem of blood stasis should not be neglected."[9]

Missed, Septic, or Incomplete Abortion

A miscarriage is always a traumatic and invasive event. It is therefore important to stabilize such women physically and psychologically with the help of TCM. In types of miscarriages that cannot be prevented—that is, in missed, septic, or incomplete abortion—the treatment after the miscarriage should be our first concern. There is a saying in TCM: "A miscarriage weighs more heavily than a birth." There is even the notion that "a miscarriage should be taken more seriously than a birth" (*xiao chan zhong yu da chan*).[12]

Habitual Abortion

The Chinese term for habitual abortion is *hua tai* ("slippery fetus"). Treatment occurs while the woman is not pregnant. This means that a woman with known habitual abortions should not pursue another pregnancy for 6–12 months and receive treatment during this time. It is important to plan this treatment in detail with the woman and convince her that the therapy has priority over a new pregnancy. In contrast to a threatened miscarriage, the main emphasis of treatment is not on quieting the fetus but on the underlying constitutional cause in the woman. The time frame of 6–12 months is necessary to effectively **stabilize the constitution**. Clinical practice

has shown that many of these women show a constitutional deficiency of kidney *qi* and blood. Kidney *qi* here loses its holding power and its ability to preserve and secure. Frequent miscarriage can damage the *chong mai* and *ren mai* and further aggravate a pre-existing kidney vacuity; therefore kidney vacuity has shown to be the most common cause of habitual miscarriages in TCM. This can be compounded by a spleen vacuity, disharmony of the *ren mai* and *chong mai*, as well as *qi* descent.

In addition to the patterns of blood stasis and blood heat, the **clinically most important therapy** in habitual abortion consists of:
* supplementing, consolidating, and strengthening the kidney and spleen
* upbearing spleen *qi*
* nourishing the blood
* harmonizing the *ren mai* and *chong mai*

There is a saying in TCM, "to treat the illness, search out the root." The energetic imbalances and disharmonies that trigger habitual miscarriages often resemble those that are responsible for infertility.

In most women, you should balance kidney *yin* and kidney *yang* before attempting another pregnancy. To achieve this, strengthen kidney *yin* after menstruation and supplement kidney *yang* after ovulation, in accordance with the menstrual cycle.

Disease Patterns

The most important disease patterns in habitual abortion include:
* kidney *yang* vacuity
* kidney *yin* vacuity
* *qi* vacuity
* blood vacuity

Kidney *Yang* Vacuity

Symptoms
The patient's history reports past miscarriages; back pain and cold symptoms, that is, cold feet, pale urine, and a pale tongue.

Causes and Disease Development
In addition to miscarriages, kidney essence is also consumed by aging. Pregnant women over 40 are therefore more likely to suffer from frequent miscarriages. In the West, we see more and more pregnant women in this age group.

Treatment Principle

It is important to warm the uterus and kidneys and also to supplement the kidneys.

Medicinal Therapy

Modifications of *Shou Tai Wan* in combination with spleen-supplementing medicinals such as in *Bu Shen Gu Chong Wan* (Kidney-Supplementing Thoroughfare-Securing Pill) have proven effective,[10,12] with medicinals like *tu si zi, xu duan, e jiao, shu di huang, lu jiao jiao* (Cervi cornus gelatinum), *bai zhu, ren shen, du zhong, gou qi zi, ba ji tian* (Morindae officinalis radix), *dang gui tou* (head of Angelicae sinensis radix), *sha ren, da zao* (Jujubae fructus), and *rou cong rong* (Cistanches herba).

For cold in the uterus, add warming medicinals like *yi zhi ren* (Alpiniae oxyphyllae fructus), *bu gu zhi*, or *ai ye*. Among the classical formulas, we treat patterns of kidney *yang* vacuity with modifications of *You Gui Wan* (Right [Kidney]-Restoring Pill)*.

Kidney *Yin* Vacuity

Symptoms

Here we find miscarriages in the patient's past history as well, combined with back pain, tinnitus, and night sweating. The tongue is reddened and without any fur.

Causes and Disease Development

Women around the age of 40 are more likely to suffer from kidney *yin* vacuity than younger women. This causes a dilemma because building up *yin* for a good development of the egg and endometrium requires a long time; at the same time, though, these women often feel that they have no time left. Nevertheless, they must be convinced under any circumstances to wait for a minimum of 4 months before another pregnancy, to strengthen *yin* sufficiently and to prepare the body for another pregnancy.

Treatment Principle

Nourish *yin* and blood, strengthen the kidneys, secure the *ren mai* and *chong mai*.

Medicinal Therapy

A commonly-used formula is *Bao Yin Jian* (Yin-Safeguarding Brew),[10,12] with medicinals like *sheng di huang* (Rehmanniae radix exsiccata seu recens), *shu di huang, bai shao yao, shan yao, huang qin*, and *huang bai*. For a classical formula, here we can use a variation of *Zuo Gui Wan* (Left [Kidney]-Restoring Pill) with *Er Zhi Wan* (Double Supreme Pill).

Qi Vacuity

Symptoms

It is typical that the cervix opens from the third month of pregnancy on as the fetus increases in size, resulting in the threat of a miscarriage.

Causes and Disease Development

A serious state of spleen *qi* vacuity can cause the uterus to drop; the cervix is no longer closed tightly to hold the pregnancy.

Treatment Principle

Supplement and upbear the *qi* of the center burner.

Medicinal Therapy

For a classical formula, we can choose a variation of *Bu Zhong Yi Qi Tang* (Center-Supplementing Qi-Boosting Decoction) to supplement and upbear spleen *qi*,[10,12] often in combination with kidney supplements.

Blood Vacuity

Symptoms

We see scant menstrual bleeding, disturbed sleep, problems with visual acuity, dry skin, and dizziness.

Causes and Disease Development

In this disease pattern, we often find a thin endometrium; this results in a failure of the egg to implant or in insufficient nourishment to the egg.

Treatment Principle

Nourish the blood and kidneys, secure the *ren mai*.

---

* Also known as Right-Restoring (Life Gate) Pill.

Medicinal Therapy

Suitable classical formulas are variations of *Si Wu Tang* or *Ba Zhen Tang* to supplement *qi* and blood. These are commonly combined with kidney supplements in any particular modification of the basic formula.[10,12]

Concluding Remarks

Similar to the treatment of infertility, the treatment of habitual and threatened abortion is an important domain of TCM as well. We can see this in the in-patient and out-patient gynecology wards of traditional Chinese hospitals. Accordingly, a great number of research projects and publications are found in this field (see p. 161).

■ Chinese Medicinal Therapy during Pregnancy

How safe is the use of Chinese medicinals during pregnancy? Where are the limits of its applications? According to US studies, roughly 25% of all women experience miscarriages as part of a **natural process**, for example, to sort out genetic defects. Miscarriages are particularly common in couples with fertility problems, late pregnancies, infectious sexually transmitted diseases, and excessive stress.

A number of babies are born with physical or mental problems. A certain percentage of these can be attributed to the consumption of medications and recreational drugs like crack, alcohol, tobacco, and coffee during pregnancy. Most women are quite aware of these connections. Many medications are not recommended during pregnancy because there is not enough proof of their safety.

The Chinese people contemplated the question of which medicinals were safe for pregnant women as early as 1800 years ago in the *Jin Gui Yao Lüe*. In the West, Chinese medicinals have only been in use for a few years. In contemporary China, pregnant women receive prescriptions for Chinese medicinals as a matter of course for many complaints. As far as we can judge without relevant statistics, there appear to be few problems.

The typical patient in the West, however, will not be prepared to accept even the smallest risk to treat a condition like a cold during pregnancy. Assuming that problems arose after the use of Chinese medicinals, these medicinals could very easily be held responsible. In mild illness or when you are unsure, it is therefore better to do without any treatment.

On the other hand, though, if the condition is so critical that the only alternative are biomedical medications that might have incalculable risks for the fetus or if the pregnancy itself is endangered by the illness, for example in threatened miscarriage, Chinese medicinal therapy is often the safer method, with fewer side-effects for mother and fetus. It is nevertheless wise to limit both the dosage and the length of usage to what is absolutely necessary.

Unfortunately, there is not enough statistical information and significant data on the safety of Chinese medicinal therapy. The experience of innumerable generations of physicians certainly counts: many Chinese medicinals and formulas are so well-tested in their application during pregnancy that they can be regarded as safe.

Medicinals like *bai zhu, huang qin, tu si zi*, or *du zhong* and formulas like *Shou Tai Wan* have a stabilizing and calming effect on the fetus in the dominant disease patterns of kidney and spleen vacuity.

Contraindications for Chinese Medicinals

The relevant materia medica texts contain lists of medicinals that are regarded as contraindicated or should be used only with caution during pregnancy (see p. 160). The category of medicinals that comes up frequently here is **blood-moving medicinals**. Some practitioners routinely warn patients against taking blood-moving medicinals during pregnancy! This category of substances is generally used quite frequently, for example, for menstrual pain or headache. Because we do not know the effect that these substances have already in the first weeks of pregnancy, we should indeed warn patients against becoming pregnant while using them.

This means that in patients who are trying to become pregnant, treatment with blood-moving medicinals can only be employed in the period from the onset of menstruation to ovulation. By all accounts contraindicated during pregnancy are strong laxative, discharging, and especially blood-moving and blood-breaking medicinals. Of course, this also applies to any other medicinals that are contraindicated during pregnancy.

But even regular foods can cause problems; hence use caution, for example, with pearl barley (Coix semen, *yi yi ren*) during pregnancy.[12]

Unfortunately, it is impossible to rule out the consumption of larger amounts of pearl barley—a popular grain in Japanese cuisine—by pregnant women. Even ginger—very popular in the treatment of morning sickness—is perhaps not without problems because one of the important essential oils in ginger—gingerol—is a mitogen that can possibly affect cell division in high dosages. In this light, even relatively "harmless" foods are not absolutely safe.[7] According to recent findings by the British MHRA (Medicines and Healthcare Products Regulatory Agency), *ren shen* and *huang lian* (Coptidis rhizoma) are also seen as problematic during pregnancy.[13]

Ultimately, all medicinal therapies are thus fraught with a certain amount of risk. Therefore, always compare and weigh risks and benefits carefully! Which therapy is really necessary during pregnancy? It is especially important to make this decision independent of how well the concerned complaints could be relieved with Chinese medicinals!

Concluding Remarks

Once you have decided to use Chinese medicinals and are certain of the diagnosis, you must make sure that the substances you are considering are not contraindicated in pregnancy. In addition, it is advisable during pregnancy to prescribe Chinese medicinals in lower dosages and only as long as necessary. Otherwise it could easily happen that you might, for example, consider treating a case of stomach heat with insatiable thirst during pregnancy with *tian hua fen* (Trichosanthis radix) to

clear the *qi* level. In an existing pregnancy, however, this would be fatal because extracts of this herb are successfully used as injections to induce artificial abortions. It is therefore regarded as contraindicated in pregnancy.

In spite of all these concerns, we should not forget that Chinese medicinal therapy can be extraordinarily effective and have fewer side-effects in threatened miscarriage and many other health problems during pregnancy!

■ Appendix

The following lists contain a selection of "commonly used" medicinals that should be prescribed with caution or are contraindicated during pregnancy.

To be Used with Caution During Pregnancy

According to Lyttleton, the following medicinals should be used with caution during pregnancy:[10]
- *bai fu zi* (Typhonii rhizoma)
- *da huang* (Rhei radix et rhizoma)
- *fan xie ye* (Sennae folium)
- *gan jiang* (Gingiberis rhizoma)
- *hou po* (Magnoliae officinalis cortex)
- *hua shi* (Talcum)
- *lu hui* (Aloe)
- *lu lu tong* (Liquidambaris fructus)
- *mu tong* (Akebiae trifoliatae caulis)
- *pu huang* (Typhae pollen)
- *rou gui* (Cinnamomi cortex)
- *san qi* (Notoginseng radix)
- *tian nan xing* (Arisaematis rhizoma)
- *tong cao* (Tetrapanacis medulla)
- *wang bu liu xing* (Vaccariae semen)
- *xue jie* (Daemonoropsis resina)
- *yi yi ren* (Coicis semen)
- *yu jin* (Curcumae radix)
- *yu li ren* (Pruni semen)
- *ze lan* (Lycopi herba)
- *zhi ke* (Aurantii fructus)
- *zhi sh* (Aurantii fructus immaturus)

In Chen,[5] the list of commonly used medicinals that should be used with caution during pregnancy also includes the following common medicinals:

- *bai guo* (Gingko semen)
- *ban xia* (Pinelliae rhizoma)
- *bing lang* (Arecae semen)
- *bu gu zhi* (Psoraleae fructus)
- *cang er zi* (Xanthii fructus)
- *da fu pi* (Arecae pericarpium)
- *dan zhu ye* (Lopatheri herba)
- *dang gui* (Angelicae sinensis radix)
- *di long* (Pheretima)
- *gou qi zi* (Lycii fructus)
- *he huan pi* (Albizziae cortex)
- *jue ming zhi* (Cassiae semen)
- *ma huang* (Ephedrae herba)
- *shen qu* (Massa fermentata medicata)
- *suan zao ren* (Ziziphi spinosi semen)
- *xiao hui xiang* (Foeniculi fructus)
- *xin yi hua* (Magnoliae flos)
- *yuan zhi* (Polygalae radix)

Contraindicated during Pregnancy

The following list presents a selection of commonly used medicinals that are contraindicated during pregnancy in Lyttleton:[10]

- *che qian zi* (Plantaginis semen)
- *e zhu* (Curcumae rhizoma)
- *fu zi* (Aconiti radix lateralis praeparata)
- *hong hua* (Carthami flos)
- *ma chi xian* (Portulacae herba)
- *mo yao* (Myrrha)
- *niu xi* (Achyranthis bidentatae radix)
- *qu mai* (Dianthi herba)
- *ru xiang* (Olibanum)
- *san leng* (Sparganii rhizoma)
- *she gan* (Belamcandae rhizoma)
- *shui zhi* (Hirudo)
- *tao ren* (Persicae semen)
- *tian hua fen* (Trichosanthis radix)
- *yan hu suo* (Corydalis rhizoma)
- *yi mu cao* (Leonuri herba)
- *zao jia ci* (Gleditsiae spina)

In Chen,[5] the list of common medicinals that are contraindicated during pregnancy additionally includes the following medicinals:

- *bai ji li* (Tribuli fructus)
- *bie jia* (Trionycis carapax)
- *da huang* (Rhei radix et rhizoma)

- *gui ban* (Testudinis plastrum)
- *hu zhang* (Arisaematis rhizoma)
- *ji xue teng* (Spatholobi caulis)
- *lu hui* (Aloe)
- *lu lu tong* (Liquidambaris fructus)
- *rou gui* (Cinnamomi cortex)
- *tu bie chong* (Eupolyphaga seu steleophaga)

Caution!
If there is any chance of pregnancy, you must not prescribe these medicinals in high doses after ovulation!

Bibliography

1. Bensky D, Barolet R. *Chinesische Arzneimittelrezepte und Behandlungsstrategien*. Kötzting: VGM Wühr; 1996.
2. Bensky D, Clavey S, Stöger E, Gamble A. *Chinese Herbal Medicine—Materia Medica*. Seattle: Eastland; 2004.
3. Chen J, Chen T. *Chinese Medical Herbology and Pharmacology*. City of Industry, CA: Art of Medicine Press; 2004.
4. Chen J, Chen T. Appendix 6—Herbs Offering Beneficial Effects to Support Pregnancy. In: Chen J, Chen T. *Chinese Medical Herbology and Pharmacology*; 2004.
5. Chen J, Chen T. Appendix 7—Cautions/Contraindications for Use of Herbs During Pregnancy. In: Chen J, Chen T. *Chinese Medical Herbology and Pharmacology*; 2004.
6. Cheung CS, Golden RS (editors). *TCM and Male and Female Infertility*. San Francisco: Harmonious Sunshine Cultural Center; 1995: 11.
7. Dharmananda S. *Chinese Herbs and Pregnancy. Where to Draw the Line?* Portland: Institute for Traditional Medicine.1996. http://www.itmonline.org/arts/pregherb.htm (accessed May 6, 2009).
8. Gerhard I, Kiechle M. *Gynäkologie Integrativ*. Munich: Urban & Fischer; 2005.
9. Jiang J et al. Clinical Observation of 41 Cases of Threatened and Habitual Abortion Treated by Blood Activation and Stasis Removal. *J Chin Med*. 1997.
10. Lyttleton J. Herbs Contraindicated During Pregnancy. In: Lyttleton J *Treatment of Infertility with Chinese Medicine*. London: Churchill Livingstone; 2004: 391.
11. Lyttleton J. *Treatment of Infertility with Chinese Medicine*. London: Churchill Livingstone; 2004.
12. Maciocia G. *Die Gynäkologie in der Praxis der Chinesischen Medizin*. Kötzting: VGM Wühr; 2000.
13. MHRA (Medicines and Healthcare Products Regulatory Agency), www.mhra.gov.uk (accessed May 6, 2009).

15 Formula *Shao Fu Zhu Yu Tang*—Decoction for Treating Infertility

Simon Becker, Young-Ju Becker

■ Introduction

Wang Qingren, a physician during the Qing dynasty, is the author of the famous book *Yi Lin Gai Cuo (Correcting the Errors in the Forest of Medicine)*. In this book, he criticized his medical predecessors for their mistakes in anatomical drawings and descriptions of physiological processes. In the introductory chapter, he wrote:

"I have studied the theories of my predecessors on zang [viscera] and fu [bowels] and their diagrams. The content is for the most part contradictory."[1]

Wang considered it impossible to treat illness without knowing the organs and their precise functions. He wrote:

"To treat illness without having any understanding of the zang and fu: How is this different from a blind person groping in the dark?"[1]

He therefore decided to focus his own studies and research on the structure and anatomy of the body.

These explorations of the body, which he described in detail in his book, formed the basis for his own understanding of anatomy and pathophysiology. Wang's theory is a colorful mixture of his own observations and traditional theories. It is an image of the body that is accepted neither by traditional nor by biomedical physicians—for the latter group it is much too imprecise. Nevertheless, Wang's theories contributed decisively to a refinement of the pathology of blood stasis. His **Zhu Yu Tang formulas** grew out of this interest. They treat **blood stasis**, which according to Wang is the central starting point of most illnesses.

Interesting and perhaps also typical for TCM as a whole is the fact that as unusual and unfounded as his theory was, it led to the creation of formulas that are now among the most frequently used in contemporary Chinese medicine. In gynecology, it is the *Zhu Yu Tang* formula for the lower burner, *Shao Fu Zhu Yu Tang* **(Lesser Abdomen Stasis-Expelling Decoction)**, which is among the most common medicinal treatments.

■ The Traditional Formula *Shao Fu Zhu Yu Tang*

In the chapter in which Wang describes *Shao Fu Zhu Yu Tang*, he states:

"[T]his formula has a seemingly magical effect on planting seeds."[1]

With this sentence, Wang describes the effectiveness of the formula for women who suffer from infertility. In accordance with this statement, the formula is commonly used today in fertility treatment. The expression "planting seeds" refers to the fertilization and implantation of the embryo.

The present chapter begins with the original description of the medicinal formula from the *Yi Lin Gai Cuo* and then deals with its modern applications in a second part. Including a detailed formula analysis, modern research reports, and case studies, it is intended to illustrate the formula's modern applications in the treatment of infertility.

The first description of *Shao Fu Zhu Yu Tang* in Wang Qingren's *Yi Lin Gai Cuo* follows:[1]

On Shao Fu Zhu Yu Tang
"This formula treats accumulations and bindings with pain in the lower abdomen*; or accumulations and

---

* Lower abdomen is the translation of *shao fu*. The *shao fu* corresponds to the lower part of the belly. The formula name *Shao Fu Zhu Yu Tang* can therefore also be translated as "Lower Belly Stasis-Expelling Decoction."

bindings without pain; or distention and fullness in the lower abdomen; or lumbar pain and distention in the lower abdomen before the onset of menstruation; or three to five menstrual periods in one month, continuously and never stopping, or coming and going. The color [of the menstrual fluid] is dark or black; or clotted; [there is] flooding and spotting* with pain in the lower abdomen; or pinkish [red-colored, chi dai] or white vaginal discharge. All this can be cured. The effect of this formula transcends any comprehensive description.

What is even more extraordinary is the fact that this formula has a seemingly magical effect on planting seeds. At the onset of every menstrual period, five preparations have to be taken consecutively. A fetus will have developed no later than after four months. To give birth to a son, the man and woman's years and months of age together must add up to an even number. If the age of the man or of the woman is an odd number and the other is an even number, you must choose an even month for the fertilization to give birth to a son. If the age of both is either odd or even, you must select an odd month [for fertilization] to give birth to a son. In the choice of the month, do not choose the first day of the lunar month as standard. You must choose the [times of the 24] seasonal changes** as standard. It is important to know that sometimes more than twenty days are necessary to conceive a fetus. In this context, make sure to make a note of the correct day. If the month [of fertilization] is not correct and a girl is born, do not say that my formula is inefficient. I have used this formula; its effects are too many to be counted on your fingers.

In the gui wei year of the reign period dao guang [1823], Su Na, civil administrator of Hebei Province and sixty years old, was in a state of great agitation because he did not have a son. He came to me to discuss this problem.

I told him that this was easy. In the sixth month, I gave this formula to his concubine,*** five preparations every month. In the ninth month, she became preg-

nant. In the following year, the year of jia shen, on the 22nd day of the sixth lunar month, a little gentleman was born. Today he is seven years old.

What is special about this formula is the fact that it is dangerous but yet not dangerous. When pregnant women have a strong body with sufficient qi and without reduced appetite, [the fetus] will certainly not be harmed. Nevertheless, in the medical literature we find a great number [of cases] who suffer a miscarriage without any reason in the third month. [When this happens,] it frequently affects several fetuses consecutively. In spite of this, effective formulas are missing from the discussions on nourishing yin and blood, strengthening the spleen and nourishing the stomach, and quieting and protecting the fetus. [The reason for this is] the lack of awareness that there is a blood stasis in the uterus and that there is no space left for the growing fetus by the time it reaches three months. The fetus falls ill from being jammed. Blood can no longer penetrate to the placenta and runs down on the side. Therefore we first see blood. Because the blood cannot penetrate into the placenta, there is no blood to nourish the fetus. This causes the miscarriage. If the miscarriage happens around the third month or if the fetus has been damaged three to five times, followed by another pregnancy, this formula should be prescribed around the second month. Three, five, or seven, eight preparations should be used to transform and to clear. The child's body will then have enough room to grow. No further miscarriage will follow.

If the miscarriage has already happened, the woman should take three to five preparations of this formula. After that, the growing fetus is certain to face no more obstacles. This formula eliminates illness, plants seeds, and quiets the fetus. Simply good and beautiful, it is truly a miraculous formula.

Rx. Shao Fu Zhu Yu Tang

- xiao hui xiang *(Foeniculi fructus)*, seven grains, stir-fried
- gan jiang *(Zingiberis rhizoma)*, 2 fen *(0.8 g)*, stir-fried
- yan hu suo *(Corydalis rhizoma)*, 1 qian *(3.7 g)*
- mo yao *(Myrrha)*, 1 qian *(3.7 g)*
- dang gui *(Angelicae sinensis radix)*, 3 qian *(11.2 g)*
- chuan xiong *(Chuanxiong rhizoma)*, 1 qian *(3.7 g)*
- guan gui *(Cinnamomi cortex tubiformis)*, 1 qian *(3.7 g)*
- chi shao *(Paeoniae radix rubra)*, 2 qian *(7.5 g)*
- pu huang *(Typhae pollen)*, 3 qian *(11.2 g)*

---

*   *Beng lou* in the original is translated into English as "flooding and spotting."

**   *Jiao jie* 交节, change of the seasons; the times of the 24 seasonal changes. The sun moves 1° every day. Fifteen days constitute one "knot" (*jie*). Thus, we find 24 seasonal changes (*jiao jie*) in one year.

*** In spite of the fact that it sounds strange, this term was a polite way of referring to the wife of a nobleman.

- wu ling zhi (*Trogopteri feces*) 2 qian (*7.5 g*), stir-fried
  Prepare as a water decoction.

Guan gui is referred to as "official cinnamon." It is the inner bark of trees that are between 6 and 7 years old. This bark contains less oils than the main substance Cinnamomi cortex (*rou gui*) and is seen as dryer. It is frequently used to warm the center and dry dampness. *Guan gui* strengthens *yang qi* less intensively than *rou gui*. Li Shizhen said that this type of cinnamon was called "official" because it was the highest grade and used exclusively for members of the government.[2]

◼ Formula Analysis

The following analysis of the composition first deals with the individual groups of similar medicinals and then evaluates the interplay of these different groups. *Shao Fu Zhu Yu Tang* is also particularly broad in its applicability because the formula is composed of so many different groups of remedies.

Acrid and Hot Substances

Xiao hui xiang, gan jiang, and *guan gui* are all acrid and warm or hot medicinals. *Xiao hui xiang* and *guan gui* enter the lower burner. *Gan jiang* warms yang, especially in the center and upper burner; because of its acrid and hot properties, this substance also disperses cold. Cold congeals and causes *qi* stagnation and blood stasis. Movement demands acridity and warmth. This first group of medicinals hence not only warms the lower burner. Because of the acrid medicinals, it also moves *qi* and disperses cold. Thereby, it supports the movement of blood.

The Combination of *Chuan Xiong* and *Dang Gui*

The *qi*-moving and stagnation-resolving function of these substances is further supported by the two acrid ingredients *chuan xiong* and *dang gui*. While these primarily move blood, they also sup-port the *qi*-moving and stagnation-resolving functions of the warming and cold-dispersing ingredients with their warm and acrid properties. This effect assists in the treatment of blood stasis.

The combination of *chuan xiong* and *dang gui* is a good fit. Both are seen as "*qi* within blood" sub-stances. *Chuan xiong*, however, is an active and slightly aggressive *yang* substance. By contrast, *dang gui* is a more nourishing but still also acrid and moving *yin* substance. The blood-nourishing properties of *dang gui* protect the blood from the stronger blood-breaking substances in this formula.

Blood-Quickening Substances

The blood-quickening ingredients are *mo yao, pu huang, wu ling zhi, chi shao*, and *yan hu suo*. With the exception of *chi shao* and *yan hu suo*, these medicinals all belong to the strongest category of stasis-eliminating substances, namely blood-breaking remedies. The combination of *pu huang* and *wu ling zhi* produces the classic basic formula for pronounced blood stasis-related pain in the epigastrium and abdomen: *Shi Xiao San* (Sudden Smile Powder). Today, this small formula is pri-marily used in the treatment of dysmenorrhea due to stasis. What is special about this formula is the fact that *pu huang* not only breaks stasis but primarily stanches bleeding. This function is sup-ported and complemented by *wu ling zhi*, which primarily breaks blood but also stanches bleeding. In addition, *gan jiang* also has a blood-stanching function. Hence, we can also use this formula for bleeding that is caused by blood stasis. Neverthe-less, *pao jiang* (blast-fried ginger) has a much stronger blood-stanching effect than *gan jiang* (dried ginger) and should be substituted in cases of bleeding.

Shi Xiao San as a pain-relieving formula is sup-ported by *yan hu suo*, also an acrid-warm sub-stance that not only quickens blood but also moves *qi*. Out of all the blood-quickening and -moving substances, *yan hu suo* is regarded as the best one for relieving pain.

Cold *Chi Shao*

Lastly, *chi shao* is also one of the blood-moving ingredients in this formula. Its thermal nature is the opposite of the temperature of the formula as a whole: while all ingredients, with the exception of a few neutral ones, are warm and many also acrid, *chi shao* is sour, bitter, and slightly cold. *Chi shao* not only assists in quickening the blood, it also prevents the formation of heat due to stasis and the presence of so many warm and hot substances. *Chi shao* thus balances out the warm and dispersing effect of the formula as a whole.

The Effect of the Combination

Altogether we can divide the ingredients into two groups that define the primary effect of the formula:

* warm and acrid, cold-dispersing substances
* blood-quickening, pain-relieving substances

Furthermore, the focus of the formula lies, as its name already expresses, in the lower abdomen. In women, this region applies to the uterus. But the formula not only breaks stasis, quickens blood, warms, and resolves stasis, it also stanches bleeding and nourishes blood. This last function is emphasized, for example, by the high dosage of *dang gui*—primarily a nourishing root with a mild blood-quickening effect.

■ The Application of *Shao Fu Zhu Yu Tang* in Modern Clinical Practice

Together with *Xue Fu Zhu Yu Tang* (House of Blood Stasis-Expelling Decoction), *Ge Xia Zhu Yu Tang* (Infradiaphragmatic Stasis-Expelling Decoction), *Shen Tong Zhu Yu Tang* (Generalized Pain Stasis-Expelling Decoction) and *Bu Yang Huan Wu Tang* (Yang-Supplementig Five-Returning Decoction), *Shao Fu Zhu Yu Tang* belongs to Wang Qingren's most famous formulas today. In the treatment of gynecological complaints, the formula and its modifications belong to the standard repertoire of Chinese medicine. The formula can, however, also have a broader application.

As we look through the modern literature for references to *Shao Fu Zhu Yu Tang*, we quickly realize that the most common application of this for-

mula is in the treatment of **dysmenorrhea** due to cold and stasis. When cold and stasis block the uterus, infertility may result. For this reason, *Shao Fu Zhu Yu Tang* is also one of the most popular formulas in fertility treatment. As the above translation from the *Yi Lin Gai Cuo* illustrates, Wang Qingren did in fact compose this formula for the specific purpose of stimulating fertility and treating spontaneous abortions.

It is important to realize that appropriate modifications of *Shao Fu Zhu Yu Tang* can extend its range of application considerably. Furthermore, such modifications are important for improving the treatment success by precisely matching the patient's disease pattern. It is one of the outstanding properties of this formula that it is very easy to modify and can therefore be used for many different disease patterns.

As the above formula analysis shows, *Shao Fu Zhu Yu Tang* has three characteristics. The formula:

* quickens blood and transforms stasis
* affects especially the lower burner
* is warm and disperses cold

The first two of these characteristics make this formula suitable for the many different gynecological and urological conditions for which it is used today. The third characteristic is more flexible. The reason for this is that its warm nature can quite easily be changed into the opposite, so that a cool formula is created. The following research and clinical reports show that *Shao Fu Zhu Yu Tang* can also treat many hot conditions. Regardless of this transformation from warm to cool, the formula always continues to quicken blood and break stasis. As such, the addition of the proper "cold" modifications makes this formula applicable for stasis with heat. This means that *Shao Fu Zhu Yu Tang* is able to treat practically all conditions with stasis in the lower burner.

Reversing the formula hierarchy can serve as one example here. If the only cold root in the formula, *chi shao*, becomes the sovereign and the acrid warm and hot ingredients *gan jiang, xiao hui xiang,* and *guan gui* become assistants and couriers, and we add a few bitter and cold substances, this medicinal combination quickly turns into a formula that clears heat and breaks stasis.

The broad range of applications for *Shao Fu Zhu Yu Tang* is also demonstrated by the fact that this formula treats not only infertility in women. Wang commented on this formula that it "has a seemingly magical effect on planting seeds." This comment can also be applied to men. Several of the following research reports describe how this formula can also be used effectively for sperm problems.

Summaries of research and clinical reports follow. The quality of the reports varies greatly. We must ask the reader not to focus primarily on the methods and results of the studies. Instead, direct your attention to the form and composition of the formulas. These describe the modern and successful application in clinic and indicate the manifold possibilities for modifying *Shao Fu Zhu Yu Tang*.

The Treatment of 41 Female Infertility Patients[8]

Study Design
In this study, 41 women with fertility problems were treated with a modification of *Shao Fu Zhu Yu Tang*. The husbands' sperm was checked and found to be normal. Thirty-four women suffered from primary infertility; seven women from secondary infertility. Twenty-eight women were between 25 and 30 years old, 13 women between 31 and 40. Twenty-six women had been trying to become pregnant for 5 years; 15 women for 6–9 years. In 11 women, the menstrual cycle was normal, 12 women had a shortened cycle, and 14 had a delayed cycle. In four cases, the periods were irregular, that is, either too early or too late.

Treatment
All women were treated only with Chinese medicine. *Shao Fu Zhu Yu Tang* was the basic formula. In women with symptoms of **qi deficiency**, *bai zhu* (atractylodis macrocephalae rhizome) and *tai zi shen* (pseudostellariae radix) were added. In women with **blood deficiency**, *shu di huang* (rehmanniae glutinosae radix praeparata) and *dan shen* (salviae miltiorrhizae radix) were added. In cases with pronounced symptoms of **vacuity cold**, *fu zi* (aconiti radix lateralis praeparata) and *xi xin* (asari herba) were added as well. For pronounced **yin deficiency** symptoms, *xuan shen* (scrophulariae radix) and *e jiao* (asini corii colla) were added as well.

Result
After treatment with this formula, 30 women became pregnant and gave birth. The longest treatment span was 1 year, the shortest 3 months.

The Treatment of Infertility Caused by Blocked Fallopian Tubes

Study Design
A total of 38 women were treated. The average age was 30.6 years. Twenty-six women suffered from primary infertility, 12 women from secondary infertility.

Treatment
All women were treated with a modification of *Shao Fu Zhu Yu Tang*. The formula consisted of the following ingredients:
* *xiao hui xiang*, 6 g
* *chi shao*, 15 g
* *chuan xiong*, 15 g
* *guan gui*, 6 g
* *mo yao*, 6 g
* *gan jiang*, 6 g
* *chao pu huang* (Typhae pollen frictus) 15 g
* *wu ling zhi*, 15 g
* *yan hu suo*, 15 g
* *dang gui*, 6 g

Additional Modifications
This basic formula was adjusted in accordance with the patients' disease patterns. For a tendency to cold, the following were added:
* *xi xin*, 3 g
* *wu zhu yu* (Evodiae fructus), 3 g

For a **tendency to heat**, *gan jiang*, *guan gui*, and *xiao hui xiang* were removed, and the following were added instead:
* *mu dan pi* (Moutan cortex), 15 g
* *bai jiang cao* (Patriniae herba), 15 g
* *zhi zi* (Gardeniae fructus) 15 g

For a **tendency to vacuity**, the following were added:
* *huang qi* (Astragali radix), 30 g
* *dang shen* (Codonopsis pilosulae radix), 15 g
* *bai zhu*, 9 g

For a **tendency to repletion**, the following were added:
* *san leng* (Sparganii rhizoma), 10 g
* *e zhu* (Curcumae rhizoma), 10 g

For a **tendency to liver *qi* stagnation** and **blood stasis**, the following were added:

* *chuan lian zi* (Toosendan fructus), 15 g
* *wu yao* (Linderae radix), 10 g

For a **tendency to cold-related coagulation with blood stasis**, the following were added:

* *xiang fu* (Cyperi rhizoma), 10 g
* *zi shi ying* (Fluoritum), 30 g

For a **tendency to *qi* stagnation with blood stasis**, *the following were added:*

* *yu jin* (Curcumae radix), 18 g
* *chuan shan jia* (Manis squama), 15 g
* *lu lu tong* (Liquidambaris fructus), 10 g

Chinese medicinal therapy was combined with biomedical treatment for tubal patency. Treatment length varied between 1 and 6 months. The average treatment length was 3.2 months.

Result
After treatment, an effect was seen in 92% of all cases and a cure in 66 patients.

Commentary
This study demonstrates vividly how *Shao Fu Zhu Yu Tang* can be modified to match all kinds of disease patterns. In particular, the treatment of heat patterns is noteworthy here. For this purpose, the warm ingredients in this essentially warm formula had to be reduced, and heat-clearing medicinals had to be added. All blood-moving medicinals were left in place! At the same time, we should emphasize that *Shao Fu Zhu Yu Tang*, a formula for cold and stasis in the lower burner, does not possess markedly hot properties. In cases of pronounced cold, we must therefore add strongly heating substances like *wu zhu yu* and *xi xin*. Incidentally, this fact can also be highlighted in the first study. In that study, the hot ingredient *fu zi* was added, for example. All in all we can thus see that *Shao Fu Zhu Yu Tang* serves as a moderate treatment for very different disease patterns. By adding the correct medicinals, the formula can be designed to fit almost any presentations.

The Treatment of 40 Female Infertility Patients[5]

Study Design
A total of 40 women suffering from infertility were treated. Their age ranged between 25 and 38. The women had been suffering from infertility for between 2 and 14 years. Twenty-four women were diagnosed with primary infertility; 16 women with secondary infertility. Twenty-one women additionally suffered from mild to medium tubal obstruction. In five women with primary infertility, uterine dysplasia was discovered; 28 women suffered from adnexitis.

Treatment
The women were treated with the following variation of *Shao Fu Zhu Yu Tang*:

* *xiao hui xiang*, 6 g
* *gan jiang*, 9 g
* *yan hu suo*, 9 g
* *dang gui*, 9 g
* *chuan xiong*, 9 g
* *rou gui*, 6 g
* *chi shao*, 12 g
* *pu huang*, 12 g
* *wu ling zhi*, 9 g
* *mo yao*, 9 g
* *dan shen*, 18 g

This prescription was started at the onset of the menstrual period and taken for 7 days. Treatment was continued for a minimum of three menstrual cycles.

Additional Modifications
For **cold pain** in the lower abdomen and a **delayed menstrual period** due to *yang* vacuity or an accumulation of cold-damp:

* the amount of *gan jiang, xiao hui xiang*, and *rou gui* was increased, and the following medicinals were added:
  – *fu zi*, 9 g
  – *cang zhu* (Atractylodis rhizoma), 9 g
  – *fu ling* (Poria), 12 g

For **stabbing pain** in the lower abdomen during the period with clots or tissue in the menstrual fluid, caused by blood stasis, the following were added:

* *tao ren* (Persicae semen), 12 g
* *hong hua* (Carthami flos), 9 g
* *yi mu cao* (Leonuri herba), 30 g

For **mild pain** after the period with pale sallow facial complexion, caused by blood deficiency, the following were added:

- *huang qi*, 30 g
- *shu di huang*, 24 g
- *e jiao*, 12 g

For **heavy menstrual periods** with red blood, internal disquietude, dry mouth, and yellow urine, the following were removed:

- *xiao hui xiang, gan jiang*, and *rou gui*

with the addition of:

- *sheng di huang* (Rehmanniae radix exsiccata seu recens), 24 g
- *huang bai* (Phellodendri cortex), 9 g
- *mu dan pi*, 12 g
- *di gu pi* (Lycii cortex), 12 g

For a **feeling of fullness in the lower abdomen** during the menstrual period with pain in the chest area and ribs and tension in the breasts, caused by *qi* stagnation, the following were added:

- *xiang fu*, 12 g
- *wu yao*, 12 g

For **cervicitis** or **adnexitis**, the following were added:

- *jin yin hua* (Lonicerae flos), 12 g
- *pu gong ying* (Taraxaci herba), 15 g
- *chuan lian zi*, 9 g
- *che qian zi* (Plantaginis semen), 12 g

Additionally, all women received biomedical treatment for tubal patency.

Result

The results were measured by whether the treated patients became pregnant or not after a certain length of treatment. Of the total of 40 patients, eight became pregnant after 1 month of treatment, 10 after 2 months, and nine after 3 months. An additional 10 were pregnant after 4–6 months. Four women failed to become pregnant even after a full year of treatment.

Commentary

Again we can see from the modifications how broadly we can use *Shao Fu Zhu Yu Tang*. The formula is used not only in cases with cold stasis, but also for adnexitis and cervicitis, which both tend to be manifestations of heat accumulation. In this study, the formula *Shao Fu Zhu Yu Tang* was mod-

ified so as either to warm or to clear heat. Furthermore, *huang qi, shu di huang*, and *e jiao* were added as strengthening substances and thereby gave *Shao Fu Zhu Yu Tang* a supplementing effect. The addition of *tao ren, hong hua*, and *yi mu cao* further increased the stasis-resolving function. By adding two or three ingredients or removing the warming and hot substances like *xiao hui xiang, gan jiang*, and *rou gui*, we can thus use this formula to treat vacuity and repletion, heat and cold.

Also interesting is the timing when the formula was dispensed: always **during** the menstrual period. The reason for this is that the effect of *Shao Fu Zhu Yu Tang* in fertility treatment is firmly rooted in its function to "cleanly" build up the uterine lining—the endometrium—as a result of which the fertilized egg is able to implant. When the formula is prescribed during the menstrual period, it can assist in the "shedding" of the endometrium and thereby facilitate the unobstructed construction of a new endometrium.

The Treatment of 12 Female Infertility Patients[4]

Study Design

The age of the 12 patients ranged between 25 and 36 years. Two women had been trying to become pregnant for more than 10 years; five women for 6–10 years; two women for 4–6 years; and the remaining three women for 3–4 years.

Treatment

The women were treated with the following prescription:

- *xiao hui xiang*, seven seeds
- *gan jiang*, 2 g
- *yan hu suo*, 5 g
- *mo yao*, 5 g
- *dang gui*, 15 g
- *chuan xiong*, 5 g
- *rou gui*, 5 g
- *chi shao*, 10 g
- *pu huang*, 15 g
- *chao wu ling zhi* (Trogopteri feces frictum), 10 g

This prescription was started on the 6th day of the menstrual cycle and taken for 7 days.

Result

This treatment lead to good results. The improvement rate was around 90%. Most patients required two or more treatment cycles.

Commentary

According to the author of this study, *Shao Fu Zhu Yu Tang* is effective in liver *qi* stagnation with internal blockage due to blood stasis. *Shao Fu Zhu Yu Tang* is indicated especially for infertility due to vacuity cold in the uterus.

The Treatment of Immune Infertility Caused by Endometriosis[9]

Study Design

A total of 94 women ranging from 24 to 38 years in age were treated for endometriosis with accompanying infertility. All women presented with the following symptoms: no pregnancy for at least 2 years, menstrual pain or a history of menstrual pain, cold in the lower abdomen, and pain relieved by the application of heat.

A gynecological check-up found tender knots on the uterosacral ligaments and in the pouch of Douglas. In the blood, antibodies against the endometrium (EmAb) were found. No anti-sperm antibodies were discovered. The fallopian tubes of the women were all patent. The length of infertility was between 2 and 10 years.

Treatment

The patients were treated with a prescription consisting of the following ingredients:

- *chao xiao hui xiang* (Foeniculi frictus fructus), 5 g
- *pao jiang* (Zingiberis rhizoma praeparatum), 5 g
- *mo yao*, 6 g
- *rou gui*, 6 g
- *chi shao*, 10 g
- *chuan xiong*, 10 g
- *chao wu ling zhi* (Trogopteri feces frictum), 10 g
- *chao pu huang*, 12 g
- *zhi shui zhi* (Hirudo praeparata), 12 g
- *dang gui*, 15 g
- *yan hu suo*, 15 g
- *zhi huang qi*, 20 g

Additional Modifications

In **blood deficiency**, the following were added:
- *ji xue teng* (Spatholobi caulis), 30 g
- *he shou wu* (Polygoni multiflori radix), 15 g

In *qi* **deficiency**, the following was added:
- *chao bai zhu* (Atractylodis macrocephalae rhizoma frictum), 15 g

This prescription was taken during the menstrual period. After three cycles, the women were checked again for antibodies against the endometrium.

Result

The antibody-test after 3 months showed negative results (i. e., no more antibodies) in 86% of the patients (81 women). The dysmenorrhea and dyspareunia had improved in 72% of all cases (73 women) and the rate of pregnancy within 6–12 months after the conclusion of treatment was around 62% (55 women).

Commentary

The authors of this study explain the disease mechanism of infertility from the perspective of TCM as follows:

"Static blood blocks the uterus and the chong mai *and* ren mai; *for this reason, infertility results. In blood stasis in the lower abdomen, the* bao mai *is blocked as well, resulting in pain. In blood stasis in the* chong mai *and* ren mai, *these two channels cannot contain any essence. This results in infertility as well. The pattern describes this."*

They comment on the addition of *huang qi* as follows:

"Huang qi strengthens right qi *and eliminates stasis. As a result, circulation in the pelvis is improved and the amount of T-cells increases. This regulates the immune function in the abdomen, and the antibodies against the endometrium are reduced."*

This statement points to the special properties of *huang qi*: not only does it boost *qi*, but it also quickens the blood. *Huang qi* is also the main ingredient for boosting *qi*, for example when *qi* vacuity leads to blood stasis.

The Treatment of 20 Patients with Semen Liquefaction Problems[3]

Study Design
Of a total of 20 men, seven ranged in age between 21 and 25, and 13 between 26 and 32. Three men came for treatment 1 year after getting married; five men after 2 years, and 12 men after 3 or more years. The Chinese disease pattern corresponded to a lack of original *yang* (*yuan yang*). All patients were tested for semen liquefaction. Missing liquefaction after 24 hours served as the criterion for treatment. In addition, pus corpuscles[*] were found in four cases.

Treatment
The men were treated with the following basic prescription:

- *xiao hui xiang*, 6 g
- *gan jiang*, 3 g
- *yan hu suo*, 6 g
- *mo yao*, 5 g
- *chuan xiong*, 6 g
- *rou gui*, 3 g
- *chi shao*, 10 g
- *pu huang*, 10 g
- *wu ling zhi*, 10 g
- *dang gui*, 12 g
- *huang jing* (Polygonati rhizoma), 30 g

Additional Modifications
For **pus corpuscles in the semen**, the following were added:

- *bi xie* (Dioscoreae hypoglaucae seu semptemlobae rhizoma), 15 g
- *shi chang pu* (Acori tatarinowii rhizoma), 10 g
- *shi wei* (Pyrrosiae folium), 20 g
- *che qian zi*, 20 g

In cases where liquefaction had normalized after the treatment but the **motility** continued to be **reduced**, the following were added:

- *huang qi*, 30 g
- *xian ling pi* (Epimedii herba), 30 g

---

[*] Pus corpuscles are decomposing, segmented granulocytes, similar to lymphocytes and monocytes. During decomposition, they release lytic ferments and thereby cause the cloudy, creamy consistency of pus.

For a **reduced sperm count**, *Wu Zi Yan Zong Wan* (Five Seeds Pills for Abundant Descendants) was administered. It consists of the five seeds *gou qi zi* (Lycii fructus), *fu pen zi* (Rubi fructus), *wu wei zi* (Schisandrae fructus), *che qian zi* and *tu si zi* (Cuscutae semen). The formula supplements the kidneys and boosts essence.

One batch of the above prescription was decocted in 400 mL and taken twice per day in doses of 200 mL. A course of treatment lasted 20 days.

Result
After one or two courses of treatment, 17 of the total of 20 patients were cured, that is, their lab values had normalized. The remaining three patients experienced an improvement after two courses of treatment. This means that liquefaction had normalized but sperm motility or sperm count continued to be reduced.

Commentary
There is a saying in Chinese medicine: "*Yang* transforms *qi*, *yin* produces form." According to the authors of this study, sperm coagulation is one of the functions associated with kidney *yin* ("produce form"), while liquefaction of semen is one of the functions associated with kidney *yang* ("transform *qi*").

The authors comment:

"A lack of original *yang* (*yuan yang*) hence causes vacuity cold in the essence chamber. As a result, *qi* transformation becomes abnormal. The essence becomes cold and coagulates. By contrast, a lack of original *yin* causes the kidney fire to flare up. Essence fluids condense."

Treatment therefore concentrated on boosting original *yang* (*yuan yang*) and regulating *qi* transformation. While *Shao Fu Zhu Yu Tang* does not have the direct effect of doing so, it still serves as a suitable formula in light of the guideline "cold leads to coagulation and warmth leads to movement." The authors explain the formula as follows:

"Xiao hui xiang, rou gui, *and* gan jiang *enter the lower burner and assist original* yang *in dispersing cold coagulation.* Yan hu suo *and* mo yao *free qi and move stasis.* Shi Xiao San, i. e., pu huang *and* wu ling zhi, *quicken the blood and resolve binds.* Dang gui *and* chuan xiong *are seen as 'yang within* yin' *and 'qi within blood' medicinals. Blood and essence share the same origin. Chi shao was added. It quickens the blood and moves* qi, *resolves cold coagulation, and regulates the essence fluid (seminal fluid). In combination, these substances warm the essence chamber and resolve coagulations. When* yang *is vitalized,* qi *transformation recovers as well. As a result, semen liquefaction is normalized and the fertilization of offspring can take place."*

Wang Qingren noted in his description of this formula:

"This is the best formula for fertilizing offspring and quieting the fetus."[1]

Although this sentence is nowadays read primarily as concerning the treatment of infertility in women, a number of studies like the one above demonstrate that *Shao Fu Zhu Yu Tang* and its variations can also treat male problems. Other studies show its effect in the treatment of male problems like delayed seminal emissions, impotence, varicoceles, hematospermia, or prostatitis.

■ Case Studies

The following five representative case studies serve to concretely illustrate the successful application of the formula *Shao Fu Zhu Yu Tang* in modern clinical practice.

Case Study 1: Infertility with Dysmenorrhea[8]

Medical History

The 25-year-old female patient had been trying for 3 years unsuccessfully to become pregnant. Examinations of her husband revealed no abnormal results. The woman had begun menstruating at age 15. Her periods lasted 5–7 days, the color of the blood was dark red, and the amount of blood was scanty. The blood also contained clots and she was suffering from premenstrual pain in the lower abdomen. Gynecological examinations showed a normal vagina, a soft cervix, and an immature,

slightly forward-tilted uterus (anteversion). The adnexas were normal on both sides.

The body of the woman was rather thin, her facial complexion was pale and colorless, and her lips were pale as well. Just recently she had lost her appetite and experienced pressure in the chest, which she attempted to release by sighing. She was also suffering from dizziness, a feeling of weakness, and disturbed sleep. Defecation and urination were both normal. The tongue was pale and enlarged, its body was relatively dark. The margins and tip of the tongue were covered with bluish-purple spots. Her pulse was thin and weak.

Diagnosis

The diagnosis was infertility and dysmenorrhea. The identified disease pattern was *qi* stagnation and blood stasis with concurrent weakness of *qi* and blood. The treatment principle was to free *qi* and quicken blood. Additionally, *qi* and blood should be boosted and nourished.

Treatment

A variation of *Shao Fu Zhu Yu Tang* was prescribed:
- *xiao hui xiang*, 6 g
- *gan jiang*, 6 g
- *yan hu suo*, 10 g
- *wu ling zhi*, 10 g
- *mo yao*, 10 g
- *chuan xiong*, 15 g
- *pu huang*, 9 g, wrapped in cloth for decocting
- *rou gui*, 6 g
- *chi shao*, 10 g
- *dang gui*, 9 g
- *bai zhu*, 15 g
- *shu di huang*, 12 g

This prescription was prepared as a water decoction. Until the onset of her next period, the patient took one package per day. Afterwards, she returned for treatment. The pain in the lower abdomen had disappeared and the clots in her menses were greatly reduced. But she still suffered from weakness, sleep problems, and lack of appetite. Therefore, the above prescription was modified by removing *shu di huang* and substituting the following instead:
- *ze lan* (Lycopi herba), 15 g
- *yi mu cao*, 24 g
- *suan zao ren* (Ziziphi spinosi semen), 15 g
- *shen qu* (Massa fermentata medicata), 10 g

Again, she was instructed to take one package per day.

By the time of her next appointment 1 month later, her problems had continued to improve. The menses no longer contained any clots, and no other symptoms manifested either. The tongue was pale with few purple spots on the tip and margins. The pulse was fine and weak. She therefore received another prescription:

- *xiao hui xiang*, 6 g
- *gan jiang*, 6 g
- *yan hu suo*, 9 g
- *wu ling zhi*, 9 g
- *dang gui*, 10 g
- *pu huang*, 9 g
- *chi shao*, 12 g
- *tai zi shen*, 15 g
- *sheng di huang*, 12 g
- *bai zhu*, 15 g
- *gou qi zi*, 10 g
- *yi mu cao*, 24 g

Result

Her menstruation became normal after 5 months. In March of the following year, she gave birth to a daughter.

Case Study 2: Infertility[8]

Medical History

The patient was a 37-year-old woman who had been trying to become pregnant for 9 years already. She had been treated unsuccessfully with Western medicine. Her menstrual period had started at age 16. Her cycle was always delayed by 10–14 days. During menstruation, she suffered from cold pain in the lower abdomen. Her blood was dark and contained clots. Her tongue was pale with a white fur, and her pulse was stringlike and slow.

Diagnosis

The diagnosis was infertility, and the pattern was identified as *qi* stagnation with blood stasis and concurrent cold stagnation in the liver channel. Treatment therefore aimed at freeing liver *qi*, transforming stasis, and warming the channels.

Treatment

The patient received the following prescription:

- Rx. *Shao Fu Zhu Yu Tang* plus
- *xi xin*
- *fu zi*
- *wu zhu yu*

This prescription was prepared as a water decoction. After the woman had taken five batches, *fu zi* was deleted from the prescription and Tetrapanacis medulla (*tong cao*) was added. Five more batches were prescribed. After this, her menstruation had become regular and the cold pain in the lower abdomen was reduced. Nevertheless, the blood continued to be dark and contain clots. The number of clots, though, was reduced. At the onset of the menstrual period, the woman stopped taking this prescription. Afterwards, another modification of the above prescription was given.

Result

After taking these medicinals for 6 months, the woman became pregnant and gave birth to a baby girl.

Case Study 3: Infertility[6]

Medical History

The 28-year-old patient had been trying to become pregnant for 3 years without success. Examinations of her husband showed no abnormal results. She had begun menstruating at age 18. Her cycle was irregular and varied between 25 and 60 days. The periods were light and lasted between 5 and 7 days. The blood was dark and contained dark clots. Menstruation was accompanied by abdominal pain, aversion to cold, cold extremities, lumbar pain, and hardness in the abdomen. Her discharge was watery and reddish-white in color. Her tongue was pale dark with a thin white fur; the pulse was deep and thin.

Diagnosis

The biomedical diagnosis was primary infertility. The Chinese pattern identification was kidney exhaustion with blood deficiency, cold in the uterus, and *qi* stagnation with blood stasis. The treatment principles were therefore to strengthen the kidneys, nourish the blood, warm the uterus, move cold and *qi*, and transform stasis.

Treatment

The patient received the following prescription:

- *shu di huang*, 20 g
- *shan zhu yu* (Corni fructus), 9 g
- *shan yao* (Dioscoreae rhizoma), 10 g
- *dang gui*, 12 g
- *chi shao*, 12 g
- *chuan xiong*, 6 g
- *guang mu xiang* (Aucklandiae radix), 6 g
- *chao zhi ke* (Aurantii fructus frictus), 9 g
- *xiao hui xiang*, 6 g
- *xiang fu*, 10 g
- *yi mu cao*, 20 g
- *chai hu* (Bupleuri radix), 6 g
- *fu zi*, 9 g
- *rou gui*, 6 g
- *tao ren*, 10 g
- *hong hua*, 10 g
- *huai niu xi* (Achyranthis bidentatae radix), 10 g
- *gan cao* (Glycyrrhizae radix), 6 g

Three to five batches of this prescription were taken during the menstrual periods in three cycles. In between, the woman received Chinese medicinals to nourish the blood and supplement the kidneys, warm the uterus, and disperse cold. This prescription consisted of:

- *shan zhu yu*, 10 g
- *bai shao yao* (Paeoniae radix alba), 10 g
- *dang gui*, 10 g
- *chuan xiong*, 6 g
- *shan yao*, 10 g
- *fu zi*, 4 g
- *rou gui*, 5 g
- *ba ji tian* (Morindae officinalis radix), 10 g
- *pu huang*, 9 g
- *gan cao*, 3 g
- *da zao* (Jujubae fructus), three pieces

Of this prescription, she took one preparation every other day.

Result

Half a year later, the woman became pregnant and 9 months later gave birth to a baby girl.

Case Study 4: Male Infertility[3]

Medical History

The 27-year-old man had already been trying for 3 years without success to have a child with his wife. His wife was examined, and no problems were found. The man therefore underwent a semen analysis. This showed that liquefaction was inadequate after 24 hours. The man felt healthy and showed no other symptoms. His tongue was pale with a thin white fur. His pulse was deep and thin.

Diagnosis

The disease pattern was identified as lack of original *yang* (*yuan yang*) with insufficient *qi* transformation. Therefore, *qi* was boosted, *yang* supplemented, and stasis transformed.

Treatment

The following prescription was administered:

- *xiao hui xiang*, 6 g
- *gan jiang*, 3 g
- *yan hu suo*, 6 g
- *mo yao*, 10 g
- *pu huang*, 10 g
- *wu ling zhi*, 6 g
- *huang jing*, 30 g

The man took one batch of this prescription every day for 20 days. Afterwards, his seminal fluid was examined again.

Result

Liquefaction had normalized and his sperm count was 80 million/mL and motility around 80%. Half a year later, his wife became pregnant.

Case Study 5: Infertility with Amenorrhea

Medical History

After the 30-year-old woman had stopped taking birth control pills in order to become pregnant, her menstrual period failed to come for 2 months. This caused her to seek Chinese medicine treatment. The woman suffered from hypothyroidism, and water easily collected in her body; this caused her to be overweight. Her nose was often congested, she had to urinate several times a night, slept only shallowly, was thirsty, had cold extremities, and experienced lumbar pain after physical exercise. She ate almost no meat, only a little chicken now and then. Her tongue was pale blue with a red tip and deep cracks in the middle. Her pulse was pale, deep, weak, and slow.

Diagnosis
The pattern was identified as kidney *yang* deficiency with blood vacuity. Hence treatment aimed at boosting *yang* and nourishing blood.

Treatment
The patient received a prescription for *You Gui Wan* (Right [Kidney]-Restoring Pill) with the addition of *fu ling*, Citri reticulatae pericarpium (*chen pi*), and *tu si zi*. The woman took this prescription for 7 days as granules. After this week, her extremities felt warmer. Hence she received a new prescription that was less supplementing, but more moving instead. This movement was intended to promote her menstrual period. Because the lower burner had to be warmed and the blood had to be quickened, the new prescription was based on the basic working principles of *Shao Fu Zhu Yu Tang* as a combination of warm, cold-dispersing substances with blood-moving medicinals. The prescription contained:

- *shu di huang*
- *dang gui wei* (Angelicae sinensis radicis extremitas)
- *bai shao yao*
- *xu duan* (Dipsaci radix)
- *du zhong* (Eucommiae cortex)
- *nü zhen zi* (Ligustri lucidi fructus)
- *fu zi*
- *wu yao*
- *ze lan*
- *tao ren*
- *hong hua*
- *chuan xiong*
- *fu ling*
- *dang shen*

This prescription was given as granules for 1 week. Subsequently, the patient reported that she suffered from abdominal fullness and distention as if she were to start her period. The prescription was therefore again adjusted to more strongly move *qi* and blood. It consisted of:

- Rx. *Xiao Yao San* (Free Wanderer Powder) plus
- *he huan pi* (Albizziae cortex)

- *ye jiao teng* (Polygoni multiflori caulis)
- *tao ren*
- *hong hua*
- *mu dan pi*
- *dang shen*
- *mu xiang*
- *shan zha* (Crataegi fructus)

Result
Two weeks later, her menstrual period started. While it was still weak, the color and duration were normal. From this point on, her menses arrived regularly. Three months later, she became pregnant and gave birth to a baby boy 9 months after that.

Commentary
This case study illustrates well that we do not always have to use the exact composition of a classic formula. Instead, we can apply its working principle as a guideline.

Shao Fu Zhu Yu Tang warms the uterus and lower burner and quickens the blood. The formula is often administered during the menstrual period in order to promote it. It is only when all the "old" blood has been discharged that a healthy uterine lining (endometrium) can be built with fresh blood. This in turn favors the implantation of a fertilized ovum. In the woman above, the menses failed to flow at all due to *yang* deficiency and blood vacuity. As such, blood, *yin*, essence, and *yang* had to be supplemented first. Her menstruation could only be promoted afterwards by applying the working principle of *Shao Fu Zhu Yu Tang* to warm the lower burner and quicken the blood. At the same time, the prescription continued to supplement the kidneys. This treatment was enough to trigger premenstrual-like feelings of fullness, a clear symptom of liver *qi* stagnation. To move liver *qi*, *Xiao Yao San* was administered. The warm and hot substances were removed to prevent heat transformation due to *qi* stagnation. The blood-moving substances were left in the prescription to promote the elimination of blood during menstruation by quickening the blood, in accordance with the working principle of *Shao Fu Zhu Yu Tang*, thereby boosting the creation of a healthy endometrium.

Even if a formula is not prescribed in its entirety and completely literally, the therapy can still be informed by its mechanisms of action. Thus, a formula is not merely a combination of different Chinese medicinals. In addition, a classic formula also represents a theoretical principle tested in practice. This principle can be developed further, and we can apply it also when using other medicinals. This opinion is, of course, also based on the presumption that a formula is effective not only when it is prescribed in its "original form." The case study above as well as the history of Chinese medicine as a whole appear to support the notion that what is most important is less the exact formula than the mechanisms of action that it is based on. The "prescription" of a formula therefore does not necessarily mean the administration of very specific substances but rather the compliance with its inherent treatment strategies and working principles.

Conclusion

Shao Fu Zhu Yu Tang is one of Wang Qingren's four famous *Zhu Yu Tang* formulas. As such, it belongs to the category of blood-moving and stasis-eliminating formulas. Blood stasis is one of the most common pathogenic factors in modern Chinese medicine. It is part of the disease pattern in most, if not all, chronic illnesses. According to a guiding principle in Chinese medicine, "long-lasting illnesses enter the network vessels." This means that chronic conditions lead to blood stasis. Treatment therefore also has to aim at least partially at resolving this stasis.

Wang Qingren was *the* master of stasis-eliminating formulas. Similar to the opinion of many modern physicians and TCM specialists, Wang also believed stasis to be a central aspect of many different illnesses. His formula *Shao Fu Zhu Yu Tang* was intended for the treatment of all types of stasis in the lower abdomen, including stasis that leads to infertility.

What makes *Shao Fu Zhu Yu Tang* so remarkable is its broad range of applications. In spite of the fact that the basic formula possesses warm blood-quickening properties, it can easily be converted into a cool blood-quickening formula. While it is a quickening formula, with few modifications it can also be used in vacuity patterns. The common denominator for the application of *Shao Fu Zhu Yu Tang* is **blood stasis**. Because a certain

amount of stasis is part of most disease patterns in infertility patients and because *Shao Fu Zhu Yu Tang* is very easy to modify, it is no surprise that this classic formula is one of the most commonly used formulas for infertility. It is hereby completely irrelevant whether the infertility presents with heat or cold, vacuity or repletion.

Shao Fu Zhu Yu Tang is used so frequently and effectively in the treatment of infertility because stasis is a key aspect in the disease mechanism of infertility. The quickening properties not only assist in restoring patency to blocked fallopian tubes, but they are also ideal for optimizing the "internal conditions" of the uterus. Optimizing these "internal conditions" means to prepare the endometrium for implantation. During the menstrual period, *Shao Fu Zhu Yu Tang* promotes contractions in the uterus and the elimination of "old and static" blood that is blocking the uterus. Afterwards, the formula assists in activating the microcirculation and thereby in the stasis-free construction of the endometrium. As a result, a mucous membrane is built in which the fertilized ovum can implant. One of the key characteristics of *Shao Fu Zhu Yu Tang* in the treatment of infertility is hence the "repair" of the endometrium, as a result of which the implantation process is supported. To benefit from this function, the formula should be taken **during the menstrual period**. During this time, it can promote the elimination of blood and the development of a new and stasis-free endometrium. This application follows the recommendations of Wang Qingren, as he already stated in his description of the formula:

"At the beginning of every menstrual period, five preparations must be taken consecutively. A fetus will have developed no later than after four months.[1]"

As some of the above cases illustrate, women can be treated with supplementing formulas in between their menstrual periods. This improves the quality of the endometrium.

In addition to the "renewal" of the endometrium, *Shao Fu Zhu Yu Tang* furthermore has the effect of resolving inflammations and reducing related tissue hyperplasia, improving the microcirculation in the pelvic area, relaxing spasms, and freeing fallopian tube blockages. In men, the formula improves microcirculation in the testicles. These are some of the properties that make this formula so effective in the treatment of many different types of infertility. These properties are partly responsible for the reason why Wang Qing-ren noted in the middle of the 19th century:

"This formula eliminates illness, plants seeds, and quiets the fetus. Simply good and beautiful, it is truly a miraculous formula."[1]

Bibliography

1. Becker S, Chung Y, Oving H. *Yi Lin Gai Cuo—Correcting the Errors in the Forest of Medicine*. Boulder: Blue Poppy; 2007.
2. Bensky D, Clavey S, Stöger E. *Chinese Herbal Medicine. Materia Medica*. Seattle: Eastland; 2004.
3. Ding Lijing. Jiang Su Zhong Yi. *Jiangsu Journal of Chinese Medicine*. 1997;8:22.
4. Guan Guixia, Sun Yaodong, Ye Doudan, Deng Zuo. Ji Lin Zhong Yi Yao. *Jilin Journal of Chinese Medicine*. 2003;11:31.
5. Guo Yugang, Dai Yachi. Shan Xi Zhong Yi Xue Yuan Xue Bao. *Journal of Shanxi University of Chinese Medicine*. 2001;6:21 – 22.
6. Hu Ailan. An Hui Zhong Yi Lin Chuang Za Zhi. *Anhui Journal of Clinical Chinese Medicine*. 1994;2:27.
7. Sun Jie. Xian Dai Zhong Xi Yi Jie He Za Zhi. *Modern Journal of Integrated Chinese and Western Medicine*. 2002;8:37.
8. Tan Huliang, Xu Yun-Ying. Bei Jing Zhong Yi Yao Da Xue Xue Bao. *Journal of Beijing University of Chinese Medicine*. 2001;1:76.
9. Zhang Yuwan, Jing Jianbo, Geng Yang. Zhong Yuan Yi Kan. *Zhongyuan Medical Journal*. 2001;6:43 – 44

Fertility Disorders and Treatment Concepts

5

Andrea A. Kaffka
Acupuncture points and combinations: Andreas A. Noll

A regular menstrual cycle is the natural prerequisite for women's fertility and therefore lies at the center of fertility treatment in TCM. In contrast to biomedicine, TCM offers numerous treatment options in this area: by means of a sophisticated differential diagnosis, it is able to harmonize a woman's cycle without any side-effects.

When a woman comes to your TCM practice for fertility treatment, her cycle and her menstrual period should be the first thing that you examine. Often, she has already made several attempts to jumpstart a pregnancy by means of modern fertility medicine. Even though it is possible to support artificial fertilization with acupuncture and medicinals, it is more important from the TCM perspective to regulate the menstrual cycle and period on the whole as the first treatment step and only afterwards, if necessary, support an artificial fertilization in accordance with the stages of the cycle. Convincing studies show that this can drastically increase the success rate.[14]

Some women who turn to TCM for help have already experienced several miscarriages. But women also frequently come because no limitations to their fertility are apparent from a biomedical perspective but they nevertheless have not been able to get pregnant. An additional problem is that women nowadays tend to decide very late, after successful partner and career choices, to start a family and have children. But fertility declines rapidly with advancing age—after age 40, it drops by about 70% and thus exposes fertility patients to time pressure as well. Nevertheless, after even one round of regulating the menstrual cycle, without any further interventions, women can either get pregnant naturally or undergo another attempt at artificial fertilization because a regulated cycle clearly increases the success rate. These experiences distinctly highlight the importance of holistic menstrual regulation in the treatment of infertility.

■ Physiology of the Menstrual Cycle

When we compare the physiology of the female organism from the biomedical perspective with the way in which TCM looks at it, we find many similarities and overlaps, but also some basic differences.

The Female Menstrual Cycle from the Biomedical Perspective

From the biomedical perspective, as a rule one egg from the pool of prenatally formed egg cells that enter a dormant stage after birth becomes fertilizable from the onset of puberty on under the cyclical influence of the hormones. In the ideal case, this hormonal cycle takes 28 days, but can deviate by 3–5 days. Around the 10th–14th day of the cycle, ovulation takes place. In this context, it is considered normal if ovulation fails to take place once or twice a year even in healthy women. The female cycle is divided into two phases in accordance with the stages of follicle formation:
- the follicular phase and
- the luteal phase (phase of the corpus luteum)

The regulation of the menstrual cycle is directed by the hypothalamus, which stimulates the hypophysis by releasing GnRH (gonatotropin releasing hormone), to secrete the follicle-stimulating hormone (FSH). In this way, the monthly cycle is set in motion.

Follicular Phase
The **follicular phase** begins with the first day of the cycle, that is, with the first day of the menstrual period. Under the influence of the FSH, a group of egg cells begins to mature in the ovaries. Among

these, the dominant follicle synthesizes the estrogen estradiol and inhibin. When a certain inhibin level is reached, this blocks FSH synthesis and thereby any additional stimulation of egg cells and their follicles. Only the dominant and most developed egg cell survives the shut-off of FSH and transforms into the Graafian follicle. The estrogen level, which has risen as well, triggers a rapid increase of luteinizing hormone (LH) from the hypophysis. This causes ovulation.

Parallel to the maturing of the ovum, estrogen is released in the uterus. This triggers the formation of a new mucous membrane, 0.8–1 cm thick and relatively poor in secretions, on top of the basal layer of the endometrium that was left over from the previous menstruation. This stage is called the proliferative phase.

Luteal Phase (Corpus Luteum Phase)

After the egg has left the ovary, the remaining tissue transforms into the corpus luteum, which now begins to produce progesterone. This is responsible for converting the endometrium by means of secretions, as a result of which the endometrium swells more strongly and at the same time becomes able, as tissue rich in glycogen, lipids, and enzymes, to nurture a fertilized ovum. This is referred to as the so-called **secretory phase**.

The fertilization of the egg takes place in the fallopian tube. While the fertilized ovum is moving down the fallopian tube to the uterus, as a trophoblast it is already secreting human chorionic gonadotropin (hCG), which preserves the function of the corpus luteum and even causes a rise in progesterone production. Without hCG, the lifespan of the corpus luteum is only 14 days. This so-called measurable pregnancy hormone indicates the additional changes of the endometrium in the case of a pregnancy, referred to as **decidualization**. Essential for the further development of the endometrium is progesterone, which causes additional changes in the stroma cells, epithelial glands, leucocytes, and arteries, making implantation possible in the first place.

If no fertilization and therefore no implantation of the ovum in the endometrium takes place, the corpus luteum disintegrates and the progesterone level drops, as a result of which the microcirculation of the endometrium is impaired. This leads to the rejection of the tissue, and the **menstrual period** begins.

Female Physiology from the TCM Perspective

In TCM, we know of four functions in which female physiology differs from male physiology:
- menstruation
- vaginal discharge
- pregnancy
- birth

The Uterus and the Extraordinary Vessels

Modern TCM pays special attention to the **uterus** (*bao gong* 胞宫). As an extraordinary organ, the uterus combines the properties of both viscera and bowels in one. In its role as a viscus, it stores essence, blood, and the fetus; as bowel, it opens during ovulation to receive sperm, as well as during menstruation and during birth.

Because of its special position, the uterus is connected neither to the viscera and bowels nor to the regular channels, but depends for its supply on:
- the eight extraordinary vessels (*qi jing ba mai* 奇经八脉)
- the uterine vessel (*bao mai* 胞脉)
- the uterine network vessels (*bao luo* 胞络)

As vessels, these structures either receive or release *qi* as needed.

The extraordinary vessels relevant for gynecology include the thoroughfare vessel (*chong mai*, 冲脉), the controlling vessel (*ren mai*, 任脉), and the governing vessel (*du mai*, 督脉), as well as the girdling vessel (*dai mai*, 带脉). The *chong mai* is regarded as the sea of blood and of the 12 channels, the *ren mai* as the sea of the *yin* channels, and the *du mai* as the sea of the *yang* channels. The *dai mai* as the girdling vessel unites all extraordinary vessels, regulates the connection between the upper and lower parts of the body as well as the connection between the fluids, and, like a belt, performs a holding function.

The *chong mai*, filled predominantly with blood (*xue* 血), nourishes the uterus and pregnancy. After pregnancy, the *chong mai* conducts the blood, which is now no longer needed for nurturing the fetus, as milk to the breast. Outside of pregnancy and lactation, it stores the blood before the menstrual period. The *chong mai* is supported in these functions by the *ren mai*. In their effect on menstruation, these two extraordinary vessels are intimately connected. The *ren mai*, which is filled with essence (*jing* 精) and *qi* (气), forms an important pair with the *chong mai*, reflecting the relationship between blood and *qi* in women. In addition, the *ren mai* also controls the timely occurrence of menstruation and is connected to the *du mai*, whose *yang* activity is balanced by the *ren mai*. The *du mai* warms the uterus by distributing the *ming men* (life gate) fire, which is important especially in the second half of the menstrual cycle.

The *ren mai*, *du mai*, and *chong mai* all originate in the uterus and thereby share the same source, while the *dai mai* rises out of the kidneys. All extraordinary vessels are connected to the *dai mai*. For this reason, we can also indirectly achieve a regulation of any functions of the other three extraordinary vessels by means of the *dai mai*.

A commonly mentioned vessel is the *bao mai* (胞脉), which links the heart and the uterus. Some schools see it as a branch of the *chong mai*, while others see it as the connection between the heart, uterus, and kidney. Additionally, it is said to play an important role in ovulation.[12]

All the above-mentioned vessels have an extremely intimate connection to the kidney. Even though they do not all originate directly from the kidney, they are indirectly linked to it via the smaller *bao luo*, which supply the uterus. The kidney itself is directly linked to the uterus via the *bao luo* and supplies it with essence.

The Relationship Between *Qi* and Blood

As we can see from most classical formulas (e. g., the formula *Dang Gui Shao Yao San* [Chinese Angelica and Peony Powder] from the *Jin Gui Yao Lüe*), treatment for regulating menstrual periods originally focused on balancing *qi* and blood. By contrast, the therapeutic approach today aims more commonly at affecting the viscera and bowels. Ultimately, the art of gynecology lies in the ability to bring these two—*qi* and blood—into harmony. *Qi* and blood regulate each other: thus, blood functions as the mother of *qi* by nourishing *qi*, while *qi* in turn forms the blood, moves and circulates it, and holds it in the channels.

If *qi* is exhausted, this can subsequently lead to blood vacuity as well, which affects menstruation in the form of delayed or reduced menstrual periods. If *qi* fails to contain the blood in the channels, the result is bleeding. If *qi* stops moving, the circulation of blood is impaired, which results in blood stasis.

Weakness in the blood, on the other hand, means that *qi* loses its foundation and consequently ascends upward and outward. Blood vacuity can lead to wind and because of reduced fluidity to blood stasis. Any form of blood stasis in turn impairs the formation of new blood. Severe blood loss is bound to also mean a loss of essence (*jing*) because essence and blood are closely connected in women.

The Viscera and Bowels

The viscera (*zang* 脏) and bowels (*fu* 腑) carry out all the physiological functions in the body. Because the viscera form *qi* and blood, they are essential also in connection with the relationship between *qi* and blood and for menstruation. This is the reason for our contemporary therapeutic approach to treat menstrual disorders primarily via the viscera and bowels. The most important viscera for the **formation of blood** are:

* the spleen
* the heart
* the kidney

The function of **controlling the blood** is performed by the following viscera:

* the spleen
* the liver
* the heart

It is always the *qi* of the relevant viscera that is responsible for these functions.

The **heart** (*xin* 心) is regarded as the ruler of the internal organs. In principle, it only plays a secondary role in gynecology, but because of the psychological strain that women with fertility problems experience and because of its role as a blood-forming organ, we should still always consider the heart as well, especially since it can affect all other organ functions. In addition, the heart is directly linked to the uterus through the *bao mai*. The notion that the *bao mai* is associated with the heart and sends the blood down to the uterus via the heart comes from the Qing period (1644–1911).

The main source of blood is the **spleen** (*pi* 脾). From excess *qi* and *yin* essence, it forms blood and postnatal essence (*jing*), with which it can in turn enrich the kidney and thereby contribute to the woman's fertility. This is all the more important because from about the age of 40 on, the kidney is exhausted and needs to be supplied with essence from the center. The prenatal source of blood is the kidney. With its essence, it provides important building blocks for the formation of blood.

The **liver** (*gan* 肝) regulates the circulation of *qi* and stores the blood. It decides how much blood is in circulation and fills the *chong mai* with blood. In its important function of blood storage, some physicans of old regarded it as the source of prenatal *qi* (*xian tian zhi qi* 先天之气) in women—a role that is normally attributed to the kidney. This makes regulating the liver a key issue in all gynecological problems.

The **kidney** (*shen* 肾) is the carrier of prenatal *qi* and thereby supports growth and reproductivity. Sharing the same *yin* root (kidney water) with the liver, the kidney supports the functions of the liver, but at the same time stabilizes the functions of the spleen by its *yang* activity (kidney fire):

> The liver, spleen, and kidney are therefore the most important viscera for female physiology.

The Heavenly Water and the Menstrual Cycle

The **heavenly water** (*tian gui* 天癸) is that part of kidney essence that is responsible for human growth and sexual maturity. The activity of the *tian gui* becomes apparent in girls when, around the age of 14, the kidney matures, the *chong mai* overflows, and the *ren mai* opens. This signifies the arrival of menarche. Menstruation is hence the result of the harmonic cooperation of the *tian gui*, the extraordinary vessels, and *qi* and blood with the uterus.

The **menstrual cycle** (*yue jing* 月经) is divided into four phases:

* the menstrual phase
* the follicular phase
* the ovulatory phase
* the luteal phase

The beginning of the monthly period also marks the end of an old and the start of a new cycle. When *yang* is at its highest level, the menstrual period begins. This means that the *chong mai* empties itself and thereby makes room for new *yin*. After as complete a discharge as possible, *yin* begins to increase and *yang* continues to decline from the fifth to the 10th day. This phase corresponds to the follicular phase in biomedicine (see p. 42ff., 178). The so-called ovulatory phase lasts from the 10th to the 14th day. During these days, *yin* reaches its peak and then transforms into *yang*. At this transition point, ovulation takes place.

The post-ovulatory and premenstrual phase describes the time from ovulation to menstruation. Here, *yang* assumes the dominant position and consumes *yin*. The activity of *yang* is reflected in a basal temperature curve and corresponds to the luteal phase. From the 25th day on, the body begins to prepare for the forthcoming menstruation whose onset concludes the cycle, if conception has not taken place.

■ Distinctive Features in Diagnosis and Treatment

Distinctive Features in Diagnosis

Questioning a female patient about her menstrual cycle is an essential prerequisite for making an accurate diagnosis and corresponding therapy in fertility treatment. A **healthy menstrual period** recurs every 28–30 days and lasts for about 5 days. The menstrual fluids should be discharged without pain and without dribbling bleeding at the beginning or end. The discharged blood can be absorbed by four to five sanitary pads or tampons per day. The blood itself should be neither too runny nor too sticky, without accumulations of lumps or phlegm. The color of normal menses is deep red, almost as if caused by a cut.

Any deviations from the description above offer clues to a woman's disease pattern and are discussed in detail in each of the corresponding menstrual disorders below. If delayed periods have occurred ever since the beginning of menarche, this can certainly constitute the individual cycle of a woman, which is then to be judged as normal.

> **In general, the following applies**: the timing of the menstrual cycle and the volume of blood indicate cold and heat; the color and consistency of the menstrual blood indicate vacuity or repletion.

As such, menstrual periods that arrive too early or are too heavy point to **heat**, while delayed and scanty menstrual periods can indicate **cold**. Irregularly appearing periods suggest *qi* **stagnation**. Brownish and runny menses are a manifestation of **vacuity**; bright red and thick menses indicate **repletion**. In clinical practice, our task lies in synthesizing the different, simultaneously occurring signs into a diagnosis.

Distinctive Features in Therapy

According to the author's personal experience, it is always important in the treatment of gynecological problems to record the exact date of the menstrual periods. This is the only way that we can ensure a precise assessment of the results of any treatment. Only after we have collected the gynecological facts (including the previous history of the patient, the date of her menarche, the entirety of symptoms related to menstruation, lower body disorders, births, etc.), can we then look at additional symptoms that represent the relationship between *qi* and blood and subsequently the functions of the viscera and bowels. For this purpose, the usual questions, for example about defecation, urination, digestion, or sweating, in combination with pulse and tongue diagnosis, offer clues to localize the disturbance more precisely. In certain cases, it can make sense to work with a basal temperature curve.

Sometimes it becomes necessary during treatment to work with the different phases of the cycle, to support the physiological processes that are natural in each specific phase instead of working against them. We point out such instances in the relevant disease patterns below.

As a rule, we can say that if you want to supplement, it is important to avoid using medicinals that are too warming or too drying. In any strategy, we have to guarantee that blood and *yin* are maintained and protected. When working with *yang*, we always have to look after *yin* at the same time. If it makes sense therapeutically to drain heat to reduce excessive menstrual bleeding, for example, we should use very cold medicinals only as briefly as necessary. Astringing substances to stanch bleeding are permissible, but may not be used at the very beginning of the period, to avoid impeding the natural discharge of blood or even

triggering a stasis. It is also important to note that long-lasting periods tend to be at least partly related to blood stasis.

One of the difficulties in presenting treatment here lies in the differences between various therapeutic approaches. Some practitioners work in accordance with the menstrual cycle and write a number of prescriptions (formulas) during one cycle; others attach less value to the cycle and only give one prescription in a single menstrual cycle, but use it deliberately with exact timing. The author tends to follow the latter practice and give a maximum of two prescriptions, usually only one. Some practitioners view the kidney as the crucial organ in the treatment of fertility disorders, others the liver. Furthermore, practitioners today often combine biomedical knowledge with TCM, which can occasionally make a lot of sense but should not distract from the Chinese perspective and diagnostics.

> Important to note: even though TCM goes out of its way to follow natural methods, if you fail to achieve results with these, the valuable diagnostic procedures of biomedicine offer the certainty of not overlooking serious disorders! Cooperating with a biomedical gynecologist in this area is therefore indispensable!

General Pathology

Menstrual disorders are related to the **timing of the cycle**, that is, menstrual periods arriving too early, too late, or irregularly, to the **volume**, that is, the heaviness and duration of the bleeding (e. g., a short or scant menstruation, a heavy or long menstruation), as well as bleeding that occurs outside of the regular time of menstruation (*beng lou* 崩漏, "flooding and spotting", see p. 192). To summarize these bleeding patterns in terms of content and therapy, the author has chosen a system that differs from common gynecology texts:

- **Excessive bleeding.** All menstrual disorders that involve excessive bleeding are treated consecutively because the relevant TCM principles repeat themselves here. This includes both an abbreviated cycle and profuse menstruation, i. e., periods that are heavier or longer than normal.

- **Dysfunctional bleeding**. By this, we mean bleeding that occurs outside the cycle, such as *beng lou*, intermenstrual bleeding, and spotting. These are discussed afterwards.
- **Insufficient bleeding**. Menstrual disorders that involve any insufficient discharge of blood, namely delayed menstruation and scant menstruation, that is, menstruation that is too scant or too short, are discussed consecutively as well. The last item in this group is amenorrhea.
- **Menstruation at irregular intervals**.
- **Dysmenorrhea**. Lastly, we cover painful menstruation.

For all these disease patterns, the author has selected representative formulas that are intended to increase our understanding of the treatment of menstrual disorders. In borderline cases, the author has oriented herself by the way in which these subjects are treated in China today. Most of the formulas mentioned in this chapter can be found in standard gynecology texts. This does not mean that there are not many other formulas that could be used. In clinical practice, though, we often find that the combination of patterns and symptoms, personal circumstances, and the causes of menstrual disorders differ greatly from patient to patient and therefore require a flexible approach to the selection of formulas and individual substances. Very famous formulas are hereby only mentioned by name, the author's personal experiences have been incorporated.

■ Excessive Bleeding

This group subsumes abbreviated cycles and menstrual periods that are too heavy or last too long. The volume of blood lost in a menstrual period is determined by its duration and heaviness. This means that the periods discussed here do not necessarily involve heavier than normal bleeding. A period that has arrived too early or lasts too long can also be very weak. From the perspective of TCM, these disturbances nevertheless all require similar treatment principles and are therefore described here in the same context.

Abbreviated Cycle—*Yue Jing Xian Qi* (月经先期)

Both TCM and biomedicine regard a menstrual cycle of up to 25 days as normal. If the cycle is shorter than that, though, this can have an effect on the woman's ability to conceive.

Causes and Disease Development

From the **biomedical perspective**, the following possibilities present themselves: an abbreviation of the follicular phase or of the luteal phase. A disturbance in the follicular phase leads to insufficient maturation of the egg cell and results in problems in the luteal phase, with reduced preparedness for pregnancy and an increased rate of miscarriages. Most of the time, though, the luteal phase is too short. It should last for at least 12 days. An abbreviated luteal phase often shows a weakness of the luteinizing hormone that resulted from a disturbance in the follicular phase even if this was not abbreviated. In cases with a weakness of luteinizing hormone, the nidation of a fertilized egg cell is no longer guaranteed. If the period arrives even earlier, it is questionable whether ovulation has taken place at all.

From the **TCM perspective**, the cycle is often shortened due to heat or to *qi* vacuity, causing an inadequate build-up of *yin* in the postmenstrual phase. Causes for abbreviated periods are:
- blood heat
- insufficiency of *qi*
- blood stasis
- damp-heat

They are listed here in the order of their frequency. Accordingly, damp-heat is the least common cause.

Blood Heat

Blood heat disturbs the regulation of the *chong mai* and *ren mai*. Blood heat is the most common cause for a shortened menstrual cycle, whereby we must distinguish between **repletion heat** (which includes stagnation heat as well) and **vacuity heat**. Medicinals should be ingested if possible at the beginning of the first half of the cycle so that we can influence a premature ovulation.

183

Repletion Heat—Shi Re (实热)

In repletion heat, heat penetrates into the blood-storing *chong mai* and causes heavy and premature bleeding. This pattern mostly affects women with a strong *yang* constitution who furthermore have been consuming heating foods and alcohol and tobacco. These "power women" do not feel nearly as exhausted after heavy bleeding as, for example, women with *qi* vacuity.

Symptoms

Thick, bright red or purple blood, increased blood flow, typically also a feeling of heat in the genital area during the discharge of blood, yellow urine, constipation, thirst, and a red face. The tongue is red with a yellow fur, the pulse is rapid and string-like or slippery.

Treatment Principle

Clear repletion heat, cool the blood, and secure the *chong mai*.

The following formulas all clear repletion heat with cold bitter drugs. For this reason, we must not prescribe them during menstruation because they can otherwise cause blood stasis and further complicate the situation. To push the onset of the menstrual period back in cases with premature bleeding, the best time for taking medicinals is in the first phase of the cycle—that is, directly after the end of the period. At this point of the menstrual cycle, formulas should be very balanced in their thermal nature. We therefore prescribe very cold formulas only after ovulation, and only until 3 days before the expected onset of menstruation, to reduce the amount of discharged blood at the very beginning of the period. During very heavy periods, you can also administer astringing or blood-stanching substances in addition, to better control the period and avoid excessive blood loss.

Medicinal Therapy

The following formula represents the classic treatment principle found in any number of gynecology texts. It gently treats repletion heat, nourishes blood, and is suitable for taking right after the menstrual period.

Rx. Qing Jing San *(Menses-clearing Powder)*[20]:
- *mu dan pi* (Moutan cortex), 6 g
- *bai shao yao* (Paeoniae radix alba), 6 g
- *sheng di huang* (Rehmanniae radix exsiccata seu recens), 6 g
- *di gu pi* (Lycii cortex), 15 g
- *qing hao* (Artemisiae annuae herba), 6 g
- *fu ling* (Poria), 3 g
- *huang bai* (Phellodendri cortex), 1.5 g

Modifications:
- If the bleeding has persisted for a long time and the *qi* is weakened, we can support the center with *dang shen* (Codonopsis radix), *bai zhu* (Atractylodis macrocephalae rhizoma), and *huang qi* (Astragali radix). Remove *fu ling* if the bleeding has persisted for a long time, because it damages the *yin* fluids.
- If the consuming heat has damaged the fluids in the blood and blood stasis has become part of the disease dynamic, we can add medicinals like *yi mu cao* (Leonuri herba) and *qian cao* (Rubiae radix). *Pu huang* (Typhae pollen) is a good choice as well. Instruct patients with heavy periods to dry-roast the powder in a skillet to increase its blood-stanching effect.
- During menstruation, we can add *yi mu cao* and *san qi* (Notoginseng radix). To stanch an overly heavy period; we can also use substances like *di yu* (Sanguisorbae radix), *qian cao, huai hua* (Sophorae flos), *xiao ji* (Cirsii herba), or *da ji* (Cirsii japonici herba seu radix).

In cases of pronounced blood vacuity due to premature menstrual periods, the following simple formula is particularly appropriate. Its application is, however, only indicated in cases with *yang ming* repletion heat, or in other words, the presence of damp-heat in the center, which the formula clears with Scutellariae radix (*huang qin*) and Coptidis rhizoma (*huang lian*).

Rx. *Qin Lian Si Wu Tang* (Scutellaria and Coptis Four Agents Decoction)[7]:
- *Si Wu Tang* (Four Agents Decoction) plus:
- *huang qin*
- *huang lian*

Additional Modifications:
- Instead of *shu di huang* (Rehmanniae radix praeparata), it certainly makes sense to use *sheng di huang* because it not only cools the blood but also stanches bleeding.
- In addition to *sheng di huang*, Maciocia additionally uses *mai men dong* (Ophiopogonis radix), to nourish *yin* and cool the blood.[13]

The following formula also combines blood-nourishing with blood-cooling substances, forcefully clears repletion heat, and stabilizes the center and the kidney. It is very effective.

Rx. *Bao Yin Jian* (Yin-safeguarding Brew)[21]:
* *shu di huang*, 9 g
* *sheng di huang*, 9 g
* *huang qin*, 9 g
* *huang bai*, 9 g
* *bai shao yao*, 9 g
* *shan yao* (Dioscoreae rhizoma), 9 g
* *xu duan* (Dipsaci radix), 9 g
* *gan cao* (Glycyrrhizae radix), 6 g

Shan yao consolidates the *chong mai*; *xu duan* enters the *chong mai* and strengthens the kidney. It is said that you can also prescribe this formula for vacuity heat.

Modifications:
* With the addition of *e jiao* (Asini corii colla), we build blood and at the same time gently stanch menstrual periods that are too heavy or too early.
* Combine with the Rx. *Er Zhi Wan* (Double Supreme Pill) for vacuity heat.

Acupuncture Points and Combinations
* LR-1, KI-2, ST-44
* SP-1 + CV-4 + SP-6 + SP-10

Depressed Heat—Yu Re (郁热)

Heat that arises due to stagnation is called depressed heat (also *mu yu hua huo*, literally: "depressed wood transforming into fire"). The liver is especially susceptible to this pattern, in which case the liver's storage function makes it quite likely that the heat might move into the blood. This condition is a repletion heat pattern as well.

Symptoms
A shortened cycle with moderate to heavy discharge of dark blood with small clots. At the same time, we may see intermittent complaints like a feeling of pressure below the ribs, dizziness, fullness in the chest, tension in the chest, and a bitter taste in the mouth. Conspicuous also are mood swings and irritability. The tongue is livid and has a thin white or yellow fur, the pulse is stringlike and possibly rapid.

Treatment Principle
Clear liver heat, regulate the *qi*, cool the blood, and regulate menstruation.

Medicinal Therapy
In cases with latent development of heat in the liver, we can prescribe standard formulas like *Jia Wei Xiao Yao San* (Modified Free Wanderer Powder) and *Jin Ling Zi San* (Toosendan Powder), in combination with *Si Wu Tang*. The specific cause determines the different indications of these two formulas: In cases with insufficient *yang*, add *chai hu* (Bupleuri radix); in cases with insufficient *yin*, increase the amount of *chuan lian zi* (Toosendan fructus). We can prescribe these formulas in the first half of the menstrual cycle if the patient is balanced, otherwise only in the second half.

Modifications:
* For very pronounced bleeding, remove *dang gui* from the formula. It is better to add *huang qin* and *sheng di huang* to the formula than to replace *bai shao yao* with *chi shao yao* (Paeoniae radix rubra), because the latter is too strongly moving.
* A proven combination for *Xiao Yao San* is *dan shen* (Salviae miltiorrhizae radix) to cool and move the blood, with *xiang fu* (Cyperi rhizoma) to move the congested *qi* even more strongly. *Dan shen* affects the *chong mai* as well.
* Very heavy periods can be cooled and stanched by adding *di yu* and *ce bai ye* (Platycladi cacumen).

Acupuncture Points and Combinations
* LR-2, LR-8, LR-14
* LR-6 + HT-4 + HT-5

Vacuity Heat—Xu Re (虚热)

Symptoms
In patients with vacuity heat, the menstrual periods are characterized by scanty amounts of blood, which are caused by an excess of heat (fire) and an insufficiency of *yin* (water). The consistency of the blood is rather thin, the color is red to dark red. Additional symptoms are: elevated temperature in the evening, hot palms and soles, disquietude, reduced thirst, a red tongue without fur, and a fine and rapid pulse.

Treatment Principle
Nourish *yin* and cool the blood.

Medicinal Therapy
The following formula supplements *yin* and the bodily fluids, to cool vacuity heat and thereby regulate menstruation. *Zeng Ye Tang* (Humor-increasing Decoction) affects the *chong mai* and forms the basis of this formula. This is complemented by *bai shao yao* (astringing and cool), *e jiao* (drawing the blood inward and thereby mildly blood-stanching), and *di gu pi* (clearing vacuity heat and affecting the blood level). The formula is outstanding for mid-cycle bleeding, which is usually caused by *yin* vacuity in combination with heat.

Rx. Liang Di Tang *(Rehmannia and Lycium Root Bark Decoction)*[20]:
• sheng di huang
• xuan shen (Scrophulariae radix)
• bai shao yao
• mai men dong
• di gu pi
• e jiao (Corii asini colla)

Modifications:
• plus *Er Zhi Wan* to stabilize kidney *yin* and stanch bleeding.

The following formula *Di Gu Pi Yin* is yet another modification of *Si Wu Tang* or *Qin Lian Si Wu Tang* (Scutellaria and Coptis). *Huang lian* and *huang qin* —which both treat repletion heat as heat dampness—are removed and replaced with *di gu pi* and *mu dan pi*, to address the vacuity heat.

Rx. Di Gu Pi Yin *(Lycium Root Bark Beverage)*[7]
• dang gui
• sheng di huang
• bai shao yao
• chuan xiong (Chuanxiong rhizoma)
• di gu pi
• mu dan pi

Acupuncture Points and Combinations
• SP-8, KI-5, KI-14, KI-2, KI-8
• CV-6 + LR-1 + KI-10 + LR-3

Insufficiency of *Qi*

Securing and holding are functions of the spleen and kidney. When we can no longer discern these functions, this can point to an insufficiency of *qi* (*qi* vacuity). An insufficiency of *qi* leads to an insecurity of the *chong mai* and *ren mai* (*chong ren bu gu* 冲任不固). We distinguish between **spleen *qi* vacuity** and **kidney *qi* vacuity**. Depending on the symptoms, we either treat the spleen, the kidney, or both organs simultaneously.

Spleen *Qi* Vacuity—Pi Qi Xu *(脾气虚)*

Most early menstrual periods related to *qi* vacuity are caused by spleen *qi* vacuity. The spleen is unable to seal the channels and hence cannot hold the blood in the channels because the spleen's *yang* function of holding blood is weakened. As a result, we see early menstrual periods with pale red blood in copious amounts, which is, however, not sticky. The longer these periods last, the more they weaken the blood and accordingly lead to lighter and lighter periods.

Symptoms
Exhaustion, shortness of breath after minor straining, reduced appetite, a feeling of pressure in the abdomen, diarrhea, a pale soft tongue with a thin white fur, and a vacuous pulse.

Treatment Principle
Strengthen *qi*, secure the *ren mai* and *chong mai*, and stanch bleeding.

Medicinal Therapy
Bu Zhong Yi Qi Tang is a very popular formula for strengthening the spleen, regaining control over the blood and the *chong mai*, and lifting *qi*. It is extremely effective in the treatment of early, but also of heavy menstrual periods. The core ingredients *huang qi*, *ren shen* (Ginseng radix), and *gan cao* have a fortifying effect on the *qi*. *Chai hu* and *sheng ma* (Cimicifugae rhizoma) lift the *qi* and bring clear *yang* back to the top. In general, this formula is modified.

Modifications of Bu Zhong Yi Qi Tang *(Center-supplementing Qi-boosting Decoction):*
• For very heavy bleeding, *dang gui* is removed from the formula because its moving effect is too strong. We can add *hai piao xiao* (Sepiae

endoconcha), *long gu* (Mastodi ossis fossilia), and *mu li* (Ostreae concha).

- For long menstrual periods, we can modify the formula by adding *xue yu tan* (Crinis carbonisatus), *zong lu tan* (Trachycarpi petioli carbonisatus), and *ai ye tan* (Artemisiae argyi folium carbonisatum).

The following formula is guided by a similar attempt to lift *qi*. It is meant to supplement the insufficiency of *qi* that leads to bleeding and resulting *yang* vacuity, and thereby fortify the blood.

Rx. Ju Yuan Jian *(Origin-lifting Brew)*:
- *huang qi*, 12 g
- *ren shen*, 9 g
- *zhi gan cao* (Glycyrrhizae radix cum liquido fricta), 9 g
- *sheng ma*, 3 g
- *bai zhu*, 9 g

Modifications:
- The formula is modified most commonly with *gan jiang* (Zingiberis rhizoma) or *pao jiang* (Zingiberis rhizoma praeparatum), *ai ye* (Artemisiae argyi folium), and *hai piao xiao*, to stanch existing bleeding more quickly and prevent premature menstrual periods. By adding *e jiao*, we likewise gently stanch bleeding, while at the same time supplementing the blood.
- For severe *yang* vacuity, we can also include *rou gui* (Cinnamomi cortex) in addition to *pao jiang*.

Comparison with Bu Zhong Yi Qi Tang
Compared with *Bu Zhong Yi Qi Tang, Ju Juan Jian* focuses more on lifting the center. Citri reticulatae pericarpium (*chen pi*) is removed from *Bu Zhong Yi Qi Tang* in order to avoid its precipitating effect. Furthermore, *e jiao* is a better choice for very heavy periods than the warm and slightly moving *dang gui*. By contrast, *Bu Zhong Yi Qi Tang* instead emphasizes the lifting (*chai hu* and *sheng ma*) and precipitating (*chen pi*) effects and thereby supports the physiological function of the center. The author herself has achieved excellent results in the treatment of premature or heavy periods with *Bu Zhong Yi Qi Tang*.

If the patient suffers not only from weakness of the spleen but also from blood vacuity in the heart, *Gui Pi Tang* is indicated. In such cases, the patient also suffers from palpitations, sleep disorders, and a tendency to brooding and anxiety.

Modifications of Gui Pi Tang *(Spleen-returning Decoction)*:
- Chronic insufficiency of *qi* is bound to result in blood stasis. In this case, we can, as mentioned above, add *xue yu tan* and *zong lu tan*, which both stanch bleeding and move the blood at the same time.

Acupuncture Points and Combinations
- SP-6, SP-8, ST-25
- SP-10 + SP-1 + ST-36

Kidney Qi *Vacuity—*Shen Qi Xu *(肾气虚)*

Kidney *qi* vacuity is a common concomitant complication, even though the literature tends to discuss it as an independent cause. Women who have experienced several miscarriages or interrupted pregnancies tend towards kidney *qi* vacuity. Young girls also often lean towards kidney *qi* vacuity. According to a treatment rule in traditional Chinese gynecology, we should treat young women via the kidney, women between the ages of 21 and 42 via the liver, and older women via the spleen. As such, we should generally treat young girls with gynecological problems via the kidney anyway.

Symptoms
Early, very runny menstrual periods that in one cycle are too heavy (inability to contain) and in the next cycle are rather too light (not enough blood and essence). Pain in the lower back, urinating at night, and a deep and vacuous pulse are typical symptoms. The tongue is pale and shows a white fur.

Treatment Principle
Replenish kidney *qi* and secure the *chong mai.*

Medicinal Therapy
Rx. Gui Shen Wan *(Kidney-returning Pill)*[22]:
- *shu di huang*
- *gou qi zi* (Lycii fructus)
- *shan zhu yu* (Corni fructus)
- *shan yao*
- *tu si zi* (Cuscutae semen)
- *du zhong* (Eucommiae cortex)
- *dang gui*
- *fu ling*

- For very heavy periods that do not contain blood clots, we can work with *long gu* and *mu li* from the second or third day of the period on. If prescribed any earlier than that, they could trigger a blood stasis.
- For constipation, which is quite common in this context, Anemarrhenae rhizoma (*zhi mu*) is suitable.

Acupuncture Points and Combinations
- SP-1, ST-25, CV-7
- KI-3 + SP-1 + BL-12 + GV-27

Vacuity Heat—Xu Re (虚热)

Vacuity heat can lead to prolonged periods that, as expected, are not profuse.

Symptoms
Dribbling red menstrual periods, a dry throat with little thirst, dry stools, a red tongue with scant fur, and a rapid and thin pulse or a superficial vacuous pulse in the *chi* position.

Treatment Principle
Cool heat, nourish *yin*, and regulate menstruation.

Medicinal Therapy
To treat this pattern, the formula *Liang Di Tang* is indicated, often in combination with *Er Zhi Wan*. You can prescribe this formula after the period, but beware that it should not be taken during the period. If the period does not stop in spite of treatment, stanch the bleeding from the sixth day on with astringing medicinals.

Modifications:
- To make the formula stronger, you can add *huang bai*.
- If the periods are accompanied by mild pain, move the blood until 3 days before the onset of the period with *yi mu cao* and *pu huang*.
- Once you have eliminated the possibility of blood stasis, you can use *long gu* and *mu li*, for example, for the purpose of containment. They have a very strong astringing effect.

Acupuncture Points and Combinations
- KI-5, KI-6, ST-25, CV-5, KI-7
- KI-1 + KI-6 + KI-10 + SP-6

Blood Stasis—*Xue Yu* (血瘀)

In blood stasis, the blood is unable to enter the channels and therefore flows irregularly. The causes of blood stasis are manifold. A typical background in such conditions is myomas or abortions and miscarriages, in which the uterus was subsequently scraped out. Depending on the severity of the blood stasis, you can start moving blood as early as 10 days before the onset of menstruation, and only prescribe the formula until the period is finished. For milder blood stasis, support the discharge of blood only during the period itself.

Symptoms
Heavy periods with dark crimson blood and blood clots, and abdominal pain that is relieved upon discharge of the blood clots. The tongue is crimson with purple spots.

Treatment Principle
Quicken the blood and eliminate blood stasis to regulate the *chong mai*.

Medicinal Therapy
Rx. Shi Xiao San *(Sudden Smile Powder), toasted, plus:*
- *yi mu cao*
- *san qi*
- *qian cao* or

Rx. Tao Hong Si Wu Tang *in combination with* Shi Xiao San.
Modifications:
- If heat in the blood is contributing to the blood stasis, replace *bai shao yao* in this formula before the onset of menstruation with *chi shao yao* and add *mu dan pi*. Both of these medicinals should, however, be removed during the menstrual period to avoid an effect that is too strongly moving.
- If the blood stasis is pronounced, balance the formulas so that you can start moving blood right after the end of the period: blood-building medicinals like *e jiao* and *bai shao yao* are very important in this case.
- For heavy periods with simultaneous heat, balance with *xuan shen* or *sha shen* (Adenophorae seu glehniae radix), for *yin* vacuity, for example, with the formula *Er Zhi Wan*.

Acupuncture Points and Combinations
- SP-8, SP-6, CV-3
- KI-8 + KI-10 + LR-3 + SP-6

Insufficiency of *Qi*

An insufficiency of *qi* leads to insecurity of the *chong mai and ren mai* (*chong ren bu gu* 冲任不固). In early menstrual periods due to insufficiency of *qi* (*qi* vacuity) and in overly heavy and long periods, the accompanying symptoms are identical (see p. 186). The kidney can be involved in this case as well. In patients with overly heavy periods, the treatment focuses on directing *qi* upward and stanching and astringing bleeding, to minimize the loss of *yin* substances as quickly as possible. Prolonged periods that are caused by *qi* vacuity are easy to treat.

Symptoms
The loss of so much pale and runny blood manifests in symptoms like dizziness, palpitations, pronounced fatigue, shortness of breath upon exertion, and paleness; a pale and dry tongue and a vacuous pulse complete the picture.

Treatment Principle
Stimulate *qi*, nourish the blood, and secure the *ren mai* and *chong mai* to regulate menstruation.

Medicinal Therapy
All the formulas mentioned in this chapter for insufficiency of *qi*, such as *Bu Zhong Yi Qi Tang, Ju Yuan Jian*, and *Gui Pi Tang* are also indicated here, but we should emphasize the *qi*-raising function in all of them.

Modifications for Overly Heavy Periods:
- To raise *qi*, add or emphasize *sheng ma, chai hu*, and *huang qi*.
- Supplement the blood with *e jiao, he shou wu* (Polygoni multiflori radix) or *shu di huang*. For weakness of the center, you can also add *sha ren* (Amomi fructus), to make *shu di huang* easier to digest and at the same time direct it into the *chong mai*.
- To stanch very heavy bleeding, we can use *ai ye, pao jiang*, and *hai piao xiao. Duan long gu* (Mastodi ossis fossilia calcinata) and *duan mu li* (Ostreae concha calcinata) are indicated as well.

Acupuncture Points and Combinations
- KI-8, ST-30, CV-7, SP-1, HT-5
- CV-7 + SP-6 + BL-20 + BL-18 + SP-1

Damp-heat

Inflammations in the lower abdomen can serve as the cause of damp-heat. In clinic, we often see this in women with IUDs. From the perspective of TCM, this pathology is understood either as damp-heat invading from the outside or in the context of weakness of the center, as a result of which the transformation of dampness is impaired. Damp-heat leads to disharmony of the *chong mai* and *ren mai* (*shi re chong ren bu tiao* 湿热冲任不调). After sinking down, dampness quickly forms heat by means of the *ming men* fire in the lower burner. If dampness is more prevalent than heat, damp-heat tends to manifest in prolonged periods because the dampness obstructs the normal flow of blood through the channels; if heat is more prevalent, we are more likely to see heavier bleeding.

Symptoms
Scant and dark menstrual periods, often malodorous, which do not stop. Before the onset of menstruation, profuse malodorous vaginal discharge and a feeling of heaviness in the body, especially in the legs. Diffuse abdominal pain also when not menstruating, a red tongue with a yellow sticky fur, and a soggy or slippery pulse, especially in the *guan* or *chi* positions.

Treatment Principle
Eliminate dampness, clear heat, and stanch bleeding.

Medicinal Therapy
We combine cold and warm medicinals to cool heat while at the same time supporting the center. This formula is prescribed while the patient is not menstruating.

Rx. Si Miao Wan (*Mysterious Four Pill*):
- *huang bai*
- *yi yi ren* (Coicis semen)
- *cang zhu* (Atractylodis rhizoma)
- *huai niu xi* (Achyranthis bidentatae radix)

Modifications:

- For inflammations in the lower abdomen, the formula is often supplemented with *ren dong teng* (Lonicerae caulis), a good medicinal for lower abdominal inflammations, with *guan zhong* (Aspidii rhizoma) to clear heat and promote uterine contractions, or with *ma chi xian* (Portulacae herba), a mild toxin-clearing medicinal. In these cases, *bai jiang cao* (Patriniae herba) is indicated as well.
- You can add *chun gen pi* (Toonae radicis cortex) when the damp-heat is almost completely cleared because of its astringent effect.
- To stanch bleeding, *di yu*, *qian cao*, and *yi mu cao* are indicated.

Acupuncture Points and Combinations

- SP-8, SP-9, CV-3
- ST-28 + CV-6 + SP-10 + KI-20

■ Dysfunctional Bleeding

This section includes the following three topics:
- acyclic bleeding
- intermenstrual bleeding
- spotting

TCM sees all these forms of vaginal bleeding as dysfunctional bleeding, even though they might fall into different categories from the biomedical perspective.

Acyclic Bleeding—*Beng Lou* (崩漏, Flooding and Spotting)

Bleeding that occurs outside of the menstrual period in roughly 2-day intervals, that is, intermittently, before or after the menstrual period and lasts for more than 7 days is referred to in biomedicine as **metrorrhagia**. Nevertheless, there are also combinations, in which, for example, a regular menstrual period might be connected to a new period by spotting, which is called **menometrorrhagia**. Hence, we often see both—menorrhagia and metrorrhagia—together and in combination,

in which case metrorrhagia is characterized specifically by the fact that it is impossible to discern any rhythmic progression.

The **cause** of such irregular bleeding can be found either in hormonal imbalance or in endometritis, myomas, polyps, malignancies, or other diseases.

In Chinese, such bleeding is called *beng lou*. *Beng* means "flooding," that is, sudden severe bleeding. *Lou* means "leaking," which points to persistent leaking of blood. Even though *beng* refers to an acute condition and *lou* to a chronic one, the cause is the same. Both conditions can, furthermore, merge into each other. As such, a *beng* condition can transform into a *lou* state after a serious loss of *qi* and blood; conversely, an untreated *lou* condition can become a *beng* state after *qi* is exhausted or blood stasis has formed.

As a rule, the appearance of *beng lou* is ascribed to blood heat due to repletion or vacuity heat, spleen vacuity, kidney vacuity, and blood stasis. The presence of heat and a pronounced weakness of center *qi* are seen as the most important disease triggers.

Disorders of metrorrhagia are complex and their treatment is accordingly difficult. Ye Tianshi and many other physicians of old developed suitable strategies for the successful treatment of *beng lou*.

In general, such treatments pursue three goals:
- **sai liu**: to dam the flood; in other words, to stanch the bleeding
- **cheng yuan**: to seek the source of the flooding, that is, to treat the root of the disorder
- **fu jiu**: to restore the old state, or to strengthen the root and consolidate the body

These three stages ultimately merge into each other and cannot be clearly distinguished. A correct diagnosis results in the application of the right treatment principle. In clinic, we tend to find that several consecutive strategies are relevant, often even at the same time. Representative medicinals are listed as examples:
- **to cool the blood**: *xiao ji* or *da ji*, *sheng di huang*, *mu dan pi*, *di yu*, *ce bai ye*, *qian cao*, *huang qin*, *chun gen pi*, *zhi zi* (Gardeniae fructus)
- **to warm the channels**: *ai ye*, *pao jiang*
- **to nourish the blood**: *e jiao*, *gui ban* (Testudinis plastrum), *lu jiao jiao*, *chao bai shao* (Paeoniae radix alba fricta)

- **to strengthen the *qi***: *ren shen, huang qi, zhi gan cao*
- **to lift the blood**: *sheng ma, chai hu*
- **to eliminate blood stasis**: *san qi, yi mu cao, qian cao, pu huang wu ling zhi* (Trogopteri feces), *mu dan pi, xue yu tan*
- **to astringe the blood**: *chi shi zhi* (Halloysitum rubrum), *long gu, mu li, hai piao xiao, xian he cao, xue yu tan, zong lu tan*

In particularly critical situations, we employ **emergency treatment** as an additional treatment strategy, carried out independently from the basic strategies discussed above. For this purpose, after severe bleeding we first consolidate *qi*, as the first step to enable us to stanch bleeding. The reason for this is that a critical loss of blood can lead to collapse, which primarily affects the *qi* of the center. Emergency treatments therefore call for large amounts of Korean ginseng (*ren shen*), to affect the original *qi* and to gain control over the blood:
- Rx. *Du Shen Tang* (Pure Ginseng Decoction) consists of nothing but *hong shen* (Gingseng radix rubra [red ginseng]), 15–30 g. Alternatively, you can prescribe:
- Rx. *Sheng Mai San* (Pulse-engendering Powder).

The following treatment patterns and associated symptoms have already been described above and are therefore not repeated here. It is important, however, to remember that *beng lou* generally involves a number of overlapping patterns. Because of the critical nature of the situation, though, other formulas are also indicated at times. The following disease patterns can be the cause of *beng lou*:
- blood heat
- spleen *qi* vacuity
- kidney vacuity
- blood stasis

Blood Heat—Xue Re (血热)
Heat is one of the key causes in the formation of *beng lou*. A constitutional tendency towards *yang* in combination with too much spicy food or emotional strain is usually the cause of this type of uterine bleeding. We distinguish between **repletion heat** and **vacuity heat**.

Repletion Heat—Shi Re (实热)
This kind of *beng lou* is characterized by a sudden onset, most commonly before the onset of the regular menstrual period.

Symptoms
The blood is thick, bright red, and profuse. This is often accompanied by rising heat sensations, thirst, constipation, nervousness, and insomnia. The tongue is red with a yellow fur; the pulse is rapid and stringlike or slippery.

Treatment Principle
Clear heat, cool and nourish the blood, and stanch bleeding.

Medicinal Therapy
Rx. Qing Re Gu Jing Tang *(Heat-clearing Menses-securing Decoction):*
- *duan long gu*
- *sheng di huang*
- *chao bai shao*
- *gui ban*
- *duan mu li*
- *zhi zi*
- *huang qin*
- *e jiao*
- *zong lu tan*
- *di yu*
- *xue yu tan*
- *xi yang shen* (Panacis quinquefolii radix)

This formula works on different levels at the same time: it cools the blood, eliminates heat and dampness, stanches bleeding, supplements blood and *yin*, and stabilizes the *qi*. Note also that most of the ingredients are prepared in such a way as to increase their blood-stanching effect.

Modifications:
- *Di gu pi* could be a good substitution here. Be careful with *mu dan pi* in this case because it has a moving effect!
- Some authors simply use *gan cao* to supplement *qi* instead of *xi yang shen*.
- To stanch bleeding, we can, of course, consider additional medicinals like: *ce bai ye*, for very profuse bleeding *ou jie*, and *xian he cao*, which seals incessant bleeding and can stanch bleeding anywhere, regardless of heat or cold, vacuity or repletion.

Acupuncture Points and Combinations

- SP-10, KI-2, TB-1, LR-14
- SP-10 + SP-1 + ST-36

Vacuity Heat Due to Yin Vacuity—Yin Xu Re (阴虚热)

This type of bleeding is more likely to occur after the end of the menstrual period and to continue dribbling for a long time.

Symptoms

Dizziness, disquietude, heat sensations toward the evening, hot palms and soles, a red dry furless tongue, and a fine and rapid pulse.

Treatment Principle

Nourish *yin* and cool the blood.

Medicinal Therapy

Under these circumstances, we recommend the above-mentioned *Bao Yin Jian* for vacuity heat, in place of *Liang Di Tang*—which is here often modified with *Er Zhi Wan* plus *gui ban*.

Modifications:

- *Gui ban* is an important medicinal in this pattern because it strongly nourishes *yin*, cools and stanches the blood, and at the same time affects the *ren mai* and *chong mai*.
- For heavy bleeding, appropriate blood-stanching medicinals are, for example: *xian he cao, ou jie,* or *hai piao xiao.*
- Dribbling bleeding can be influenced with *san qi* and roasted *pu huang.*

Acupuncture Points and Combinations

- KI-6, CV-4, CV-5
- KI-10 + LR-3 + SP-6

Spleen Qi Vacuity—Pi Qi Xu (脾气虚)

Spleen *qi* vacuity can lead to very heavy bleeding. The spleen is no longer able to seal the channels; the *chong mai* loses its hold and must be secured again.

Symptoms

The blood is runny and bright red. In addition, we see unformed loose stools, fatigue, paleness, and a tendency to bruising.

Treatment Principle

Supplement spleen *qi*, secure the *ren mai* and *chong mai*, and stanch bleeding.

Medicinal Therapy

The formula *Ju Yuan Jian* has an uplifting function, but must be further modified for *beng lou* conditions of bleeding with blood-stanching medicinals (see modifications). The following formula strengthens the blood and stanches bleeding.

Rx. Gu Ben Zhi Beng Tang *(Root-securing Flood-stanching Decoction):*

- *huang qi*
- *shu di huang*
- *bai zhu*
- *pao jiang*
- *dang shen*
- *dang gui*

Modifications:

- Important! Remove *dang gui* from the formula for *beng lou* disorders because it is too strongly moving. In its place, use *e jiao* or *he shou wu*.
- To stanch bleeding in heavy periods, add *xian he cao* and *hai piao xiao; ai ye tan* is also appropriate—it has a warming effect while at the same time stanching bleeding.
- For dribbling bleeding, you can add *jing jie tan* (Schizonepetae herba et flos carbonisatae) and *yi mu cao*.
- For uplifting, you can add *sheng ma* and *chai hu* and also increase the dosage of *huang qi*.

Acupuncture Points and Combinations

- CV-6, CV-7, SP-6, TB-6
- LU-7 + SI-1 + PC-7 + CV-17

Kidney Vacuity—Shen Xu (肾虚)

Medicinal Therapy

The following formula, which is related to *Zuo Gui Wan* (Left [Kidney]-restoring Pill), supplements the kidney, replenishes the *qi*, secures the *chong mai*, and regulates menstruation.

Rx. Gu Yin Jian *(Yin-securing Brew):*

- *tu si zi*
- *shu di huang*
- *shan zhu yu*
- *ren shen*

- *shan yao*
- *zhi gan cao*
- *wu wei zi* (Schisandrae fructus)
- *yuan zhi* (Polygalae radix)
- *fu pen zi* (Rubi fructus)
- *lu jiao jiao*

This formula addresses the *ren mai, chong mai, du mai*, and *dai mai* with specific medicinals. *Fu pen zi* supplements the *ren mai, shan yao* secures the *chong mai, lu jiao jiao* strengthens the *du mai*, and *wu wei zi* secures the *dai mai*.

Modifications:
- If you want to emphasize *yang* more strongly, you can add *xu duan* and *du zhong*.
- You can replace *lu jiao jiao* with *lu jiao shuang*.

Acupuncture Points and Combinations
- KI-6, CV-3, CV-5, KI-27
- KI-15 + CV-4 + BL-32 + SP-6

Blood Stasis—*Xue Yu* (血瘀)

Symptoms
In addition to the already mentioned blood clots and pain, another typical sign of blood stasis is interrupted menstruation. The period stops for 1 or 2 days and then resumes. The tongue is dark; the pulse is rough or stringlike.

Treatment Principle
Nourish the blood and eliminate blood stasis.

Medicinal Therapy
The formula *Shi Xiao San*, already recommended above for the category of early or profuse menstruation, is indicated in combination with *Si Wu Tang*.

Modifications:
- *Yi mu cao, san qi*, and *qian cao* are proven medicinals that support the blood-stanching effect of the above-mentioned formulas in addition to their cooling and moving influence.
- In cases of blood stasis due to cold, *ai ye tan* is the ingredient of choice. For heat, you can consider *di yu*. For very strong periods, we can always consider *xian he cao*.

- You can also give your patients *Yun Nan Bai Yao* (Stop Bleeding Powder) to take at home, thereby conveying the impression that they can take something else on their own to control their periods. This is particularly effective if they are indeed suffering from blood stasis.

Acupuncture Points and Combinations
- SP-8, LU-7, LR-14
- KI-14 + BL-17 + BL-22 + ST-36

Intermenstrual Bleeding—*Jing Jian Qi Chu Xue* (经间期出血)

Intermenstrual bleeding refers to regularly occurring bleeding at the time of ovulation. Traditionally, this symptom is also called **mid-cycle bleeding**. It is characterized by an extremely scanty amount and only lasts for 1 or 2 days at the most. It arises from a temporary decline in estrogen during the rupture of the follicle.

From the perspective of TCM, bleeding during ovulation suggests the presence of heat. Experience shows that this heat in intermenstrual bleeding is most often rooted in an existing *yin* or blood vacuity. The literature often mentions liver heat, dampness with heat, and blood stasis as well, in addition to vacuity heat. When *yin* transforms into *yang* during ovulation, the hyperactivity of *yang* in women with *yin* vacuity can cause the channels to break, resulting in bleeding. In general, we speak of an insecurity of the *chong mai*.

In treatment, we give any indicated formulas from the ninth day of the cycle for 1 week, to prevent the bleeding.

The following disease patterns can be involved:
- vacuity heat
- liver heat due to *qi* stagnation
- damp-heat
- blood stasis

Vacuity Heat in Liver *Yin* Vacuity—*Shen Yin Xu Re* (肾阴虚热)

Experience shows that *Liang Di Tang* is an extremely effective base formula when we add other medicinals in accordance with presenting symptoms.

Symptoms

The light bleeding is intensely red and without clots. Disquietude, lower back pain, and a dry mouth complete the picture.

Treatment Principle

Supplement *yin*, strengthen the kidney, clear vacuity heat, and regulate menstruation.

Medicinal Therapy

Rx. Liang Di Tang *plus* :
* *Er Zhi Wan*
* *gui ban*
* *e jiao*

Modifications:
* To give additional support to kidney *yin* while at the same time securing the *chong mai*, you can also add *shan yao*.
* Dark roasted *jing jie tan* is an excellent substance for stanching the bleeding.

Some practitioners also give the formula *Wu Ji Bai Feng Wan* (literally "white phoenix, black chicken pills"), a patent remedy for building blood and *yin*, which is, however, not able to stanch bleeding. The formula *Liu Wei Di Huang Wan* (Six-ingredient Rehmannia Pill) is commonly used as well, to strengthen *yin* and thereby treat the root.

Acupuncture Points and Combinations
* KI-6, KI-27, LR-8
* LR-9 + CV-4 + BL-67 + SP-6

Depressed Heat—*Yu Re* (郁热)

If the flow of *qi* in the liver is blocked, heat can develop quite easily. In particular, *yin* or blood vacuity often facilitate the development of stasis heat. *Yang* is no longer balanced by *yin* and blood and hence harms the channels. The most popular formula for this pattern is *Jia Wei Xiao Yao San*, often modified with *huang qin* and Prunellae spica (*xia ku cao*).

Acupuncture Points and Combinations
* LR-2, LR-3, LR-8, GV-2
* LR-14 + LR-2 + SP-10

Damp-heat—*Shi Re* (湿热)

During menstruation or while lying in, damp-heat can penetrate into the extraordinary vessels (especially the *chong mai*) because they are vacuous and vulnerable during this time. Alternatively, damp-heat can arise from a weakness of the spleen, as a result of which the transformation of dampness is impaired. Absorbed by the *dai mai*, this dampness flows downward, stagnates in the lower burner, and easily transforms, also often due to the activity of the *ming men* fire, into damp-heat. At the time of ovulation, which is characterized by intense *yang* activity, the presence of damp-heat reinforces *yang qi*, further injuring the channels.

Symptoms

Regularly occurring intermenstrual bleeding with a slow onset and dark slimy blood; dark urine, vaginal discharge, fatigue and heavy extremities, a red tongue with a slimy yellow fur, and a slippery pulse.

Treatment Principle

Eliminate dampness, clear heat, and regulate menstruation.

Medicinal Therapy

Rx. Si Miao San *(Mysterious Four Powder) plus:*
* *zhi zi*
* *ma chi xian*
* *guan zhong*
* *chun gen pi*

Here, *zhi zi* is supposed to clear heat above the triple burner, *guan zhong* clears heat in the lower abdomen, and *ma chi xian* addresses toxic heat. *Chun gen pi* consolidates the *dai mai* and should therefore not be added to the very first prescription but only after the damp-heat is mostly cleared.

Acupuncture Points and Combinations
* LR-5, KI-13, SP-8, SP-9, CV-3
* ST-40 + CV-5

Blood Stasis—*Xue Yu* (血瘀)

Blood stasis impairs the function of the *chong mai* and leads to bleeding. Experience shows that this is more likely to be an accompanying pathology.

Symptoms
Mild bleeding with very dark blood and blood clots. The pulse is wiry and the tongue is crimson.

Treatment Principle
Move the blood, disperse the stasis, and regulate menstruation.

Medicinal Therapy
Rx. Zhu Yu Zhi Xue Tang (Stasis-expelling Blood-stanching Decoction)*[8]:
- *sheng di huang*
- *dang gui wei* (Angelicae sinensis radicis extremitas)
- *zhi ke* (Aurantii fructus)
- *da huang* (Rhei radix et rhizoma)
- *chi shao yao*
- *mu dan pi*
- *gui ban*
- *tao ren* (Persicae semen)

Modifications:
- Instead of the medicinal *tao ren*, which is part of the original formula, use *yi mu cao*.
- *Chai hu* is used for upbearing.

Acupuncture Points and Combinations
- LR-2, LR-5, CV-5
- CV-7 + SP-6 + CV-3 + SP-10

Spotting—*Lou* (漏)

Premenstrual spotting suggests a progesterone deficiency, while spotting after the period points more towards an estrogen deficiency.

An incomplete breakdown of the corpus luteum before the menstrual period can lead to spotting that occurs before the onset of menstruation. Occasionally, the basal temperature even fails to drop in spite of the beginning of menstruation. This would then suggest that we are dealing with a luteal deficiency whose cause in turn is found in the first phase of the cycle.

Spotting after the period indicates that the endometrium is detaching only reluctantly during menstruation. For this reason, the period continues dribbling. Sometimes new spotting recurs already after the end of the period. From the biomedical perspective, this suggests that the formation of the endometrium was not promoted sufficiently as a result of estrogen deficiency. We therefore see secondary hemorrhaging. Myomas or polyps can lead to spotting as well.

To carry out the differential diagnosis described above, a basal temperature curve is necessary. Experience shows that spotting is most often caused by **blood stasis**, but can also be related to **yin vacuity**.

Blood Stasis—*Xue Yu* (血瘀)

Premenstrual spotting with dark red blood frequently indicates blood stasis. Nevertheless, you should not move *qi* and blood before the basal temperature has dropped, after you have eliminated the possibility of a pregnancy. Any blood-moving formula that corresponds to the energetic situation of a woman, such as *Tao Hong Si Wu Tang* will then solve this problem. To promote the normal breakdown of the corpus luteum, begin the formula 3 to 4 days before the expected onset of menstruation. To support the breakdown of the endometrium, continue the formula into the first few days of the menstrual period.

Acupuncture Points and Combinations
- LR-2, LR-3, ST-25, SP-10
- SP-10 + SP-1 + ST-36

Yin Vacuity—*Yin Xu* (阴虚)

After menstruation is over, that is, on the fourth day of the cycle, we can begin to strengthen *yin*.

Symptoms
Bright red spotting indicates a *yin* vacuity. Additional symptoms like heat in the palms and soles, a red tongue with no fur, and a thin and rapid pulse should support this diagnosis.

Treatment Principle
Nourish *yin* and the blood, stanch the bleeding.

---

* Formula by Fu Qingzhu, originally for injuries of the *ren mai* and *chong mai*.[8]

Medicinal Therapy

Rx. Zhi Bai Di Huang Wan *(Anemarrhena, Phellodendron, and Rehmannia Pill)*

Modifications:

- It is important to add *gui ban* to this base formula, as well as other supplementing medicinals like *tu si zi, bai shao yao*, and the formula *Er Zhi Wan*.
- Important: if the woman could possibly be pregnant (high basal temperature), you must not prescribe medicinals that stanch bleeding, like *dan shen*, to cool and move the blood!

Acupuncture Points and Combinations

- KI-6, CV-3, CV-4, CV-5
- CV-5 + CV-7 + LR-3

■ Insufficient Bleeding

Subsumed under this heading are menstrual cycles that are too long and menstrual periods that are either too short or characterized by a scant amount of blood. Here as well, the principle that we mentioned above applies: this categorization is based on treatment strategy, even if a long cycle does not necessarily always mean a reduced loss of blood.

Delayed Menstruation—*Yue Jing Hou Qi* (月经后期)

A period that begins only after 32–35 days or even later is clinically referred to as **oligomenorrhea**. The delay is most commonly caused by a prolonged first phase of the cycle. The endometrium requires more time to form than the usual 14 days. One of the most common causes from the biomedical view is an ovarian disturbance, which points to hormonal problems and can be recognized, in addition to the basal temperature curve, by an incomplete formation of cervical mucus (disturbed follicular maturation, prolactinemia, polycystic ovary syndrome, reduced response of the ovaries to FSH, or other hormonal malfunctions). Nevertheless, eating disorders and hyperthyroidism can also result in a prolonged menstrual cycle.

From the perspective of TCM, either **vacuity** or **stagnation**, both of which prevent the regular onset of menstruation, is responsible for oligomenorrhea. Delayed menstrual cycles are caused by:

- blood vacuity
- kidney vacuity
- cold
- stagnation

They can, however, sometimes also be the result of phlegm stagnation.

Blood Vacuity—*Xue Xu* (血虚)

Blood vacuity is the most common cause of delayed menstrual cycles. As a rule, we say in TCM that women are more prone to suffer from blood vacuity than men. In women with blood vacuity, the body is unable to form sufficient blood within the regular 28 days to fill the sea of blood (*chong mai*) and the uterus for menstruation. Previous disorders, severe blood loss, long breastfeeding, or insufficient generation of blood due to spleen *qi* vacuity, often caused by excessive worrying or a long-term vegetarian diet, can lead to blood vacuity and thereby affect the sea of blood. In cases of spleen *qi* vacuity, it is important to pay attention to a good digestion and a healthy appetite. The reason for this is that the prescribed medicinals must be absorbed and transformed by the center. For this reason, we must sometimes stabilize digestion first.

Symptoms

The menstrual period, which starts only after 32 days or even later, is thin and pale pink or watery and brownish. The patient is pale, suffers from stupor or dizziness, dry skin or dry eyes, and physical weakness, is thin, and fails to gain weight. Sleeping disturbances may be present as well. Dull pain in the lower abdomen that is relieved by pressure is always mentioned in the literature but has rarely been observed in clinic so far. The tongue is pale red, without any fur, and dry; the pulse is floating and vacuous or fine. Loose stools and a reduced appetite indicate that the center is not functioning properly.

Treatment Principle

Nourish the blood (and supplement *qi*), to fill the *chong mai* and regulate menstruation.

Medicinal Therapy

Rx. Xiao Ying Jian *(Minor* Construction *Decoction):*
- *dang gui*
- *shu di huang*
- *bai shao yao*
- *shan yao*
- *gou qi zi*
- *gan cao*

In patients with delayed menstrual periods, you can prescribe this formula as the basis for supplementing blood immediately after menstruation from the fifth day on, to strengthen the reconstruction of the endometrium. It directs its focus clearly to the extraordinary vessels. *Dang gui*, the best medicinal for filling the extraordinary vessels, fills the *chong mai*, while *gou qi zi* directs the supplementing formula additionally to the *ren mai* and *du mai. Shan yao* secures the *chong mai.* In cases with *qi* vacuity, however, add *qi*-supplementing substances to the formula.

It is also obvious that the formula addresses the blood as the *yin* aspect. As in the following formulas, the most important blood-building formula *Si Wu Tang* is here represented as the base formula.

Modifications:
- For existing spleen *qi* vacuity: *dang shen* and *bai zhu.* Both of these supplement the function of the spleen.
- For loose stools: *sha ren.*
- For insomnia and low-quality sleep: *suan zao ren* (Ziziphi spinosi semen), *wu wei zi*, and *yuan zhi.*
- For blood vacuity that is compounded by *yin* vacuity, the formula *Er Zhi Wan: nü zhen zi* (Ligustri lucidi fructus), *han lian cao* (Ecliptae herba), and *di gu pi.*
- For blood vacuity that is connected to *qi* stagnation: see p. 201.
- For the presence of cold: *du zhong, rou gui*, and *huai niu xi.*

The following formula puts its main emphasis on the center and the heart. Use it in cases where states of disquietude and the longing for a child have begun to affect and impair blood formation. It is based on the formulas *Si Jun Zi Tang* (Four Gentlemen Decoction), *Dang Gui Bu Xue Tang* (Chinese Angelica Blood-supplementing Decoction),

and *Si Wu Tang*, without *chuan xiong* but with the addition of *rou gui, yuan zhi*, and *wu wei zi.*

Rx. Ren Shen Yang Rong Tang *(Ginseng Construction-nourishing Decoction)*[7]:
- *ren shen*
- *huang qi*
- *dang gui*
- *bai shao yao*
- *shu di huang*
- *rou gui*
- *chen pi*
- *bai zhu*
- *fu ling*
- *wu wei zi*
- *yuan zhi*
- *gan cao*

The following formula treats blood vacuity by addressing the spleen and kidney:

Rx. Ren Shen Zi Xue Tang *(Ginseng Blood-enriching Decoction):*
- *ren shen*
- *shan yao*
- *fu ling*
- *chuan xiong*
- *bai shao yao*
- *shu di huang*
- *dang gui*

Modifications:
- The addition of *huang qi*, which increases the supplementing effect on spleen *qi*, stimulates blood formation even more strongly; by adding *he shou wu* and *ji xue teng* (Spatholobi caulis), we can supplement the blood and gently move it in the network vessels.

Acupuncture Points and Combinations
- LR-9, LR-11, CV-6, ST-36
- KI-8 + KI-10 + LR-3 + SP-6

Kidney Vacuity—*Shen Xu* (肾虚)

If the body's ability to supply substances from the kidney for the blood is impaired, this affects liver blood as well as the *chong mai* and thereby also the menstrual period.

Symptoms

Delayed periods with scanty amounts of blood. Depending on the condition of the kidney, the blood is either bright red (*yin* vacuity) or pale (*yang* vacuity). Pain in the lower back or knees, tinnitus, a pale (or red) tongue, and a thin and deep pulse are additional signs of a weakness in the kidneys.

Treatment Principle

Supplement the kidney and liver, nourish essence and blood, and regulate menstruation.

Medicinal Therapy

Rx. Dang Gui Di Huang Yin *(Chinese Angelica and Rehmannia Beverage)*[1]:
* *dang gui*
* *shu di huang*
* *shan zhu yu*
* *du zhong*
* *shan yao*
* *zhi gan cao*
* *huai niu xi*

This modification of the formula *Liu Wei Di Huang Wan* supplements the kidney primarily in its *yin* aspect. Nevertheless, the kidney has not yet formed heat, otherwise the arrival of the menstrual period would not be delayed but premature. Kidney vacuity always involves both aspects. If the kidney is too weak, it is unable to build up substances without the necessary *yang*. It is also for this reason that the formula contains *du zhong*, which supplements the kidney, the liver, and the *chong mai*, while *dang gui* fills the *chong mai* and *shan yao* supplements the kidney and stabilizes the acquired essences in the *chong mai*. You can prescribe this formula right away after the end of the menstrual period.

Modifications:
* To strengthen the effect of the formula on the *yang* aspect, you can add *xu duan* and *tu si zi*.
* In cases with concurrent blood stasis, replace *huai niu xi* with *chuan niu xi* (Cyathulae radix).

Acupuncture Points and Combinations
* CV-3, KI-13, GV-3
* CV-6 + CV-3 + SP-10 + SP-8
  - LU-7 + KI-6
  - KI-3, CV-4 moxa
  - BL-23, GV-4

Cold—*Han* (寒)

Cold in the *chong mai* and *ren mai* leads to *qi* stagnation and blood stasis. As a result, we see delayed menstruation with rather scanty amounts of dark thick blood, possibly containing clots. If the blood is pale, this indicates **vacuity cold**; bright dark or even black blood indicates **repletion cold**.

Vacuity Cold—Xu Han (虚寒)

Symptoms

The pain that occurs during menstruation is relieved by pressure and warmth; the patient additionally suffers from aversion to cold, cold extremities, cold buttocks and back, pain and tension in the abdomen, and weakness. The menstrual period is runny and dark without clots. The tongue is pale with a thin white fur; the pulse is deep and vacuous, but also fine and slow.

Treatment Principle

Strengthen *yang* to regulate menstruation.

Medicinal Therapy

Rx. Ai Fu Nuan Gong Wan *(Mugwort and Cyperus Palace-warming Pill)*:
* *ai ye*, 9 g
* *wu zhu yu* (Evodiae fructus), 4.5 g
* *rou gui*, 6 g
* *xiang fu*, 9 g
* *dang gui*, 9 g
* *chuan xiong*, 6 g
* *bai shao yao*, 6 g
* *huang qi*, 6 g
* *sheng di huang*, 6 g
* *xu duan*, 6 g

In vacuity cold, the stomach and spleen produce less *qi* and blood. For this reason, vacuity cold occurs together with *qi* and blood vacuity. This formula promotes the generation of *qi* and blood by means of *ren shen*, *dang gui*, *bai shao yao*, and *chuan xiong*. *Huang qi* supports blood formation. *Ai ye*, *wu zhu yu*, and *rou gui* warm the uterus and support *yang*. *Xu duan* supplements *yang* and moves the blood.

Acupuncture Points and Combinations
* KI-13, CV-3, CV-4—moxa with cigar or box!
* KI-6 + CV-3 + SP-6 + *zi gong* (3 *cun* lateral to CV-3)—moxa with cigar or box!

Repletion Cold in the **Chong Mai** *and* **Ren Mai**—
Chong Ren Shi Han *(*冲任实寒*)*

Like a river slowed down by ice, repletion cold in the blood causes delayed, scanty menstrual periods that are dark in color. Cold tends to invade women during the menstrual period when the *chong mai* is emptied and blood vacuity exists there. We find cold more often than we would expect. The following formula is one of the most commonly used formulas in gynecology. As the result of blood stasis, we find heat in the upper body at the same time. *Wen Jing Tang* is a pronounced *chong mai* formula.

Symptoms
The period is delayed, dark, and clotty, accompanied by cold and pain in the lower abdomen, which are relieved by the local application of warmth but sensitive to pressure. This pathology presents with a pale blue tongue and a sunken, slow, and tight pulse.

Treatment Principle
Eliminate cold, warm the *ren mai* and *chong mai*, and regulate the blood.

Medicinal Therapy
Rx. Wen Jing Tang *(Menses-warming Decoction):*
- *wu zhu yu*, 9 g
- *gui zhi* (Cinnamomi ramulus), 6 g
- *dang gui*, 9 g
- *chuan xiong*, 6 g
- *bai shao yao*, 6 g
- *e jiao*, 6 g
- *mai men dong*, 9 g
- *mu dan pi*, 9 g
- *ren shen*, 6 g
- *gan cao*, 6 g
- *sheng jiang* (Zingiberis rhizoma recens), 6 g
- *ban xia* (Pinelliae rhizoma), 6 g

Modifications:
- If cold has caused a more serious blood stasis with severe pain and large clots, you can add *e zhu* (Curcumae rhizoma) to break the blood.

Acupuncture Points and Combinations
- KI-13, CV-3, CV-4—warm needle!
- KI-6 + CV-3 + SP-6 + *zi gong* (3 *cun* lateral to CV-3)—warm needle!

Stagnation—*Yu Zheng* (郁证)

Stagnation by necessity always leads to blood stasis. The blood becomes thicker (a sign of excess) and blood clots form. Small clots in the menstrual blood point more towards *qi* **stagnation**, while large dark clots suggest **blood stasis**.

Qi Stagnation—*Qi Zhi* (气滞)
Blood vacuity is an ideal breeding ground for the development of *qi* stagnation. The liver, which regulates the *qi*, requires a lot of blood for this function. Alternately, though, emotions can also constrain the *qi*. If *qi* stagnation results, this in turn affects the blood-forming function of the spleen.

Symptoms
Symptoms associated with a delayed menstrual period due to *qi* stagnation manifest most clearly shortly before the onset of menstruation. Pulling pain in the rib-sides, mood swings, and tension in the breasts are usually important signs that *qi* stagnation is involved. The tongue color is inconspicuous or slightly livid, the fur is thin, and the pulse is stringlike, or also very thin when blood vacuity is present.

Treatment Principle
Regulate *qi*, strengthen the spleen, nourish the blood, and regulate menstruation.

Medicinal Therapy
Depending on the pathology, we can employ different formulas to harmonize the flow of *qi*. As a rule, you can prescribe these formulas throughout the entire cycle up to the onset of menstruation, whenever the volume of blood is sufficient. Otherwise you have to supplement *yin* and blood, when you begin taking the formula directly after the period.

Xiao Yao San (Free Wanderer Powder) is the formula indicated for liver *qi* stagnation with spleen *qi* vacuity and liver blood vacuity. It treats the liver and regulates the connection to the spleen, which is important for gynecology. This is certainly one of the reasons why *Xiao Yao San* is one of the most popular formulas in gynecology.

Modifications:
- For pronounced blood vacuity, add *Si Wu Tang* to this formula.

- The formula is called *Hei Xiao Yao San* (Black Free Wanderer Powder) if you add either *shu di huang* for the blood or *sheng di huang* to nourish the fluids more effectively.
- *Xiang fu*, *mu xiang* (Aucklandiae radix), *yu jin* (Curcumae radix), *zhi ke*, and *fo shou* (Sacrodactylis fructus) are important *qi*-regulating medicinals that can be added as needed.

For patients with chronic *qi* stagnation without blood vacuity, *Chai Hu Shu Gan San* (Bupleurum Liver-coursing Powder) is an important formula that can also deliver good results in the treatment of premenstrual symptoms.

Acupuncture Points and Combinations
- LR-3, LR-8, CV-3
- LU-7 + BL-18 + BL-23 + BL-17 + SP-6

Blood Stasis—Xue Yu (血瘀)

The mechanisms that lead to blood stasis vary. In all cases of blood stasis, it is important to find the cause. Blood stasis that occurs in the context of delayed menstruation tends to be rooted either in blood vacuity or in cold. The body is not strong enough to eliminate the stasis via the blood, as a result of which menstruation is delayed.

Symptoms
When the menstrual period finally arrives, the patient discharges large dark clots in dark menstrual blood, accompanied by stabbing pain that is relieved upon discharge of the clots. The pain is often worse at night. The tongue is purple, the pulse is typically rough.

Treatment Principle
Move the blood, resolve the stasis, and regulate menstruation.

Medicinal Therapy
Prescribe any formulas up to 7 days before the onset of menstruation as well as during the period, so that the uterus is emptied completely and blood formation is no longer impaired by blood stasis.

The most important formula for blood stasis in patients with blood vacuity is *Tao Hong Si Wu Tang* (Peach Kernel and Carthamus Four Agents Decoction). The formula *Wen Jing Tang* is indicated for blood stasis due to cold in patients with existing blood vacuity. It is indicative of *Wen Jing Tang* that we see signs of cold in the lower body and signs of heat in the upper body. Alternatively, you can also prescribe the formula *Sheng Hua Tang* (Engendering Transformation Decoction).

For very severe blood stasis due to cold without blood vacuity, the following formula is indicated:

Rx. Jiang Huang San *(Turmeric Powder):*
- *jiang huang* (Curcumae longae rhizoma)
- *e zhu*
- *gui zhi*
- *dang gui*
- *chuan xiong*
- *yan hu suo* (Corydalis rhizoma)
- *mu dan pi*
- *hong hua*
- *bai shao yao*

Acupuncture Points and Combinations
- PC-5, LR-2, LR-14, KI-2
- KI-14 + BL-17 + BL-22 + ST-36 + SP-6

Phlegm Stagnation—*Tan Zhi* (痰滞)

Sometimes women mention that they discharge phlegm during the menstrual period. Occasionally, this discharge of phlegm occurs only after menstruation. This is a key sign that we must also treat phlegm in such cases. If the period is delayed because of polycystic ovaries, we should always consider the involvement of phlegm stagnation. Phlegm can be treated at any time other than during the menstrual period.

Symptoms
Fatigue and unwillingness to move, heavy extremities, and overweight (**beware**: slender women can also suffer from phlegm!), can arise. In spite of sufficient sleep, such women feel quite exhausted and dazed when they get up in the morning, a condition that often only improves 1–2 hours after getting up. Key signs for diagnostic purposes are thick and scanty menses and a sticky white tongue fur, but especially a slippery pulse in the *guan* position.

Treatment Principle
Transform phlegm, eliminate dampness, move *qi* and blood.

Medicinal Therapy

The two formulas below are the standard formulas found in the literature for the treatment of phlegm stagnation in connection with the blood. In clinical practice, we often incorporate this strategy into other formulas, or at least it is rare to give one of these formulas alone in this form.

Rx. Dan Xi Shi Tan Tang *(Danxi's Damp-phlegm Decoction:*
- *cang zhu*
- *bai zhu*
- *ban xia*
- *fu ling*
- *dang gui*
- *chuan xiong*
- *hua shi* (Talcum)
- *xiang fu*

This formula treats phlegm stagnation with an aspect of *qi* stagnation. *Dang gui* and *chuan xiong* are supposed to gently move the blood. *Hua shi* opens the lower body through the urine and is commonly used in cases with blood stasis as a phlegm-eliminating medicinal (Zhang Jiebin's strategy).

Rx. Xiong Gui Er Chen Tang *(Chuanxiong and Chinese Angelica Two Matured Ingredients Decoction):*
- *chuan xiong*
- *dang gui*
- *chen pi*
- *fu ling*
- *zhi gan cao*

Acupuncture Points and Combinations
- LR-2, LR-5, SP-8, KI-13
- ST-40 + CV-5
- ST-40 + LU-7
- SP-9, CV-12, ST-29

Scant Menstruation—*Yue Jing Guo Shao* (月经过少)

Menstrual periods that occur regularly in terms of the cycle but are scant in volume or last for less than 3 days are referred to as **hypomenorrhea**. Even though affected women often experience these as normal, they can be one of the causes of infertility. As a result of low estrogen production, the endometrium is too thin and therefore insufficient for the successful implantation of a fertilized ovum.

The endometrium develops after the menstrual period and should be approximately 8 mm thick, according to biomedicine. If the endometrium is too thin, the period will be correspondingly scant or short. If the body is unable to build up enough *yin* and blood, it cannot transform into *yang*. An abundance of *yin* energy is the prerequisite for the birth of *yang*. From the biomedical perspective, this situation can lead to insufficiently developed egg cells or even a lack of ovulation. Insufficient secretion in the middle of the cycle would also point in this direction.

From the TCM point of view, the same factors that cause delayed menstruation also lead to scant, short, or light menstrual periods. They are here again listed in the order of frequency:
- blood vacuity
- kidney vacuity
- cold
- blood stasis
- phlegm-damp obstruction

Blood Vacuity—*Xue Xu* (血虚)

Blood vacuity is the most common pattern in short or scant menstruation. The causes of blood vacuity are found primarily in the center or the kidney, which has consumed too much essence. In the treatment of vacuity conditions, we therefore always look at the function of the blood-forming organs. Under certain circumstances, you may have to remove sticky medicinals like *shu di huang* from a formula to avoid straining the function of the center unnecessarily. It would be overburdened in its function of separating the turbid and the clear. Blood-moving medicinals should not be too aggressive in their effect, so as not to do additional harm to the already weakened blood.

Symptoms
In addition to the sign of weak menstrual periods with pale and rather thin blood, affected women present with paleness in the face, a tendency to stupor and dizziness, dry skin, and possibly also dry eyes. The tongue is pale with a thin white fur; the pulse is thin and vacuous.

The application of the following formulas starts already on the fifth day of the cycle and is continued until the 14th day of the cycle. Blood vacuity responds very well to treatment. In most cases, the menstrual period clearly becomes longer or heavier already in the first treatment cycle.

Treatment Principle
Nourish the blood, supplement *qi*, and regulate menstruation.

Medicinal Therapy
Si Wu Tang is probably the most important and well-known formula for building blood. As already discussed in the section on delayed menstruation, *Xiao Ying Jian* is also a good formula, supplementing the blood via the liver and entering the extraordinary vessels. Both of these can easily be modified, depending on the cause of blood vacuity.

Ba Zhen Tang (Eight Gem Decoction) is a standard formula that supplements blood and *qi* on a general level. If the blood vacuity is rooted in a weak digestive system, *Liu Jun Zi Tang* (Six Gentlemen Decoction) is indicated. This is a particularly effective combination of *Si Jun Zi Tang* with *dang gui* and *bai shao yao* for the purpose of supplementing the blood. With the addition of *chen pi, mu xiang*, and *sha ren*, this formula becomes *Xiang Sha Liu Jun Zi Tang* (Costusroot and Amomum Six Gentlemen Decoction), which brings blood and *qi* into the *ren mai* and *chong mai*, and has proven extremely effective. The formula *Ren Shen Yang Rong Tang* incorporates the heart as the ruler of blood into its strategy.

Modifications:
- Blood vacuity always carries with it the danger of blood stasis; for this reason, *dan shen* is particularly appropriate because it enters the *chong mai* and easily supplements the blood.
- *ze lan* (Lycopi herba) or *yue ji hua* (Rosae chinensis flos) are particularly well-suited for gently circulating the blood without injuring it. Both work more by moving *qi* within the blood and can thereby move stasis. *Yue ji hua* additionally has a positive effect on the emotions as well.

Acupuncture Points and Combinations
- ST-30, CV-3, SP-6, ST-25, GV-7
- LR-11 + CV-4 + ST-29 + SP-6

Kidney Vacuity—*Shen Xu* (肾虚)

Symptoms
Scant, pale, and watery menstrual periods and other kidney signs like pain in the lower back, tinnitus, frequent urination, a pale swollen tongue, and a sunken, vacuous, or fine pulse.

Treatment Principle
Nourish the kidney and liver, supplement essence and blood, and regulate menstruation.

Medicinal Therapy
The formula that we use most frequently for this pattern is *Dang Gui Di Huang Yin* (for the formula, see p. 200), which we have already mentioned above for delayed menstruation. Again, we prescribe it immediately after menstruation to take advantage of the body's natural impulse in the first phase of the cycle to strengthen *yin* and the blood.

Acupuncture Points and Combinations
- KI-13, KI-5, CV-4
- KI-8 + KI-10 + LR-3 + SP-6

Cold—*Han* (寒)

Symptoms
Dark blood that is discharged only hesitatingly and in small amounts, as well as a feeling of cold in the lower abdomen, desire for warmth, which clearly eases the bleeding, cold extremities, a pale face with a pale or sometimes (in concurrent blood stasis) even dark tongue, and a sunken and tight pulse.

Treatment Principle
Warm the menses and the channels, dissipate cold, nourish the blood, and eliminate blood stasis.

Medicinal Therapy
Rx. Variation of *Wen Jing Tang (Menses-warming Decoction)*:
- *dang gui*
- *chuan xiong*
- *rou gui*
- *e zhu*
- *ren shen*
- *mu dan pi*
- *bai shao yao*
- *chuan niu xi*

Modifications:
- To bring the warming ingredients of this formula into the smaller channels as well, we can further supplement the formula with *hong hua* and *ji xue teng.*

Acupuncture Points and Combinations
- KI-13, KI-14, CV-3, CV-4—moxa with cigar or box!
- KI-6 + CV-3 + SP-6 + *zi gong* (3 *cun* lateral to CV-3)—moxa with cigar.

Blood Stasis—*Xue Yu* (血瘀)

Just as blood stasis can lead to profuse menstrual periods, it can also lead to scant menstruation when the *qi* is not strong enough to eliminate the stasis via the blood. Under these circumstances, the blood stasis inhibits the blood flow, as a result of which we see only scant menstrual periods. Blood stasis that persists for a longer period of time furthermore prevents the generation of new blood, a problem that resolves itself when the blood stasis is eliminated. In this picture, blood stasis is often caused by *qi* stagnation, heat, or cold.

Symptoms
Menstrual periods with scant amounts of tar-like blood, containing clots. The blood is discharged only hesitatingly and the period is accompanied by pain in spite of its lightness. The tongue is dark and the typical pulse is rough and often also stringlike.

Treatment Principle
Nourish the blood and eliminate blood stasis.

Medicinal Therapy
Unlike in the other patterns, we give the blood-moving formulas also after the menstrual period in this pattern. *Tao Hong Si Wu Tang* is the all-purpose formula for moving blood. It is especially suitable in this context. It nourishes and moves the blood while at the same time protecting it from the acrid moving medicinals.

Modifications:
- In cases with more severe blood stasis, you can replace *bai shao yao* with *chi shao yao.* For additional stagnation heat that has damaged the blood fluids, replace *shu di huang* with *sheng di huang.*

- *Chuan niu xi* is added to direct the medicinals downward.
- To regulate the *qi* in concurrent *qi* stagnation, we can add *zhi ke, xiang fu,* and Linderae radix (*wu yao*).

Acupuncture Points and Combinations
- LR-2, LR-8, GB-26, KI-15, CV-7
- CV-7 + SP-6 + CV-3 + SP-10

Phlegm-damp Obstruction

Phlegm-damp leads to obstruction in the uterus (*bao gong tan shi zu zheng* 胞宫痰湿阻证). Phlegm that causes scant menstruation, on the other hand, is rarer.

Symptoms
The menstrual period is scant, the patient has profuse vaginal discharge, a physical feeling of heaviness, and in the mornings phlegm in the throat. The tongue is swollen and has a thick fur; the pulse can be sunken and fine if the pathology has already entered deeply into the network vessels, or otherwise slippery and stringlike.

Treatment Principle
Disperse phlegm, transform dampness, strengthen the center, and regulate menstruation.

Medicinal Therapy
You can prescribe the formulas any time other than during menstruation. The treatment principle of nourishing and moving blood during menstruation runs counter to the treatment of phlegm—namely, to dry.

Rx. *Xiong Gui Er Chen Tang* (Chuanxiong and Chinese Angelica Two Matured Ingredients Decoction):
- Rx. *Er Chen Tang* plus:
- *dang gui*
- *chuan xiong*

Modifications:
We can modify this formula in numerous ways. Instead of or in addition to the blood-building ingredients, we can:
- add the formula *Si Jun Zi Tang* to strengthen the center
- modify with *dan shen* to bring the formula into the *chong mai*

- add *tao ren* to simultaneously move blood and promote the elimination of phlegm via the stool
- increase the effect of the formula with *cang zhu* and Magnoliae officinalis cortex (*hou po*)
- in almost completely absent menstruation due to stasis, complement the formula with *e zhu, xiang fu*, and *mu xiang.*

Acupuncture Points and Combinations
- LR-5, PC-5, CV-3
- SP-6 + SP-10 + CV-4 + TB-6

Amenorrhea—*Bi Jing* (闭经)

A menstrual period that occurs in longer intervals than normal (i.e., more than 28 days) is called **oligomenorrhea**. If the menstrual period is completely absent for more than 3 months, we speak of amenorrhea. **Primary amenorrhea** refers to cases where a woman has never had a menstrual period, that is, menarche never arrived in the first place. **Secondary amenorrhea** means that menstruation has stopped for at least 3 months, after initially beginning at the appropriate age.

The causes of this disorder are manifold:[15]
- 61% hypothalamic-hypophysic disorders
- 18% hyperprolactemia
- 9% ovarian disorders (hyperplasia, PCOS, tumors)
- 5% secondary uterine disorders (loss of endometrium after curettage)
- 7% extragenital disorders

It is interesting that hypothalamic-hypophysic disorders in secondary amenorrhea are very often regarded as functional disorders, as long as no organic disorder in the form of tumors is present. This type of amenorrhea is more common in anorexia, professional athletes, or after psychological trauma. In hyperprolactemia, the high levels of prolactin inhibit follicular maturation and thereby cause the absence of both ovulation and menstruation.

Ovarian disorders like polycystic ovary syndrome (PCOS) cause immature egg cells to accumulate in the ovaries without any concurrent release of FSH and subsequent ovulation. Instead we see an increase in the secretion of testosterone (increased growth of hair, acne, ovarian fibrosis), and of LH. The luteal phase fails to appear, and the

ovaries may increase in size (see p. 42ff. and Chapter 21).

Problems of the endometrium itself are particularly common in China, where abortions are part of women's daily lives and can lead to fertility disorders later on. In our culture, the sustained use of birth control pills time and again causes secondary amenorrhea after the woman stops taking them.

From the TCM perspective, this is related either to a vacuity state or to stagnation, which is impeding the flow of blood. Translated into biomedical language, this could mean: a follicle does not reach complete maturity due to a deficiency state, or ovulation fails to take place because it is blocked in one way or another.

Biomedical clarification is especially important in amenorrhea. In a patient with polycystic ovary syndrome, for example, we can proceed in a much more deliberate way than if we do not know the disorder that has led to the absence of menstruation.

From the TCM point of view, the **causes** correspond to the causes of delayed menstruation:
- blood vacuity
- kidney vacuity
- *qi* stagnation and blood stasis
- cold
- phlegm-damp

Because amenorrhea is a very complex subject, we can only present the basic treatment principles here. To achieve diagnostic clarity, the time of menarche and the course of previous menstrual periods can offer information on a woman's constitutional situation. If menarche only arrived at the age of 15 or 16 (this number is measured in light of today's circumstances where some girls get their period at age 11), this reflects a kidney vacuity. Periods that were weak or irregular already from the start also show that the body needs support through the kidney. Suddenly interrupted periods, on the other hand, point more clearly toward stagnation than periods that slowly become lighter and lighter and eventually stop altogether as the result of a vacuity state.

More important than in the previously discussed menstrual problems is the **institutionalization of a cycle**. If the woman senses a cycle in spite of absent menstruation, as, for example, from tension in the breasts, this provides the rhythm for therapy. If no signs of a cycle are discernible at all, you can orient therapy towards the lunar cycle because it corresponds to women's physiological cycle.

Keeping track of the basal temperature curve during treatment can be very useful for matching treatment to a gradually forming cycle, if you are unsure of your pulse diagnosis. At the beginning of any treatment, focus the formula on the existing pathology and try to lay the foundations for a cycle: this means sufficient *yin* and blood. The next step can then be to promote ovulation. When the desired ovulation finally takes place, it is important to change the treatment principles to strengthening *yang* and subsequently to moving blood, to promote the elimination of blood.

Blood Vacuity—*Xue Xu* (血虚)

In the prehistory of a patient with amenorrhea based on blood vacuity, we often find only scant, pale red menstrual periods that were initially delayed and gradually stopped altogether. The *chong mai* and *ren mai* are no longer filled sufficiently, and menstruation stops. Sometimes, menstruation fails to reappear after childbirth, miscarriage, or lactation, because the woman has lost too much blood. If breastfeeding did not last for more than 6 months, this suggests a weak constitution. In this context, it is especially important to regulate the center because it is the main source of blood formation and over time in vacuity conditions also exhausts the kidneys.

Symptoms
Paleness in the face, stupor, dizziness, a pale tongue, and a fine and vacuous pulse.

Treatment Principle
Nourish the blood, supplement *qi*, and regulate menstruation.

Medicinal Therapy
Formulas like *Shi Quan Da Bu Wan* (Perfect Major Supplementation Pill) or *Ba Zhen Tang* are intended to supplement *qi* and blood in order to fill the *ren mai* and *chong mai*. Hereby we often have to exercise a little patience before we can see results. Furthermore, you must never disregard the connection between the spleen and the liver because blood vacuity very often also causes stagnation (see case study p. 216).

Modifications:
- After the patient has reached a healthy blood level and the pulse has become stronger, you can add medicinals like *ji xue teng* and *xiang fu* to the formula above, to gently move *qi* and blood and to stimulate ovarian activity.
- The following medicinals can also be added to the above-mentioned formula: substances that build kidney *yin* are intended to support the transformation from *yin* to *yang*. Suitable choices here are, for example, Loranthi seu *sang ji sheng* (visci ramus) and *tu si zi*.
- For a weak digestion and reduced appetite, *Xiong Gui Liu Jun Zi Tang* is an important formula that stimulates activity in the center and regulates digestion, before you can specifically treat the blood vacuity:

Rx. Xiong Gui Liu Jun Zi Tang *(Chuanxiong and Chinese Angelica Six Gentlemen Decoction)*:
- *dang gui*
- *chuan xiong*
- *dang shen*
- *bai zhu*
- *fu ling*
- *ban xia*
- *chen pi*
- *gan cao*
- *sha ren*
- *mai ya* (Hordei fructus germinatus)
- *xiang fu*

Sha ren enters the *chong mai*. *Mai ya* stimulates the transformative function of the center and moves liver *qi*, is an important medicinal for cysts and raised prolactin levels, but can also stop lactation and lead the blood back to the lower body.

The desire for children often triggers deep emotions. Women feel pressured and are afraid that their longing will not be fulfilled. If these factors affect blood formation, it is essential to add medicinals that quiet the spirit (see p. 209 heart *qi* stagnation).

Acupuncture Points and Combinations
- LR-1, SP-4, ST-30, GV-7
- CV-6 + CV-3 + SP-10 + SP-8

Kidney Vacuity—*Shen Xu* (肾虚)

Kidney vacuity always means a relative weakness of *yin* or *yang*.

Kidney Yin *Vacuity*

Symptoms

Late menarche, always rather scant menstrual periods until menstruation finally stops completely, dizziness, tinnitus, soreness or pain in the lower back, or other signs of kidney *yin* vacuity, with a red or pale tongue and a sunken and fine or vacuous pulse. If you see constipation and thirst, this indicates heat, which exhausts the blood and fluids and often announces itself by overly frequent menstrual periods that turn into absent ones.

Treatment Principle

Strengthen *yin* and essence, reduce the heat, connect the heart to the uterus, and regulate menstruation.

Medicinal Therapy

We can treat amenorrhea caused by kidney *yin* vacuity with formulas like *Zuo Gui Yin* (Left-restoring [Kidney *Yin*] Beverage) or *Dang Gui Di Huang Yin* (see p. 200 for the formula). In cases with more obvious vacuity heat that is affecting the heart, *Bu Shen Di Huang Wan*, a formula related to *Tian Wang Bu Xin Dan* (Celestial Emperor Heart-supplementing Elixir), is a better choice.

Rx. Bu Shen Di Huang Wan *(Kidney-supplementing Rehmannia Pill):*
- Rx. *Zhi Bai Di Huang Wan* plus:
- *fu shen* (Poria cum pini radice)
- *xuan shen*
- *mai men dong*
- *gui ban*
- *dan zhu ye* (Lophatheri herba)
- *suan zao ren*
- *yuan zhi*
- *sang piao xiao* (Mantidis ootheca)

This formula primarily supplements kidney *yin* and essence, eliminates heat from the lower burner, and establishes the connection to the heart. In addition, the formula works through the lung to strengthen water and thereby control the fire from the kidney.

Modifications:
- In the application of *Zuo Gui Yin* or *Dang Gui Di Huang Yin* in cases with vacuity heat, we add *mu dan pi* and *di gu pi* as well as *dan shen* to cool and move the blood.
- Treat heat with concurrent blood vacuity by means of *Bai Zi Ren Wan* (Arborvitae Seed Pill).
- If ovulation still fails to appear after several weeks of this therapy, use *Gui Shen Wan* with *chuan niu xi* and *ze lan*, to promote the change from *yin* to *yang*, or in other words, ovulation.[12]

Acupuncture Points and Combinations
- KI-5, KI-13, CV-4, GV-3
- KI-8 + BL-23 + CV-6 + CV-4 + SP-6

Kidney Yang *Vacuity* (Shen Yang Xu 肾阳虚)

Kidney *yang* vacuity often occurs in combination with spleen vacuity.

Symptoms

Absent menstruation, sensitivity to cold, cold feet, frequent urination, diarrhea, and fatigue. The tongue is pale and moist, the pulse sunken and vacuous.

Treatment Principle

Replenish *yang* and regulate menstruation.

Medicinal Therapy

Frequently used formulas are *You Gui Wan* (Right-restoring [Life Gate] Pill)* or *Gui Shen Wan* (for the formula, see p. 187).

Acupuncture Points and Combinations
- CV-4, BL-23, KI-27
- KI-11 + BL-23 + CV-4 + SP-6

Stagnation—*Yu Zheng* (郁证)

Liver Qi *Stagnation*—Gan Qi Yu (肝气郁)

Amenorrhea as the result of *qi* stagnation is most common after the use of birth control pills or in conjunction with elevated prolactin levels. In such patients, we often also find blood vacuity that promotes the formation of *qi* stagnation. In clinic, the development of heat is particularly common. The period generally returns already after 2–3 weeks of regulating liver *qi*. Results are not as good in cases with elevated prolactin levels due to adeno-

---

* Also known as Right [Kidney]-restoring Pill.

mas. While we succeed in relieving the symptoms like secretion of breast milk and tension in the breasts, it is often impossible to substantially lower the prolactin values.

Symptoms
Mood swings, pronounced frustration, tension in the breasts, pulling pain in the lower abdomen. Normal or reddish or livid tongue color with normal tongue fur. The pulse is stringlike or fine.

Treatment Principle
Regulate *qi*, nourish the blood, and regulate menstruation; if necessary, also clear heat.

Medicinal Therapy
The famous formulas like *Si Wu Tang* in combination with *Xiao Yao San, Chai Hu Shu Gan San*, and *Jia Wei Xiao Yao Tang* (Supplemented Free Wanderer Decoction) are very effective.

Modifications:
- To place more emphasis on treating the emotions, you can add medicinals such as Albizziae cortex (*he huan pi*) to gently move *qi*, harmonize the liver and spleen, and quiet the spirit; this is also good in combination with *yu jin*, which moves *qi*, also in the blood.
- In cases with developing heat, use *chi shao yao* instead of *bai shao yao*, to cool and to move, often in combination with *mu dan pi* to cool the liver.
- We can lower prolactin levels with high doses (20–30 g) of *mai ya*.

Acupuncture Points and Combinations
- LR-8, GB-26, CV-24, ST-30, LR-1
- LR-11 + CV-4 + ST-29 + SP-6

Heart Qi Stagnation—Xin Qi Yu (心气郁)

The involvement of the psyche is extremely important in women with the desire for children. It affects ovulation as well. Some authors believe that a stagnation of heart *qi* affects the *bao mai*, which is responsible for opening the uterus for ovulation, and thereby prevents ovulation.[12] We know for certain that the emotional component in fertility problems plays an important role in clinical practice and can affect the formation of blood and the flow of *qi*, to say nothing of the connection between the heart and the kidney.

Symptoms
Insomnia, palpitations, profuse dreaming, disquietude, great sadness because of existing childlessness, and fear that this will remain so.

Treatment Principle
Stabilize the *shen*, regulate heart *qi*, and regulate menstruation.

Medicinal Therapy
A few of the important heart-regulating medicinals follow:
- *he huan pi*—moves *qi* and quiets the spirit
- *gou teng*—relaxes, loosens, and quiets the spirit
- *suan zao ren*—nourishes the blood of the heart and liver and leads the blood into the *bao mai*
- *dan shen*—moves the blood and cools the heart
- *yuan zhi*—opens the heart, in anxiety and when heart and kidney fail to communicate with each other
- *long gu*—for very strong heat and resulting disquietude

When prescribed together, *suan zao ren* and *yuan zhi* are very important medicinals in the treatment of infertility, used with the intention of bringing heart *qi* down into the uterus.

Acupuncture Points and Combinations
- KI-27, HT-5, LU-7, CV-24
- KI-5 + HT-5 + LR-1

Blood Stasis—Xue Yu (血瘀)

It is not uncommon for blood stasis to develop after surgical interventions, but other unknown inflammations can also lead to adhesions that obstruct the blood flow. As a cause of amenorrhea, however, blood stasis is rarer. The following formula can also be modified for *qi* stagnation that leads to blood stasis.

Rx. Xue Fu Zhu Yu Tang (*House of Blood Stasis-expelling Decoction*)
Modifications:
- *Xiang fu* and *yi mu cao* are proven medicinals for focusing the formula more strongly on the lower abdomen when you remove *jie geng* (Platycodonis radix).

Acupuncture Points and Combinations
- LR-1, LR-14, LR-2, PC-5
- CV-7 + SP-6 + CV-3 + SP-10

Cold—*Han* (寒)

When cold penetrates into the uterus, blood stasis results. The female organism is particularly sensitive to cold influences right before and during menstruation. Cold foods like ice-cream or raw foods, going outside with wet hair, or swimming during the menstrual period are common causes that can lead to amenorrhea due to cold.

Symptoms
Complaints that can be relieved completely by warmth. The tongue is pale and the pulse is slow.

Treatment Principle
Warm the menses, eliminate cold, nourish the blood, and eliminate blood stasis.

Medicinal Therapy
Rx. Wen Jing Tang *(Menses-warming Decoction):*

Acupuncture Points and Combinations
- ST-28, CV-4, CV-3, KI-5
- KI-8 + BL-23 + CV-6 + CV-4 + SP-6

Phlegm-damp—*Shi Tan* (湿痰)

This pathology develops especially in the context of polycystic ovary syndrome (PCOS) and ovarian cysts, which are treated separately in this book (see Chapter 21). Phlegm-damp here sinks into the *dai mai* and blocks the functions of the *ren mai* and *chong mai*.

Acupuncture Points and Combinations
- LR-2, LR-5, SP-8, CV-5, PC-5
- ST-40 + CV-5

■ Menstruation at Irregular Intervals

Irregular menstrual periods are periods that fail to occur at regular intervals. They can arrive earlier or later than expected. This condition results from a disharmony between *qi* and blood, or in gynecological terms, a disharmony between *ren mai* and *chong mai*. In most cases, we find the cause in **liver**

qi **stagnation** or less frequently in a disharmony that is the result of **kidney or spleen vacuity**.

Liver *Qi* Stagnation—*Gan Qi Yu* (肝气郁)

In most cases, it is younger women who suffer from menstruation at irregular intervals. Experience shows that they commonly suffer from chronic tension that eventually manifests also in the menstrual periods. Liver *qi* stagnation on the one hand causes delayed menstruation because the stagnation obstructs the free flow of *qi* and blood. With the onset of the menstrual period, the body can eliminate the stagnation, but then tends to develop heat in the next cycle, which leads to the next period arriving too early. In this way, the cycle swings back and forth.

Symptoms
Irregular menstruation with dark blood containing small clots, pulling pain during menstruation, premenstrual complaints with persistent mood swings, very depressed, then in turn very irritated, an inconspicuous tongue, and a stringlike pulse.

Treatment Principle
Harmonize the liver and regulate the blood.

Medicinal Therapy
The formulas are taken after the end of the menstrual period during the entire cycle. Experience has shown that we do not have to treat cycles of different lengths differently.

Rx. Xiao Yao San *(Free Wanderer Powder)*
Modifications:
- To regulate liver *qi* and the blood even more strongly while at the same time cooling the heat, add *xiang fu, chuan xiong, chuan lian zi,* and *yu jin*.
- *Fo shou* moves *qi*, but at the same time also harmonizes the center, which is suffering from excessive tension in the liver.

Fu Qingzhu's formula describes the same scenario on the basis of the connection between the liver and kidney.[20] Due to their mother–child relationship, liver *qi* stagnation also leads to stagnation in the kidney and thereby to an impairment of its opening and closing function. When the stagnation is resolved, menstruation naturally returns to its regular cycle.

The following formula focuses on replenishing the kidney and liver and treats the stagnation only secondarily.

Rx. Ding Jing Tang *(Menses-stabilizing Decoction):*
- *tu si zi*
- *bai shao yao*
- *dang gui*
- *shu di huang*
- *shan yao*
- *fu ling*
- *chao jing jie* (Schizonepetae flos frictus)
- *chai hu*

Acupuncture Points and Combinations
- LR-2, LR-5, ST-30, SP-6
- LR-9 + CV-4 + BL-67 + SP-6

Kidney Vacuity—*Shen Xu* (肾虚)

In kidney vacuity, we are always dealing with the relative balance of *yin* and *yang*. These two aspects can swing back and forth. If the balance swings towards kidney *yin* vacuity, we see early menstrual periods, in which the heat is discharged. The periods are characterized by bright shiny blood. The resulting relative kidney *yang* vacuity leads to delayed menstruation.

Symptoms
Scant but runny periods without clots, fatigue and pain in the back, dizziness, and tinnitus. The tongue is pale with little fur; the pulse is vacuous, especially in the *chi* position.

Treatment Principle
Replenish the kidney and liver, regulate menstruation.

Medicinal Therapy
The following formula focuses on replenishing the kidney and liver and treats the stagnation only secondarily.

Rx. Gu Yin Jian *(Yin-securing Brew):*
- *ren shen*
- *shu di huang*
- *shan yao*

- *shan zhu yu*
- *yuan zhi*
- *zhi gan cao*
- *tu si zi*
- *wu wei zi*

Acupuncture Points and Combinations
- KI-2, KI-5, KI-8, KI-14
- KI-13 + BL-23 + CV-6 + SP-6

■ Dysmenorrhea

From the biomedical view, painful menstrual periods—**dysmenorrhea**—develop as the result of increased contractility of the endometrium. The **causes** of this condition are largely unknown, but we suppose that in addition to organic causes like endometriosis, uterine adenomyosis, myomas, polyps, and STDs (sexually transmitted diseases), psychological factors are particularly instrumental. Studies have shown that daughters whose mothers suffered from pain during menstruation also have a tendency to experience these uncomfortable side-effects. In addition, some authors believe that an overly close relationship to the father might favor the development of menstrual pain.[16] Painful menstruation appears in some way to document a "lack of being completely in touch with one's feminine side."

Pain that surfaced already at the beginning of menarche is referred to as **primary dysmenorrhea**; menstrual pain that arises later is called **secondary** or **acquired dysmenorrhea**. Here we assume that organic disorders like endometriosis, myomas, abortions, or inflammations in the lower abdomen contribute to the development of pain. Nowadays, many young girls already receive prescriptions for the birth control pill to relieve menstrual pain. An additional frequent indication for the early use of the birth control pill is acne in puberty.

Based on our knowledge that TCM can treat not only the body but also energetically the woman's psyche, the following paragraphs discuss the **diagnosis** of dysmenorrhea.

Pain (*tong* 痛) develops due to a lack of or blocked flow of energy, that is, a **stagnation**. Stagnation can come from **repletion** or **vacuity**. Repletion-related stagnation is rooted either in the presence of cold or heat, or of phlegm. Stagnation due to vacuity is caused by a lack of *qi* or a lack of moistening by blood or the bodily fluids (*jin ye* 津液), as a result of which the *chong mai* and *ren mai* no longer receive sufficient nourishment and the person therefore experiences dull pain.

Stagnation, blood stasis, and cold, as well as vacuity of *qi*, blood, and of fluids can disrupt the normal flow of energy and lead to blockage, which manifests in pain before, during, or after the menstrual period.

In conjunction with menstrual pain, numerous **symptoms** can manifest such as diarrhea, nausea, vomiting, headache, pulling pain in the thighs, or pronounced shivering. These symptoms can often give us an indication of the overall energetic state of the patient, which we then need to incorporate into the therapy.

Menstrual Pain from *Qi* Stagnation—*Qi Zhi* (气滞)

In *qi* stagnation, we can differentiate between conditions caused by vacuity and conditions caused by repletion, even though they ultimately always constitute a repletion state. On the basis of this distinction, we must treat them differently. For this purpose, we can subdivide all cases roughly into:
- *qi* stagnation with vacuity
- *qi* stagnation with heat

In general, we can say that menstrual pain due to *qi* stagnation has a tendency to arise **before menstruation** and to disappear with the onset on the 1st or 2nd day. Menstruation is often associated with premenstrual complaints like tension in the breasts, increased sensitivity, or the desire for physical activity before the beginning of the period. Most of the time, *qi* stagnation is treated in the second half of the cycle.

Symptoms
The period is either scant or normal in volume, starts only slowly, and tends to be dark in color. There may be small clots. Patients are sensitive to pressure, which indicates repletion. The pain comes and goes. The pulse is stringlike, in existing blood vacuity also fine.

Qi Stagnation with Vacuity—*Xu Qi Zhi* (虚气滞)

Dysmenorrhea due to *qi* stagnation responds well to treatment with formulas like *Xiao Yao San*, especially when the cause of the pain is related more to psychological factors and the stagnation has developed as a result of internal tension against the background of *qi* and blood vacuity. The relationship of blood and *qi* in the liver is the key to a harmonious *qi* flow. To a certain extent, the blood controls *qi* to make it soft and even.

Treatment Principle
Nourish the blood and regulate liver *qi* to regulate menstruation.

Medicinal Therapy
There are many formulas that can regulate liver *qi*. If the stagnation enters more deeply into the blood but has not yet developed into blood stasis, *Chai Hu Shu Gan San* is an excellent formula.

Modifications:
- To relax the patient emotionally as well, we can add other medicinals like *he huan pi* and *yu jin*.
- If heat develops as the result of the stagnation, *mu dan pi* and *zhi zi* are the most important medicinals; we refer to this modification as *Jia Wei Xiao Yao San*. *Xia ku cao* and *huang qin* are important medicinals for liver heat as well.
- Painful diarrhea during menstruation is treated with additions like Saposhnikoviae radix (*fang feng*) and *chen pi*, according to the formula *Tong Xie Yao Fang* (Pain and Diarrhea Formula). Mild diarrhea without pain can often be regulated with *bai zhu* alone.
- If the liver invades the stomach, we can consider *wu zhu yu*, *ban xia*, and *chen pi*. These medicinals bring down stomach *qi* and thereby restore the normal flow of energy.

Acupuncture Points and Combinations
- LR-8, SP-8, LU-7, KI-4
- CV-6 + CV-7 + LR-1

Qi Stagnation with Depressed Heat—*Qi Zhi Re Yu* (气滞热郁)

When *qi* stagnation becomes more chronic, it tends to engender heat. The most commonly used formula for this pattern is the above-mentioned *Jia Wei Xiao Yao San*. The formula *Jin Ling Zi Tang* (Toosendan Decoction) regulates liver *qi* in cases where mild heat signs are present; it is an important formula in gynecology as well. Fu Qingzhu developed the formula *Xuan Yu Tong Jing Tang* (宣郁痛经汤) for this pattern. It is frequently used in China.

Symptoms
If stagnation leads to heat, we often see symptoms like headache, insomnia, disquietude, or acne in conjunction with the well-known signs of *qi* stagnation. These appear before the period and recede with the onset of menstruation.

Treatment Principle
Nourish the blood, cool the liver, and regulate *qi* to regulate menstruation.

Medicinal Therapy
Rx. Xuan Yu Tong Jing Tang *(Stagnation-diffusing Menstruation-promoting Decoction)*
- *dang gui*
- *bai shao yao*
- *mu dan pi*
- *zhi zi*
- *bai jie zi* (Sinapsis albae semen)
- *chai hu*
- *xiang fu*
- *chuan yu jin* (Curcumae radix sichuanensis)
- *huang qin*
- *gan cao*

Acupuncture Points and Combinations
- LR-8, SP-8, LU-7, KI-4
- CV-6 + CV-7 + LR-1

Blood Stasis—*Xue Yu* (血瘀)

Blood stasis is, like phlegm, always a secondary pathology. This means that we must consider different formulas, depending on the cause of the blood stasis. Because the uterus is located in the lower burner, cold is the most common trigger of blood stasis. We generally treat blood stasis from about 1 week before menstruation on and during menstruation itself, to free the uterus from the stasis. In cases of severe blood stasis, you can also treat throughout the entire cycle, as long as you nourish the blood itself sufficiently and protect it from the acrid medicinals. Otherwise you could easily set off premature menstrual periods.

The causes of blood stasis can be manifold. The condition develops from:
- *qi* stagnation
- vacuity cold
- cold-damp
- damp-heat
- *qi* and blood vacuity

Symptoms
The key symptom of menstrual pain due to blood stasis is large blood clots. After their discharge, the pain disappears. While the pain can also arise before the period, it primarily occurs during the 2nd and 3rd day, worsens at night, and has a lancing characteristic. The tongue is purple with stasis macules; the pulse is rough, stringlike, and in severe pain tight.

Treatment Principle
The nature of the pain often offers important clues to the therapeutic approach: pain that is felt only in the center of the abdomen suggests that the stagnation is located in the uterus, while pain on the sides points to an involvement of the liver channel. Pain in the back indicates an involvement of the kidney, and downward-pulling pain suggest *qi* vacuity, which we must treat with uplifting medicinals like *sheng ma*, *huang qi*, or *chai hu*, in spite of the blood stasis. Sudden knife-like pain indicates blood stasis.

Acupuncture Points and Combinations
- SP-8, SP-10, SP-6
- KI-14 + BL-17 + BL-22 + ST-36 + SP-6

Blood Stasis due to *Qi* Stagnation—*Qi Zhi Xue Yu* (气滞血瘀)

Symptoms
In addition to the symptoms mentioned above, pain and premenstrual complaints arise already in the run-up to the menstrual period.

Treatment Principle
Regulate the *qi*, move the blood, and eliminate the blood stasis to regulate menstruation.

Medicinal Therapy
To treat blood stasis from *qi* stagnation, we can consider any *qi*-regulating formula to which the appropriate blood-moving medicinals have been

added. In the literature, we always find here the formula *Xue Fu Zhu Yu Tang*.

Modifications:
- It is important to remove *jie geng* from the formula and add medicinals such as *xiang fu*, which bring the formula into the lower burner.
- For pain that occurs primarily in the lumbus, we can add ingredients like *xiao hui xiang* (Foeniculi Fructus) and *ju he* (citri reticulatae semen).
- Pain in the thighs can be treated with *qin jiao* (Gentianae macrophyllae radix).
- Besides *tao ren* and *hong hua*, other important medicinals for moving blood with great clinical relevance are: *yi mu cao, yan hu suo, ze lan, e zhu,* and *san leng* (Sparganii rhizoma).

Acupuncture Points and Combinations
- LR-3, SP-6, SP-10, TB-6
- CV-7 + SP-6 + CV-3 + SP-10

Blood Vacuity with Blood Stasis—*Xue Xu Xue Yu* (血虚血瘀)

Symptoms
Severe pain during the menstrual period, which is rather scanty. Even though the blood clots are quite small, we find typical signs of blood stasis. The tongue is pale and livid, the pulse stringlike and fine or rough.

Treatment Principle
Nourish the blood and eliminate the blood stasis to regulate menstruation.

Medicinal Therapy
Rx. Tao Hong Si Wu Tang
Modifications:
- If *qi* stagnation exists as well, we can supplement this formula effectively for corresponding symptoms with the addition of *xiang fu, yi mu cao,* and *mu xiang.*

Acupuncture Points and Combinations
- LR-8, LR-2, SP-8, BL-17
- LU-7 + BL-18 + BL-23 + BL-17 + SP-6

Blood Stasis due to Vacuity Cold in the *Ren Mai* and *Chong Mai*—*Chong Ren Xu Han Xue Yu* (冲任虚寒血瘀)

It is a mistake to believe that cold is practically non-existent in our latitudes and in our lifestyle with central heating. A large number of our female patients who seek treatment for dysmenorrhea do in fact get treated with a warming formula like *Wen Jing Tang.*

Symptoms
Pain that occurs already before or only during menstruation, dark blood with clots, scant amounts of blood with a tendency to delayed onset, pain that is relieved by warmth. The pulse is sunken, rough, and fine.

Treatment Principle
Eliminate the cold and the blood stasis and nourish the blood to regulate menstruation.

Medicinal Therapy
Rx. Wen Jing Tang *(Menses-warming Decoction)*
Modifications:
- For concomitant headaches, *chong wei zi* (Leonuri fructus) is an important medicinal.
- We can treat a feeling of tension in the lower abdomen with *wu yao* and *xiao hui xiang.*
- For very severe pain, we can add the formula *Shi Xiao San.*

Acupuncture Points and Combinations
- SP-4, SP-8, ST-30, ST-28
- SP-4 + SP-30 + CV-4

Blood Stasis due to Cold-damp—*Han Shi Xue Yu* (寒湿血瘀)

Symptoms
Pain before or during menstruation, scant sticky blood with clots, pain that is sensitive to pressure but relieved by warmth, cold and heavy extremities, and other signs of excessive dampness, a pale tongue with a white sticky fur, and a sunken and slippery pulse.

Treatment Principle

To regulate menstruation, warm the channels to dispel cold, eliminate dampness, and expel the blood stasis.

Medicinal Therapy

Rx. Gui Zhi Fu Ling Wan *(Cinnamon Twig and Poria Pill)* or

Rx. Shao Fu Zhu Yu Tang *(Lesser Abdomen Stasis-expelling Decoction) plus:*

- *cang zhu*
- *fu ling*

Shao Fu Zhu Yu Tang is warming; we must add medicinals for treating the dampness.

Modifications:

- *Yi yi ren, che qian zi* (Plantaginis semen), and *gan jiang* can be added as well to complement the treatment of dampness.

Acupuncture Points and Combinations

- CV-2, CV-3, KI-14, KI-2
- ST-25 + CV-9 + SP-6

Blood Stasis due to Damp-heat—*Shi Re Xue Yu* (湿热血瘀)

Symptoms

If the patient has a pre-existing damp-heat constitution or if cold-damp transforms into damp-heat, we will see prolonged and malodorous menstrual periods and yellow vaginal discharge. In more chronic conditions, we find symptoms that affect the whole body like dry stool due to the development of heat in the blood, vaginal eczema, or dark urine. The tongue is red with a yellow fur, and the pulse is slippery and rapid.

Treatment Principle

Clear the heat, expel the dampness, and eliminate the blood stasis to regulate menstruation.

Medicinal Therapy

Rx. Qing Re Tiao Xue Tang *(Heat-clearing Blood-regulating Decoction):*

- *mu dan pi*
- *sheng di huang*
- *huang lian*
- *dang gui*
- *bai shao yao*
- *chuan xiong*
- *hong hua*
- *tao ren*
- *e zhu*
- *xiang fu*
- *yan hu suo*

Modifications:

- To emphasis the heat-clearing action of this formula even more, we can add *hong ten* (Sargentodoxae caulis) and *bai jiang cao*, and for the dampness, *yi yi ren* and *che qian zi*.

Acupuncture Points and Combinations

- LR-8, CV-2, PC-5
- KI-5 + SP-6 + CV-3

Blood Stasis due to *Qi* and Blood Vacuity—*Qi Xue Xu Xue Yu* (气血虚血瘀)

After the end of the menstrual period, the *chong mai* is empty. If the patient is weak, we will now see dull pain and exhaustion. Simple formulas like *Ba Zhen Tang* or *Shi Quan Da Bu Tang* (Perfect Major Supplementation Decoction) are indicated here as well.

Symptoms

The pain appears either after menstruation or during the last days of the period, when the *ren mai* and *chong mai* are already empty. The patient has a desire for physical touch, the menstrual period is weak, pale, and runny. The tongue is pale with a thin white fur; the pulse is vacuous or fine.

Treatment Principle

Supplement *qi* and nourish blood.

Medicinal Therapy

Rx. Sheng Yu Tang *(Sagacious Cure Decoction):*

- Rx. *Si Wu Tang* plus:
- *huang qi*
- *dang shen*

Here, *huang qi* is the main ingredient to promote the movement of blood.

Modifications:
Depending on the symptoms, we can add many medicinals:

- For pain in the back, *du zhong, sang ji sheng, xu duan*, and *tu si zi* are suitable.
- For dizziness and palpitations, consider *gou qi zi* and *ye jiao teng* (Polygoni multiflori caulis).

Acupuncture Points and Combinations

- LU-7, TB-6, CV-6
- LU-7 + BL-18 + BL-23 + BL-17 + SP-6

■ Commonly Used Acupuncture Points and their Combinations in Modern TCM

Almost all of the points and combinations listed in the paragraphs above have been obtained from the classical acupuncture texts. The absence or minor significance of points that are widely used in the context of menstrual disorders today, like LR-3. LI-4, and GV-20, is conspicuous. **Table 16.1** gives an overview of the points used in modern TCM. In

this table, both selection and evaluation (e.g., as "main point") result also from the author's personal experience.

■ Case Studies

The case studies considered here illustrate common problems in clinic, like amenorrhea and infertility with a relevant prehistory, and substantiate the efficacy of simple formulas.

Case Study 1: Female Patient, Age 24 (Amenorrhea)

First Consultation

A slender woman, she seems downcast and is very unhappy with her skin, which is shiny and has a tendency to blackheads. Before menstruation stopped 9 months ago, she menstruated at irregular intervals, with a tendency to longer cycles. She is very exhausted.

Table 16.1 Commonly used acupuncture points and their combinations in modern TCM

Disharmony	Main Point	Possible Combinations With	Qi Jing Ba Mai (Eight Extraordinary Vessels)
Spleen *qi* vacuity	SP-6	CV-6, LU-7, GV-20, BL-20	–
Qi stagnation	LR-3	LI-4, SP-10, LR-14, KI-14, TB-6, SP-6, CV-4, CV-6, PC-7, PC-6, GB-34	SP-4/PC-6
Blood stasis	SP-10	LR-3, BL-17, SP-8, SP-6, CV-6, KI-14, ST-29, ST-30	SP-4/PC-6
Blood vacuity	BL-17	KI-13, LR-8, ST-36, SP-6, BL-20, BL-23, BL-18	–
Blood heat	SP-10	LI-11, BL-17, LR-2, ST-44, KI-2	SP-4/PC-6
Qi vacuity	LU-7	CV-6, CV-4, ST-36, SP-6, SP-8, BL-20	–
Kidney *yin* vacuity	KI-6	KI-3, LR-8, SP-6, KI-2, CV-7, KI-5, KI-13, SP-8, BL-52	LU-7/KI-6
Kidney *yang* vacuity	GV-4	BL-23, KI-2, CV-4, ST-36, SP-6, BL-20, SP-6, SP-8	–
Kidney *qi* vacuity	KI-7	BL-23, ST-36, GV-20, BL-20, CV-6, CV-4	LU-7/KI-6
Cold	CV-4	CV-6, ST-29, SP-8, ST-36, GV-4, ST-25	LU-7/KI-6
Dampness and phlegm	SP-9 (dampness) ST-40 (phlegm)	CV-6, ST-28, CV-9, BL-22, BL-32, SP-6, CV-12, BL-20, CV-4, SP-8	LU-7/KI-6 GB-41/TB-5

Medical History

Menarche at age 15, regular at the beginning but with pain. At age 16, the birth control pill for 3 years; after she stopped taking it, initially a return to regular menstrual periods. Gradually prolonged cycles. The most recent menstrual periods lasted for 4 days, with rather bright, sometimes stretchy blood, light bleeding (three tampons) that began with spotting, accompanied by lower abdominal pulling that was relieved by warmth and rest.

Very greasy skin and many blackheads, but no acne. Always cold hands and feet, suddenly occurring hot flashes about twice a week. Frequent hunger but little appetite, thirst, wakes up in the night with a dry mouth, feels very exhausted, and has a hard time getting going in the morning. Always different stools, without complete elimination.

Tongue: pale with white fur

Pulse: liver, stringlike; middle, vacuous; generally very fine

Diagnosis

Spleen *qi* vacuity and blood vacuity with liver *qi* stagnation, damp-heat, and some phlegm. Based on the menstrual signs, a spleen and blood vacuity is in the foreground. The initially delayed onset of menstruation shows the existing stagnation, which is reflected also in the pulse and psyche.

Therapy

Because the amenorrhea arose roughly at the same time as her life as a single woman and the liver showed a stringlike pulse, she received *Xiao Yao San* as her first prescription.

First prescription: *Xiao Yao San*, modified for 5 days, plus:
* *mu dan pi*, 4 g
* *chen pi*, 4 g
* *yi yi ren*, 8 g
* *bi xie* (Dioscoreae hypoglaucae seu semptemlobae rhizoma), 4 g
* *sha ren*, 4 g

Second Consultation (Day 4 of the Cycle)

The period arrived after 3 days, hesitatingly but without pain. Level of energy clearly improved but still not satisfying. Always complete elimination in defecation, skin unchanged.

Second prescription: *Ba Zhen Tang* in pill form for the next 10 days.

Third Consultation (Day 18 of the Cycle)

Repetition of the first formula: *Xiao Yao San* (without *yi yi ren*, *bi xie*, and *bai shao*):
* *chi shao yao*, 4 g
* *mu dan pi*, 3 g
* *zhi zi*, 3 g
* *huang bai*, 4 g
* *ze lan*, 6 g
* *chuan xiong*, 3 g

After the period, she should again take the formula *Ba Zhen Tang*.

Fourth Consultation (Day 20 of the Cycle)

The period came after 33 days, with heavier bleeding after one day; before that, slight irritation but now feeling well in terms of mood and energy level. Good skin.

Rx. *Dang Gui Shao Yao San* (Chinese Angelica and Peony Powder):
* *xiang fu*, 6 g
* *huang bai*, 3 g
* *mu dan pi*, 3 g
* *chen pi*, 4 g
* *chai hu*, 3 g
* *sha ren*, 6 g

Result

The menstrual period came regularly every 33–35 days. Because the skin had improved, the patient stopped treatment due to financial reasons, even though she would have had to continue treatment in order to stabilize menstruation. It is foreseeable that amenorrhea will develop again.

Case Study 2: Female Patient, Age 36 (Infertility with Dysmenorrhea and Tendency to Miscarriage)

First Consultation (Day 12 of the Cycle)

The patient had already had 16 inseminations and had been pregnant three times, twice miscarrying in the ninth week, once in the sixth week. No pregnancy in the past year.

Medical History

She had received homeopathic treatment in the past year, as a result of which her menstrual pain had improved. The period used to come every 26–28 days (as the result of acupuncture by a colleague, the period now comes every 32 days), lasts 4–5 days, noticeably stronger on the second day, with hard dark clots and pain. From the third day on, only residual bleeding. Severe PMS, moodiness, weeps easily, at times very extreme feelings, but no tension in the breasts, tendency to feel cold very quickly, in addition to cold hands and feet also ice-cold legs and buttocks. She also complains of tension in the shoulders. She has difficulty falling asleep and has a tendency to brooding. The tongue is slightly orange with a very fine tongue body, the pulse is fine, in the liver position string-like, and soft in the center.

Diagnosis

Blood vacuity with *qi* stagnation and blood stasis, with kidney *yang* vacuity.

Therapy

The patient was encouraged to stop the inseminations for three cycles, to optimize conditions first. The patient received

Rx. *Dang Gui Shao Yao San* (Chinese Angelica and Peony Powder) plus:

* wu yao, 4 g
* yin yang huo (Epimedii herba), 2 g
* huang qin, 3 g

The period arrived after 26 days, with little pain but still with discharge of clots. The therapy was continued for an additional month.

Second Consultation (Day 10 of the Cycle)

To stabilize the kidneys, the patient received acupuncture. To open *ren mai*: LU-7, KI-6.

In the next menstrual period, the discharge of clots was clearly reduced, the pain had almost completely disappeared, and the patient had a comfortable feeling of warmth in the abdomen. As a result of this, she wanted to make another attempt at insemination.

Third Consultation (Day 13 of the Cycle)

On the previous day, the patient had had an insemination. For the second half of the cycle (after the insemination), she is now receiving:

Rx. Zhu Yu Tang *(Stasis-expelling Decoction)*, *Modified:*

* dang gui, 4 g
* bai shao yao, 6 g
* shan yao, 6 g
* mu dan pi, 4 g
* fu ling, 4 g
* tu si zi, 8 g
* xu duan, 4 g
* yin yang huo, 2 g
* chai hu, 3 g
* he huan pi, 6 g

Result

The patient becomes pregnant. In the first weeks of pregnancy, she continues to receive treatment because of her tendency to abortion and severe morning sickness. She gives birth to a healthy son.

Literature

1. Bensky D, Barolet R. *Chinesische Arzneimittelrezepte und Behandlungsprinzipien*. Kötzting: VGM Wuhr; 1996.
2. Bensky D, Clavey S, Stöger E. *Chinese Herbal Medicine—Materia Medica*. Washington: Eastland; 2004.
3. Clavey S. *Fluid Physiology and Pathology in Traditional Chinese Medicine*. London: Churchill Livingstone; 1998.
4. Flaws B. *A Handbook of Menstrual Diseases in Chinese Medicine*. Boulder: Blue Poppy; 1997.
5. Flaws B. *A Handbook of Traditional Chinese Gynecology*. Boulder: Blue Poppy; 1994.
6. Flaws B. *Schwester Mond*. Kötzting: VGM Wuhr; 1994.
7. Fu Ke Xin Fa Yao Jue. In: *Golden Mirror of Orthodox Medicine*. Taos: Paradigm; 2005.
8. Fu,QZ. *Fu Qing-Zhu's Gynecology*. Boulder: Blue Poppy; 1999.
9. Kaffka A. *Zu den Quellen Weiblicher Kraft*. Oy-Mittelberg: Joy; 2003.
10. Kirschbaum B. *Die 8 Außerordentlichen Gefäße in der Traditionellen Chinesischen Medizin*. Uelzen: ML; 1995.
11. Liu FW. *The Essence of Liu Feng-Wu's Gynecology*. Boulder: Blue Poppy; 1998.
12. Lyttleton J. *Treatment of Infertility with Chinese Medicine*. London: Churchill Livingstone; 2004.

13. Maciocia G. *Obstetrics & Gynecology in Chinese Medicine.* London: Churchill Livingstone; 1998.
14. Paulus W, Zhang M, Strehler E. A Study from the Christian Lauritzen Institute, Ulm, Germany. *Fertility and Sterility.* 2002;77:4.
15. Pfleiderer A, Breckwoldt M, Martius G. *Gynäkologie und Geburtshilfe.* Stuttgart: Thieme; 2001.
16. Schmidt-Matthiesen H, Hepp H. *Gynäkologie und Geburtshilfe.* Stuttgart: Schattauer; 1998.
17. Shen Y. *A Heart Approach to Gynecology: Essentials in Verse.* Taos: Paradigm; 1995.
18. Tang J. *Chinesische Medizin in der Gynäkologie.* Munich: Urban & Fischer; 2000.
19. Wing TA, Sedlmeier ES. Measuring the Effectiveness of Chinese Medicine in Improving Female Fertility. *J Chinese Medicine.* 2006;80:22.
20. Yang SZ, Liu DW. *Fu Qing-Zhu's Gynecology.* Boulder: Blue Poppy; 1998.
21. Zhang J. Complete Works of Jingyue, 1624. In: Gongwang L *Fundamentals of Formulas of Chinese Medicine.* Beijing: Huaxia Publishing; 2002.

Stefan Englert

■ Introduction

Western Diagnosis

When menopausal symptoms occur long before the age of 50, it is standard practice from the perspective of Western medicine to order a gynecological hormone diagnosis. Occasionally, this might be only a temporary phase of menopausal complaints, which subsequently recede again; such patients then return to a normal menstrual cycle for any number of years. In this context, typical complaints of early menopause are hot flashes and irregular and/or weakening menstrual periods. A complete absence of menstruation is not rare either. Furthermore, we see occasional night sweating, mood swings, and internal disquietude. In combination with these typical symptoms, the diagnosis is made by means of key laboratory parameters: a lowered estradiol-2 level in conjunction with an elevated FSH level. In pathophysiological terms, this means a decrease in ovarian function in women who are markedly younger than 45–50.

Symptoms

In so-called early menopause, the key symptoms are typically an absent or markedly irregular menstrual period. Alternatively, the period can arrive in very large intervals only and be very weak.

Additional symptoms can be sensation of internal heat, hot flashes, sudden sweating or night sweating, general signs of increasing dryness like dry skin, hair loss, a dry vagina, or dry constipation.

Differentiation from the TCM Perspective

From the TCM perspective, early menopause can have a variety of causes. Accordingly, different types of **disharmony patterns** can be at the root of these complaints. We distinguish between **vacuity patterns** and **repletion patterns**:

Vacuity Patterns
- insufficiency of blood (and *qi*)
- insufficiency of kidney *yin*
- insufficiency of kidney *yang*
- insufficiency of essence

Repletion Patterns
- liver *qi* stagnation
- blood stasis
- damp-heat in the lower burner
- phlegm accumulation

It is not uncommon that we find a combination of two patterns in a single patient; for example, we commonly see insufficiency of blood in conjunction with liver *qi* stagnation. Alternatively, a residual pathogenic factor can exist in the lower burner in conjunction with simultaneous exhaustion of kidney energy.*

---

* Energy and *qi* are not the same and should not be confused. Kidney energy includes the whole different aspects of the kidney—*yang* and *yin*. In this sense a depletion of kidney energy should indicate a kidney *yin* and *yang* vacuity.

■ Vacuity Patterns

Insufficiency of Blood (and *Qi*)

Causes and Disease Development
Exhaustion of the blood (*xue*) is often rooted in chronic overwork. Especially when subjected to permanent hectic or stress, women clearly use up more blood than men. The female physiology is a "physiology of blood," as is stated in many Chinese texts. Women of childbearing age are furthermore especially in need of a healthy and individually targeted diet. The spleen is tied closely to the production of blood in its function of transforming food into new *qi* and clarified juices. Women who, for example, start their day without breakfast in the morning run the risk of gradually steering their body into blood vacuity. In addition, strict vegetarians occasionally develop an insufficiency of blood if they fail to pay attention to the type, composition, preparation, and timing of their diet.

In the psychological arena, a possible cause of blood vacuity can be a pronounced loss of self-esteem. Because every person's self-confidence resides in the blood, hurtful separations from a partner can result in blood vacuity in women.

Symptoms
In the system, the blood has the function of "nurturance." Insufficiency of blood can therefore lead to symptoms like paleness with a withered lusterless complexion, exhaustion, tendency to internal disquietude, and weakened self-esteem. An insufficiency of blood and the resulting insufficient nurturance affects all aspects of the body, for example, dry skin, lusterless dull hair, hair loss, brittle nails, tendency to constipation, tendency to a dry vagina, muscle cramps, feeling of numbness, and weak, delayed, or absent menstrual periods.

Tongue and Pulse Signs
● Tongue body: pale, possibly small or flat.
● Tongue fur: normal to reduced.
● Pulse: fine, forceless.

Therapy

Acupuncture

Table 17.1 Recommended acupuncture points in insufficiency of blood (and *qi*)

Points	Name	Indication/Effect
SP-6	*San yin jiao*—Three *Yin* Intersection	Spleen-stomach points support the transformation of food into new *qi* and blood
ST-36	*Zu san li*—Leg Three *Li*	One of the most important points for increasing *qi*; also supports blood production indirectly
SP-10	*Xue hai*—Sea of Blood	Stimulates blood production, moves blood
LR-8	*Qu quan*—Spring at the Bend	Promotes the production of liver blood
CV-6	*Qi hai*—Sea of *Qi*	Increases the *qi* in the body, strengthens kidney energy, also supports blood production indirectly

Needle Manipulation
Supplement at all points.

Medicinal Therapy
Rx. Ba Zhen Tang *(Eight Gem Decoction):*
● *ren shen* (Ginseng radix), 3 g or *dang shen* (Codonopsis radix), 9 g
● *bai zhu* (Atractylodis macrocephalae rhizoma), 9 g
● *fu ling* (Poria), 9 g
● *gan cao* (Glycyrrhizae radix), 4 g
● *shu di huang* (Rehmanniae radix praeparata), 12 g

● *dang gui* (Angelicae sinensis radix), 6 g
● *bai shao yao* (Paeoniae radix alba), 6 g
● *chuan xiong* (Chuanxiong rhizoma), 4 g

Effect
Supplements *qi* and nourishes blood.

Indication
Combined insufficiency of *qi* and blood.

Suggested Use
Dosage for 2 days, decocted twice: take one cup three times a day at body temperature.

Insufficiency of Kidney *Yin*

Causes and Disease Development

Insufficiency of kidney *yin* constitutes exhaustion on a fundamental level. Kidney energy represents our *yin* pool in the system. As a rule, such a lack of energy can develop in women as the result of numerous births that were spaced too close together. In addition, the functional system kidney is weakened by years and years of continuous overstrain, sleep deficit, or chronic disease. This far-reaching exhaustion is often connected to a feeling of internal disquietude and a lack of feeling rooted in the body, and to a tendency to internal heat.

The mood is often easily frightened. It is possible that long-lasting fears or a single shock event or trauma have damaged the energy of the kidneys. In reverse, an energetic vacuity of the kidney leads to an increase in fears. One patient realized, for example, after childbirth, which had greatly weakened her kidney energy, that she now disliked going into the dark basement, even though it had never bothered her before. In this sense, changes in a patient's emotional balance are valuable diagnostic hints pointing to the functional system of the kidney.

Symptoms

When it is primarily the weakened functional system of the kidney that lies at the root of early menopause, specific symptoms of kidney vacuity tend to complete the clinical picture: typical symptoms of kidney vacuity are located in the area of the lower spinal column and the lower extremities. Patients therefore often complain of symptoms in the area of the lumbar spinal column (LSC) or the knee. The kidney supplies the ears. Impaired hearing and tinnitus are therefore typical kidney symptoms. In insufficiency of kidney *yin*, we see great dryness because the kidney is seen as the "lower source of water." Typical manifestations are hence dry skin and mucous membranes, constipation, dry throat, and thirst. The kidney supplies the hair on the head. Hence, hair loss may arise. The unbridled and no longer rooted *yang* leads to ascending heat sensations, a red face with hot flash symptoms, and disquietude. This heat is classically known as the "fire of the five hearts": a sensation of heat in the soles, palms, and the center of the chest. This feeling of internal heat typically increases in the late afternoon or night. In addition, we frequently find a tendency to night sweating. In patients with an insufficiency of kidney *yin*, the hot flashes, disquietude, and night sweating are most pronounced.

Tongue and Pulse Signs
- Tongue body: reduced, shrunken, and cracked.
- Tongue fur: reduced or often completely absent.
- Pulse: fine, as well as forceless especially in the third position; pulse tends to be accelerated and in some cases superficially palpable.

Therapy

Acupuncture

Table 17.2 Recommended acupuncture points in insufficiency of kidney *yin*

Points	Name	Indication/Effect
KI-6	*Zhao hai*—Shining Sea; "opening point" of the *yin qiao mai*	Nourishes kidney *yin*, quiets and restrains the ascent of vacuity heat, clears dry throat
CV-4	*Guan yuan*—Pass Head	Nourishes blood and *yin*, strengthens kidney energy
BL-23	*Shen shu*—Kidney Transport (*shu* point of the kidney)	Supplements the kidney; even in *yin* vacuity, it is important to strengthen the active energies of the kidney
SP-6	*San yin jiao*—Three *Yin* Intersection	Has a general supporting effect, especially on the lower abdomen
KI-7	*Fu liu*—Recover Flow (supplementing point)	Supplements kidney *yin* and *yang*

Needle Manipulation
Supplement at all points.

Medicinal Therapy
Rx. Liu Wei Di Huang Wan *(Six Ingredient Rehmannia Pill):*
- *shu di huang,* 12 g
- *shan zhu yu* (Corni fructus), 6 g
- *mu dan pi* (Moutan cortex), 6 g
- *shan yao* (Dioscoreae rhizoma), 6 g
- *ze xie* (Alismatis rhizoma), 6 g
- *fu ling,* 6 g

Effect
Supplements kidney *yin.*

Indication
Insufficiency of kidney *yin.*

Suggested Use
Dosage for 2 days, decocted twice: take one cup three times a day at body temperature.

Insufficiency of Kidney *Yang*

Causes and Disease Development
Insufficiency of kidney *yang* is closely related to insufficiency of kidney *yin.* In the kidney's functional system, *yin* and *yang* are intimately interconnected; hence a weakness of one of them over time always leads to a weakness of the other side. If the lack of *yang* forces predominates, we primarily see cold symptoms.

The causes are again similar to those of insufficiency of kidney *yin*: numerous or very exhausting pregnancies and births, long-term overstrain, lack of sleep, or chronic disease. Kidney *yang* is also very specifically affected negatively by excessive physical exertion, as is common in competitive sports.

Symptoms
Patients with an insufficiency of kidney *yang* suffer from a weakened ministerial fire. The kidney is the source of all *yang* in the body and is also referred to as the "lower fire" of life. Such women therefore suffer from great inner cold, which is particularly pronounced in the area of the lower half of the body. This leads to cold feet and to a feeling of cold in the LSC area or buttocks. Additionally, the fire is lacking in the realm of sexuality, which results in apathy and lacking libido. Because the kidney constitutes the will (*zhi*), we often see a weakened willpower.

Other typical symptoms of kidney *yang* vacuity concern three areas in particular:
- the LSC area and the lower extremities
- urination
- the genital area

Especially common complaints of kidney *yang* insufficiency are therefore lumbar pain, weakness, cold, or pain in the lumbar region that can also radiate outwards, knee problems, cold feet, also weakness of the lower extremities, and frequent urination with large amounts of clear and unconcentrated urine. Occasionally, this is accompanied by incontinence, that is, the inability to hold urine or stool, because the kidney governs the two "lower openings." In the genital area, the weakened fire is especially noticeable. In women, this results in reduced libido with a tendency to increased whitish vaginal discharge. Possibly premature graying of the hair on the head. In patients with early menopause due to kidney *yang* vacuity, we find only a minor tendency to hot flashes. Instead, the lack of libido and internal cold are emphasized.

Tongue and Pulse Signs
- Tongue body: can still look relatively normal, but tends to be pale and swollen.
- Tongue fur: relatively normal to slightly more whitish.
- Pulse: especially in the third position weak and forceless, as well as slow.

Therapy

Acupuncture

Table 17.3 Recommended acupuncture points in insufficiency of kidney *yang*

Points	Name	Indication/Effect
KI-3	*Tai xi*—Great Ravine; *yuan* source point	Nourishes kidney *yin*, quiets and restrains the ascent of vacuity heat, clears dry throat
GV-4	*Ming men*—Life Gate	Supplements kidney *yang* and original *qi*
CV-4	*Guan yuan*—Pass Head	Strengthens kidney energy
BL-23	*Shen shu*—Kidney Transport (*shu* point of the kidney)	Supplements the kidney
SP-6	*San yin jiao*—Three *Yin* Intersection	Has a general supporting effect, especially on the lower abdomen
KI-7	*Fu liu*—Recover Flow (supplementing point)	Supplements kidney *yin* and *yang*

Needle Manipulation
Supplement at all points.

Moxibustion
In this pattern, moxibustion on all points—especially BL-23, GV-4, and CV-4—is highly recommended.

Medicinal Therapy
Rx. Jin Gui Shen Qi Wan *(Golden Coffer Kidney* Qi *Pill):*
- *shu di huang*, 12 g
- *shan zhu yu*, 6 g
- *mu dan pi*, 6 g
- *shan yao*, 6 g
- *ze xie*, 6 g
- *fu ling*, 6 g
- *rou gui* (Cinnamomi cortex), 2–6 g
- *fu zi* (Aconiti radix lateralis praeparata), 1–6 g

Effect
Supplements kidney *qi* and *yang.*

Indication
Insufficiency of kidney *yang.*

Suggested Use
Dosage for 2 days, decocted twice: take one cup three times a day at body temperature.

Insufficiency of Essence

Causes and Disease Development
Insufficiency of essence is a form of energetic kidney deficiency. A deficiency of essence manifests differently in children and adults.

In **children**, insufficiency of essence is very often congenital, which is to say that the child is born with it. Essence deficiency can be traced back to a weakness of parental *jing* at the time of conception. A difficult pregnancy can contribute to an insufficient development of the embryo as well. After birth, the essence controls development and growth. The kidney is responsible for the marrow and brain: children with insufficient essence are therefore characterized by delayed bone growth and neurological development.

In **adults**, *jing* depletion is generally the result of chronic long-lasting intensive overwork or sport-related extreme strain. *Jing* depletion in adults thus represents rather a premature consumption of essence.

Symptoms
Typical symptoms of essence insufficiency are in **children**: delayed fontanel closure, "weak" fragile bones, and a delay in motor and linguistic development.

In **adults**, the following are symptoms of essence depletion: infertility, weakness of the lower spinal column, and loss of teeth. In men, we see insufficient sperm production, in women ovarian insufficiency with lacking or reduced maturation of the egg cells. In addition, amenorrhea. Most of the time, essence depletion appears in conjunction with a certain level of *yin* and *yang* vacuity. In this context, a predominant *yang* vacuity, but also a *yin* vacuity can further emphasize the symptoms, depending on which of the two aspects of kidney energy is affected more strongly.

Therapy

Acupuncture

Tongue and Pulse Signs
- Tongue body: can look relatively inconspicuous. If the *yang* aspect of the kidney is affected more strongly, the tongue tends more towards paleness and dampness. If the *yin* aspect is more involved, the tongue tends more towards redness and shrinking.
- Tongue fur: can be normal
- Pulse: forceless in the third position.

Table 17.4 Recommended acupuncture points in insufficiency of essence

Points	Name	Indication/Effect
CV-4	*Guan yuan*—Pass Head	Nourishes blood and *yin*, strengthens kidney energy
GV-4	*Ming men*—Life Gate	Supplements kidney *yang* and original *qi*
KI-7	*Fu liu*—Recover Flow (supplementing point)	Supplements kidney *yin* and *yang*
BL-23	*Shen shu*—Kidney Transport (*shu* point of the kidney)	Supplements kidney energy, especially the *yang* aspect
BL-32	*Ci liao*—Second Bone-hole	Supplements the kidney and strengthens the essence
SP-6	*San yin jiao*—Three *Yin* Intersection	Has a general supporting effect, especially on the lower abdomen

Needle Manipulation
Supplement at all points.

Medicinal Therapy
Rx. Zuo Gui Yin *(Left-restoring [Kidney* Yin*] Beverage)*:
This formula represents a modification of *Liu Wei Di Huang Wan*:
- *shu di huang*, 12 g
- *shan zhu yu*, 6 g
- *shan yao*, 6 g
- *gou qi zi* (Lycii fructus), 6 g
- *fu ling*, 6 g
- *gan cao*, 4 g

Effect
Supplements kidney essence, kidney *qi*, and kidney *yin*.

Indication
Insufficiency of kidney essence.

Suggested Use
Dosage for 2 days, decocted twice: take one cup three times a day at body temperature.

■ Repletion Patterns

Liver *Qi* Stagnation

Causes and Disease Development
The most common cause of liver *qi* stagnation is emotional strain, which can disrupt the free flow of *qi* in the liver. When such strain persists over a longer period of time, it begins to manifest in the physical realm as well.

Symptoms
Typical symptoms of liver *qi* stagnation are feelings of pressure and oppression. These result from the blocked flow of *qi*, which is no longer able to move freely. Frequent complaints include pressure on the right or left costal arch, cramping or colic in the abdominal space, pulling on the lumbus, and lateral headaches. Cold extremities and a general feeling of exhaustion can also be manifestations of the blocked flow of *qi*.

In the psychological realm, we see an irritated or frustrated basic mood, which is often projected outwards and hence leads to various forms of assigning blame to the person who might have caused the patient's own misfortune.

If menstruation still occurs, this pattern frequently leads to PMS complaints.

Tongue and Pulse Signs
- Tongue body: prominent and reddish on the margins; the margins are often slightly "rolled up" and tensed.
- Tongue fur: mostly normal.
- Pulse: stringlike, tight, as well as forceful.

Therapy

Acupuncture

Table 17.5 Recommended acupuncture points in liver *qi* stagnation

Points	Name	Indication/Effect
LR-3	*Tai chong*—Supreme Surge; *yuan* source point	Regulates liver *qi*, harmonizes the flow of energy in the liver
LI-4	*He gu*—Union Valley; *yuan* source point	Regulates and opens
GB-34	*Yang ling quan*—*Yang* Mount Spring; *hui* meeting point of the sinews	Strengthens the sinews, relieves pain and cramping in the muscles and sinews
BL-18	*Gan shu*—*shu* transport point of the liver	Supports the liver, regulates the energy flow
SP-6	*San yin jiao*—Three *Yin* Intersection	Has a general supporting effect, especially on the lower abdomen

Needle Manipulation
Harmonize at all points.

Medicinal Therapy
Rx. Chai Hu Shu Gan San (*Bupleurum Liver-coursing Powder*):
This formula constitutes a modification of *Si Ni San* (Counterflow Cold Powder):
- *chai hu* (Bupleuri radix), 6 g
- *bai shao yao*, 6–9 g
- *chen pi* (Citri reticulatae pericarpium), 6 g
- *zhi ke* (Aurantii fructus), 6 g
- *xiang fu* (Cyperi rhizoma), 6 g
- *chuan xiong*, 6 g
- *gan cao*, 3 g

Effect
Regulates liver *qi*.

Indication
Liver *qi* stagnation.

Suggested Use
Dosage for 2 days, decocted twice: take one cup three times a day at body temperature.

Blood Stasis

Causes and Disease Development
Blood stasis can develop out of chronic *qi* stagnation because the *qi* moves the blood. Blood stasis is also facilitated by blood deficiency since this means that only a limited amount of blood is available, which is more likely to be blocked than a large full stream. In addition, blood stasis patterns can arise after surgery or due to injury or the use of an IUD.

Symptoms
Typical symptoms of blood stasis are severe to very severe pain. If the patient still has occasional menstrual periods, the menstrual blood is dark, livid, and clotted. The nature of the pain is typically piercing or stabbing and often localized.

Tongue and Pulse Signs
- Tongue body: livid, the sublingual network vessels are congested.
- Tongue fur: rather unchanged and only reduced in concomitant blood vacuity.
- Pulse: stringlike, rough, forceful.

Therapy

Acupuncture

Table 17.6 Recommended acupuncture points in blood stasis

Points	Name	Indication/Effect
SP-10	*Xue hai*—Sea of Blood	Regulates the blood and relieves pain
SP-6	*San yin jiao*—Three *Yin* Intersection	Has a general harmonizing effect, especially on the lower abdomen
ST-30	*Qi chong*—*Qi* Thoroughfare; intersection with the *chong mai*	Regulates the blood and menstruation
CV-3	*Zhong ji*—Central Pole; *mu* alarm point of the bladder	Regulates the lower burner
BL-17	*Ge shu*—Diaphragm Transport; *hui* meeting point of the blood	Regulates the blood flow, disperses blood stasis
LR-3	*Tai chong*—Supreme Surge; *yuan* source point	Regulates liver *qi*, harmonizes the flow of energy in the liver

Needle Manipulation
Harmonize at all points.

Medicinal Therapy
Rx. Xue Fu Zhu Yu Tang *(House of Blood Stasis-expelling Decoction):*
* *dang gui*, 6–9 g
* *chi shao yao* (Paeoniae radix rubra), 6 g
* *sheng di huang* (Rehmanniae radix exsiccata seu recens), 6 g
* *tao ren* (Persicae semen), 3–9 g
* *hong hua* (Carthami flos), 6–9 g
* *chuan xiong*, 3–6 g
* *huai niu xi* (Achyranthis bidentatae radix), 6–9 g
* *chai hu*, 3 g
* *zhi ke*, 6 g
* *jie geng* (Platycodonis radix), 6 g
* *gan cao*, 3 g

Effect
Regulates the blood and resolves blood stasis.

Indication
Blood stasis.

Suggested Use
Dosage for 2 days, decocted twice: take one cup three times a day at body temperature.

Modifications
The following formula is a modification of this formula. It targets the lower abdomen in particular and expels cold from the inside.

Rx. Shao Fu Zhu Yu Tang *(Lesser Abdomen Stasis-expelling Decoction):*
* *xiao hui xiang* (Foeniculi fructus), 3–6 g
* *rou gui*, 2–6 g
* *gan jiang* (Zingiberis rhizoma), 26 g
* *dang gui*, 6–9 g
* *chuan xiong*, 3–6 g
* *mo yao* (Myrrha), 3 g
* *wu ling zhi* (Trogopteri feces), 3–9 g
* *yan hu suo* (Corydalis rhizoma), 3–6 g
* *chi shao yao*, 6 g
* *pu huang* (Typhae pollen), 3–9 g

Effect
Regulates the blood, disperses blood stasis, and expels cold from the inside.

Indication
Blood stasis and cold.

Suggested Use
Dosage for 2 days, decocted twice: take one cup three times a day at body temperature.

Damp-heat in the Lower Burner

Causes and Disease Development

Heat and dampness are pathogenic factors that can arise externally and internally. Damp-heat frequently develops out of residual dampness. This results in a blocked energy flow, which over time can gradually cause the formation of heat. Dampness usually arises internally in the center burner, as the result of a faulty diet or weakened spleen. When dampness is compounded by heat, the pathogens often "sink" into the lower burner. Furthermore, emotional factors like stress cause a blocked *qi* flow. Any stagnation that persists for a longer period of time can generate heat and impede the downward drainage of the waterways. This means that dampness can cause heat and that heat can also conversely cause dampness.

Symptoms

A typical symptom in patterns affected by the pathogens heat and dampness is white to yellow vaginal discharge. This can often lead to itching and burning. The external genitals are reddened. In addition, genital eczema can arise as well. In this pattern, the heat leads to sensations of warmth and burning, while the dampness aspect leads to sensations of heaviness or localized fullness or pressure. Internal inflammations in the genital and lower abdominal area can also arise in this context, as well as adnexitis or inflammatory bowel disease.

Tongue and Pulse Signs

- Tongue body: reddened and swollen; possibly dental impressions on the margins.
- Tongue fur: increased and yellowish.
- Pulse: stringlike, forceful.

Therapy

Acupuncture

Table 17.7 Recommended acupuncture points in damp-heat in the lower burner

Points	Name	Indication/Effect
CV-3	*Zhong ji*—Central Pole; *mu* alarm point of the bladder	Regulates the lower burner, drains damp-heat
SP-6	*San yin jiao*—Three *Yin* Intersection	Affects especially the lower burner, drains damp-heat
GB-26	*Dai mai*—intersection with the *dai mai*	Regulates the uterus and menstruation, drains damp-heat
ST-40	*Feng long*—Bountiful Bulge; *luo* network point	Regulates the *qi* and drains dampness
Non-channel point: Ex-CA-18	*Zi gong*—Infant's Palace; point of the uterus	Regulates menstruation and drains damp-heat

Needle Manipulation
Harmonize at all points.

Medicinal Therapy

Rx. Jia Wei Er Chen Tang *(Supplemented Two Matured Ingredients Decoction):*
- *ban xia* (Pinelliae rhizoma), 6 g
- *chen pi*, 6 g
- *fu ling*, 6 g
- *bai zhu*, 6 g
- *huang bai* (Phellodendri cortex), 6 g
- *huang qin* (Scutellariae radix), 5 g
- *huang lian* (Coptidis rhizoma), 4 g
- *dang gui*, 5 g

- *bai shao yao*, 5 g
- *gan cao*, 3 g

Effect
Drains dampness, clears heat, transforms phlegm, and gently supports the spleen and blood.

This is the recommended treatment for collection of damp-heat when heat and dampness are present in relatively equal amounts.

Suggested Use
Dosage for 2 days, decocted twice: take one cup three times a day at body temperature.

Phlegm Accumulation

Causes and Disease Development
Phlegm disorders are frequently rooted in spleen pathologies. Spleen *qi* vacuity is rooted in years of malnourishment. Especially energetically and physically cold foods like raw foods or an excessive consumption of dairy products can harm the spleen's ability to transform. In addition, sweets, alcohol, and late night dinners strain the spleen. Phlegm is often referred to as a so-called "secondary pathogen." Phlegm frequently blocks the free flow of energy.

Symptoms
Typical symptoms of phlegm accumulation are feelings of pressure and fullness in the thorax and upper abdomen. We often also see increased phlegm in the throat area. These symptoms tend to be compounded by continuous increased white vaginal discharge. The spirit (*shen*) is dull, lethargic, and dazed. Dizziness occurs and the face can appear swollen. In the extremities, swelling and edemas arise in combination with a feeling of heaviness.

Tongue and Pulse Signs
- Tongue body: enlarged; shows dental impressions on the margins.
- Tongue fur: thick and sticky.
- Pulse: slippery, stringlike, forceful.

Therapy

Acupuncture

Table 17.8 Recommended acupuncture points in phlegm accumulation

Points	Name	Indication/Effect
SP-9	*Yin ling quan*—*Yin* Mound Spring; water point of the spleen channel	Regulates the spleen and resolves and drains dampness
ST-40	*Feng long*—Bountiful Bulge; *luo* network point	Eliminates dampness and transforms phlegm
CV-9	*Shui fen*—Water Divide	Drains dampness and disperses accumulations
SP-6	*San yin jiao*—Three *Yin* Intersection	Has a general harmonizing effect, especially on the lower abdomen
BL-20	*Pi shu*—*shu* transport point of the spleen	Supplements the spleen and its ability to transform; thereby reduces dampness and phlegm

Needle Manipulation
Harmonize at all points, supplement at BL-20.

Medicinal Therapy
Rx. Er Chen Tang (Two Matured Ingredients Decoction):
- *ban xia*, 12 g
- *chen pi*, 12 g
- *fu ling*, 8 g
- *gan cao*, 4 g

Effect
Eliminates dampness, transforms phlegm, and regulates *qi*.

Indication
Collection of phlegm-damp.

Suggested Use
Dosage for 2 days, decocted twice: take one cup three times a day at body temperature.

Modifications
A common modification and expansion of this formula is presented by the following formula:

Rx. Xiang Sha Liu Jun Zi Tang (Costusroot and Amomum Six Gentlemen Decoction):
- *ren shen*, 3 g or *dang shen*, 9 g
- *bai zhu*, 9 g
- *fu ling*, 8 g
- *ban xia*, 12 g
- *chen pi*, 12 g
- *mu xiang* (Aucklandiae radix), 6 g
- *sha ren* (Amomi fructus), 6 g
- *gan cao*, 4 g

Effect
Strengthens the spleen, eliminates dampness, transforms phlegm, and regulates *qi*.

Indication
Accumulation of phlegm-damp, with a weakness of spleen *qi* at the root of the condition.

Suggested Use
Dosage for 2 days, decocted twice: take one cup three times a day at body temperature.

■ Conclusion

It is often possible to reestablish the menstrual cycle by means of Chinese medicine. Nevertheless, it is important to recognize that this requires time. Two to 3 months of treatment are often the minimum time needed. During this period, the predominant pattern can gradually change. Therefore, the practitioner should carefully reevaluate the patient's state in each session. If done correctly, the supplementation of deficiencies or elimination of pathogens will eventually show effects and, if possible, sometimes reestablish the menstrual cycle.

Literature

1. Bensky D, Barolet R. *Chinesische Arzneimittelrezepte und Behandlungsstrategien.* Kötzting: VGM Wühr; 1997.
2. Bensky D, Clavey S, Stöger E. *Chinese Herbal Medicine. Materia Medica.* Seattle: Eastland; 2004.
3. Chen S, Li F. *A Clinical Guide to Chinese Herbs and Formulae.* London: Churchill Livingstone; 1993.
4. Clavey S. *Fluid Physiology and Pathology in Traditional Chinese Medicine.* London: Churchill Livingstone; 1995.
5. Deadman P, Al-Khafaji M. *A Manual of Acupuncture.* Seattle: Eastland; 1998.
6. Deadman P. *Großes Handbuch der Akupunktur.* Kötzting: VGM Wühr; 2001.
7. Ehling D. *The Chinese Herbalist's Handbook.* Santa Fe: High Mountain; 1994.
8. Englert S. *Großes Handbuch der Chinesischen Phytotherapie, Akupunktur und Diätetik.* Kötzting: VGM Wühr; 2003.
9. Englert S. *Kleines Handbuch der Chinesischen Phytotherapie.* Munich: Müller & Steinicke; 2007.
10. Flaws B, Bürgel H. *Schwester Mond.* Kötzting: VGM Wühr; 1994.
11. Focks C. *Leitfaden Traditionelle Chinesische Medizin.* 4th ed. Munich: Urban & Fischer; 2002.
12. Focks C. *Atlas Akupunktur.* Stuttgart: Fischer; 1998.
13. Hempen CH. *Akupunktur.* Stuttgart: Thieme; 1995.
14. Hempen CH, Fischer T. *Leitfaden der Chinesischen Phytotherapie.* Munich: Urban & Fischer; 2001.
15. Him-Che Y. *Chinese Herbs.* 2nd ed. Rosemead: Institute of Chinese Medicine; 1995.
16. Him-Che Y. *Handbook of Chinese Herbal Formulas.* Rosemead: Institute of Chinese Medicine; 1983.
17. Johns F. *Die Kunst der Akupunkturtechniken.* Kötzting: VGM Wühr; 2000.
18. Jong-Chol C. *Japanese-English Dictionary of Oriental Medicine.* Tokyo, Iseisha: Oriental Medicine Research Center of Kitasato Institute; 1993.
19. Kaptchuk T. *Das Große Buch der Chinesischen Medizin.* Munich: Heyne; 1983.
20. Kirschbaum B. *Atlas und Lehrbuch der Chinesischen Zungendiagnostik.* Kötzting: VGM Wühr; 2001.
21. Kubiena G. *Praxishandbuch Akupunktur.* 3rd ed. Munich: Urban & Fischer; 2004.
22. Li X, Zhao J. *Acupuncture—Patterns & Practice.* Seattle: Eastland; 1993.
23. Macocia G. *Die Grundlagen der Chinesischen Medizin.* Kötzting: VGM Wühr; 1994.
24. Macocia G. *Die Praxis der Chinesischen Medizin.* Kötzting: VGM Wühr; 1997.
25. Macocia G. *Die Gynäkologie in der Praxis der Chinesischen Medizin.* Kötzting: VGM Wühr; 2001.
26. Macocia G. *Tongue Diagnosis in Chinese Medicine.* Seattle: Eastland; 1995.
27. Neeb G. *Das Blut-Stase-Syndrom.* Kötzting: VGM Wühr; 2001.
28. Ou M. *Chinese-English Dictionary of Traditional Chinese Medicine.* Hongkong: Joint Publishing; 1988.
29. Paulus W, Zhang M, Strehler E, Danasouri I, Sterzik K. Influence of acupuncture on the pregnancy rate in patients who undergo assisted reproduction therapy. *Fertility and Sterility.* 2002;77:4.
30. Porkert M. *Klinische Chinesische Pharmakologie.* Heidelberg: Verlag für Medizin Dr. Ewald Fischer; 1978.
31. Porkert M. *Klassische Chinesische Rezeptur.* Zug: Acta Medicinae Sinensis; 1984.
32. Ross J. *Akupunktur Punkt Kombinationen.* London: Churchill Livingstone; 1995.
33. Schmidt H. *Konstitutionelle Akupunktur.* 3rd ed. Stuttgart: Hippokrates; 1988.
34. Shibata Y, Wu J. *Kampo Treatment for Climacteric Disorders.* Taos: Paradigm; 1997.

35. Song W. *Das Praxis-Handbuch der Chinesischen Akupunktur und Moxibustion.* Kötzting: VGM Wühr; 2001.

36. Teeguarden R. *Chinese Tonic Herbs.* Tokyo: Japan Publications; 1985.

37. Terasawa K, Bacowsky H (translator). *Kampo—Japanese-Oriental Medicine.* Tokyo: K.K. Standard McIntyre; 1993.

38. Weixin J, Wenxin N (translator). *Diagnosis of Sterility and its Traditional Chinese Treatment.* China: Shandong Science and Technology Press; 1999.

39. Wiseman N, Ellis A, Zmiewski P. *Fundamentals of Chinese Medicine.* Taos: Paradigm; 1985.

40. Wiseman N. *Dictionary of Chinese Medicine (English-Chinese/Chinese-English).* Beijing: Foreign Language Press; 1995.

18   Infertility and Sexual Disorders

Andreas A. Noll

Formulas: Jacqueline Peineke

This chapter is concerned with the effects of sexual disorders in the context of fertility treatment. On the one hand, such disorders can be regarded as a priori, that is, they impede the success of fertility treatment from the start. On the other hand, these disorders also arise in the course of fertility treatment. Most commonly, we differentiate these disturbances by means of the *wu xing* (five phases) and *zang fu* (viscera and bowels) theories.

The Three Dimensions of Sexuality

Regardless of the fact that we now deal with problems of sexuality much more openly and liberally than in the past (for example, the use of Viagra), it is probably still true most of the time that we fail to consciously reflect on either sexuality or fertility. In both of these subject areas, we do not ask "Why?" but assume that they are a given from the start. Just like the topic of childbearing, the desire for and performance of sexual intercourse "is simply one of those things…" Problems with sex quickly lead to bafflement, self-doubt, and intense crises of identity, for both women and men. In view of the technological possibilities in biomedicine, sexual disorders appear to have been pushed into the background when we are dealing with insemination, ICSI, IVF etc. It is fatal, however, that only one side—the reproductive dimension—is taken into consideration. The reason for this is that sexuality has at least three different dimensions that are intimately connected to each other:
- the communicative, social dimension
- the reproductive dimension
- the pleasure dimension

First, there is the **communicative, social dimension**. This covers the need for emotional and physical closeness, for love and reciprocation of love, as well as for deep social relations; it goes far beyond the time of pure reproductivity. Because Confucian thought, which is socially minded as well, has left a clear mark on the attitudes of Chinese medical philosophy, we find aspects of this social level, for example, in all five phases of correlative thinking:
- compassion (wood)
- honesty (metal)
- ritual (fire)
- wisdom (water)
- trust (earth)

The **reproductive dimension**, on the other hand, is limited by arbitrariness and time-related factors (reproductivity). What gives it meaning is the creative act that finds its fulfillment in the birth of a new being. In the course of fertility treatment, when childbearing is therefore no longer normal and taken for granted, couples ask themselves the existential questions of the ultimate "Why?" And the motivation provides decisive, often all the more pressing impulses to the "project" and life as such: it is the wish to recognize oneself (and one's partner), to pass on one's own life, so to speak, and to be able to leave a trace in the world beyond one's existence (see also Chapter 4). After we have recognized these motives, the inability to fulfill this existential desire can lead to equally existential crises if the meaning of life —or at least of the relationship—is questioned due to the failure of this creative power. From the view of TCM, these are disorders of the water phase, which can then conversely lead to dwindling sexual desire and fear and panic.

The **pleasure dimension** is the level of sexuality that finds fulfillment in subjective experience. While the experience of pleasure in turn motivates the reproductive and social-communicative dimensions, due to autoeroticism and introversion it is not primarily oriented towards relationships and the social dimension. In TCM, this level of sexuality is again associated with the water phase and the kidneys: in kidney *yin*, as the elemental experience of pleasure and corporeality; in

232

kidney *yang*, especially in the *ming men*, as a life-fulfilling and directive power.

Yin and *yang*—these are the two fundamental and original aspects in the worldview of the ancient Chinese that determine and define the entire existence, in all its dimensions of the macro- and microcosm. The duality of heaven and earth, day and night, sun and moon, are mirrored on earth in the duality of man and woman. On the basis of the division of labor, in society as well as in the home, and extending to the shape of the sexual organs and the most commonly practiced form of sexual intercourse, the man is *yang*, oriented outward, giving, and moving. The woman, on the other hand, is *yin*, oriented inward, taking and receiving—whereby any *yang* contains the root of *yin* and any *yin* contains dynamic *yang*. When these two come together, when *yin* and *yang* unite, new life is created. *He yin yang*—the union of *yin* and *yang*—is the Chinese term for sexual intercourse. Both unite in *yin*, and the new *qi* is formed from the dynamism of the movements during sexual intercourse. Without this *qi*—the movements of both man and woman—new life is possible only with difficulty.

The difference in the energetics of both partners in this creative play also results in a difference in their susceptibility to disturbances. While kidney energy in the broadest sense can become exhausted in both partners, this affects primarily kidney *yin* in the man and kidney *yang* in the woman. Wood, or the liver, manifests in the man decisively in the erection of the penis, in accordance with the male attributes of activity, movement, and extroversion. The spleen and lung as levels of the emotions and introversion, on the other hand, are in the foreground for the woman. Regardless of all possible disharmonies and especially of individual differences—which in the context of sexual intercourse can certainly also lead to a complete reversal of these initial "roles"—the goal is for *yin* and *yang* to come together and thereby complement or support each other. The differences and mutual support of *yin* and *yang* also become clear when we look at the reactions in the union of man and woman: the man is *yang* and agitates during sex with his *yin*; this is where he wants to be approached. The woman is *yin* and acts during sex initially with the *yang*, with the head—she initially wants to be touched with the eyes and with language. Then, the woman's *yang* sinks into *yin* and thus causes the fluids to move.

The man's *yin*, on the other hand, is lifted up by the woman's *yang* and starts moving.

■ Disorders of Male Fertility— Exhaustion of Water (Kidney) and Wood (Liver)

Fear creates blockage—especially men who are very achievement-oriented are blocked in their sexuality by their expectations and fear of failure. We also find erectile dysfunctions as a sort of self-fulfilling prophecy in the context of certain basic disorders like diabetes or as a described side-effect of medications. These fears—as an expression of weakness in the kidney—often multiply in the course of fertility treatment. Associated with this fear is the pressure to perform and also the fulfillment of the so-called "mythical" assumption: men can and want to do it at any time. Satisfying and above all pleasurable sex then becomes very difficult, especially in the context of fertility treatment when the sexual myths—which still control many men—are compounded by time pressure and the narrow medical framework.

Sexual Myths
- We are sophisticated people and take pleasure in sex.
- A real man doesn't need "sissy things" like emotions and constant conversation.
- Every touch is sexual or should lead to sex.
- Men can and want to do it at any time.
- During sex, a real man shows what he can do. Sex concerns a stiff penis and what you can do with it.
- Sex equals sexual intercourse.
- A man must make his partner experience an earthquake.
- Good sex includes an orgasm.
- In sex, men should not listen to women.
- Good sex is spontaneous, there is nothing to plan or talk about.
- Real men have no sexual problems.[14]

◾ Disorders in the Sexuality of Men and Women

In **men,** it is mostly the pressure to perform and **fear of failure** that cause problems in sexuality. In **women,** on the other hand, corresponding **fear of reaction** plays an important role: the fear of not being able to react appropriately, also due to individual experiences like feelings of guilt, self-sacrifice, or possibly even experiences of abuse. For women, the fear of failure multiplies in fertility treatment with every failed attempt at fertilization and can lead to a striking loss of identity as a woman. This means, while the field of tension in **men** is located in the area **kidney-liver** (fear and pressure), in **women** it is located in the area **lung-kidney** (emotion and fear). The following disease patterns can occur:

- liver *qi* congestion
- weakness of spleen *qi*
- dampness/damp-heat
- additional blockages
- kidney vacuity
- weakness of kidney *yang*
- weakness of kidney *qi*
- weakness of lung *qi*
- weakness of heart *yang*

Always under Pressure—Liver *Qi* Congestion

Causes and Disease Development

Zheng—the regular, targeted flow of energies—from the TCM perspective, this is the responsibility of the liver. *Qi,* the life force, is directed outward for the development of the person, the fulfillment of the inborn potential and destiny. In terms of *qi,* sexuality means that the male or female partner is "conquered," in accordance with one's own wishes and expectations, but also with one's "urges" that seek this goal. Pressure builds, which seeks release and fulfillment. If this is not achieved, *qi* becomes blocked, especially if the liver is unable to provide for the necessary flexibility and adaptability.

Pressure from the outside or inside or exaggerated demands on oneself greatly strain the function of the liver. The pressure can also be overwhelming from the outside, for example, the pressure in the context of fertility treatment, which manifests monthly during the time of ovulation, or which can result from personal and professional planning. The pregnancy is supposed to be planned, after all. Every plan, however, can strain our adaptability—which, according to TCM, is guaranteed by the liver—to the breaking point. The risk of obstacles, of areas of life that are incalculable because they are beyond human control, is too great. Trusting in the coincidences of creation collides with the constraints of biomedicine and life, such as, for example, the termination of human, especially female, fertility, but also the reimbursement practices of medical insurances in attempted artificial fertilization. The liver regulates the relationship between human desires and the adversities of life. In this function, it should resemble—a very beautiful image—bamboo, which is hard, solid, and stable, single-mindedly growing upward, bending in the storm without breaking. The liver should not—to stay with this image—be like an oak, which is solid and has strong roots, but breaks in the storm.

If there is no open communication between the partners in the relationship, hidden feelings can frequently also lead to blockages and thereby to sexual disturbances. When they fail to communicate about their wishes, aversions, and expectations, this can lead to blockages of the *qi* flow, and from there also of the flow of the fluids and blood, in either the man or the woman.

Consequently, the blood fails to move from the liver into the sexual organs, and likewise, on the microscopic level, the sperm cells are unable to move correctly. Alternatively, the woman's menstrual blood congeals, causing cramping and pain. To resolve this pressure, TCM regards the social component of liver-wood as key: *ren*—benevolence. Helpful for resolving blockages are open discussions and putting oneself in the partner's place.

The penis is the "sinew of the liver." Its much-mentioned strength and "steadfastness" demonstrate the strengths and weaknesses of wood. The liver channel, its muscle channel, and its *luo* network vessels supply the penis in the man, but also the external genitals and the uterus in the woman, with blood and *qi.*

In the *jue yin* layer, the liver is connected to the *xin bao* (pericardium). This "protector of the heart" guarantees the opening and closing of the personality in emotional injuries. This function regulates the person's "role play" in social situations, that is, the extent to which the heart as the "ruler" in the person should open or close. Attacks on a person's "soul" can thus also lead to disturbances in the liver and kidney, especially on the sexual level.

The liver's *yang* aspect is represented in the function of the gallbladder, which is responsible for doing the right thing in the decisive and correct moment.

Symptoms

When liver *qi* stagnates, we can see this in **blockages** of all kinds—emotional, spiritual, and physical. The pressure manifests in a pronounced tendency to irascibility, on the muscular level in

tension, and in the inability to express one's emotions, opinions, and desires.

All liver disorders improve with movement and worsen under (time) pressure—this is a key symptom! This means that love play that is not limited in time can resolve these blockages, especially also playful engagement with different sexual techniques. According to TCM, we can recognize any involvement of the gallbladder in problems with putting ideas and expectations into practice. Fear and despondency as well as high spirits and the related tendency to infringe on others are signs of disharmony in this bowel.

Tongue: tense, dark, also with red margins (ascending liver *yang*)

Pulse: tight

Table 18.1 Key symptoms for sexuality and reproduction: liver *qi* congestion

	Woman	**Man**
Sexuality and reproductive organs	Vaginitis, dyspareunia	Inability to achieve an erection and penetration, especially under pressure; "erections (in one's sleep, from masturbation) are normal
Reproduction and menstruation	Premenstrual tension, painful menstruation, no or irregular ovulation With blood stasis, cold/dampness/phlegm: myoma, polycystic ovaries (PCO)	Reduced sperm motility With blood stasis: sperm antibodies

Therapy

Regulate and soothe liver *qi*.

Acupuncture

Table 18.2 Acupuncture points in liver *qi* congestion

Points	**Name**	**Indication/Effect**
LR-3	*Tai chong*	Quickens the spirit and the eyes, improves the flow of *qi*, quiets the spirit, resolves *qi* blockages
LI-4	*He gu*	Especially in combination with LR-3: frees the surface, regulates *qi* and blood, disinhibits the channels and network vessels, quiets the spirit, resolves blockages
SP-6	*San yin jiao*	Regulates the chamber of blood (uterus) and the essence palace (testicles), softens hardenings, regulates menstruation, lifts *qi*
PC-6	*Nei guan*	Especially for insecurity, vulnerability: regulates the *qi* in the center burner, quiets the spirit, harmonizes the stomach, gives a "thick skin"
KI-1	*Yong quan*	Rage that rises into the head, disquietude, when heart fire is unable to sink
LR-6	*Zhong du*	Stagnations in the liver channel, after vasectomy
LR-1	*Da dun*	Blockages, stagnations of blood and *qi* in the penis, also lack of sensitivity

Medicinal Therapy

Rx. Xiao Yao San *(Free Wanderer Powder);*
Modification for the Treatment of Infertility and
Sexual Disorders:

- *chai hu* (Bupleuri radix), 4–6 g—strongly raises *qi*, soothes liver *qi*
- *dang gui* (Angelicae sinensis radix), 4–6 g—supplements and quickens blood, quiets the *shen*, moistens the intestine
- *bai shao yao* (Paeoniae radix alba), 9–12 g—nourishes liver blood, quiets the liver
- *bai zhu* (Atractylodis macrocephalae rhizoma), 6–9 g—supplements the spleen, strengthens *qi*, dries dampness, stabilizes *wei* (defense)
- *fu ling* (Poria), 6–9 g—strengthens the spleen, harmonizes the center, eliminates dampness, quiets the spirit
- *sheng jiang* (Zingiberis rhizoma recens), three slices—warms the spleen and stomach
- *da zao* (Jujubae fructus), three pieces—supplements the center, strengthens the spleen and stomach, supplements blood, quiets the spirit, harmonizes the formula
- *du zhong* (Eucommiae cortex), 6–9 g—supplements the liver, kidney, and essence, downbears ascending liver *yang*
- *tu si zi* (Cuscutae semen), 6–9 g—supplements kidney *yang*, contains essence, supplements liver *yin*
- *bo he* (Menthae herba), 2–3 g—regulates liver *qi*, circulates *qi* (lung *qi* by downbearing, liver *qi* by upbearing)

Modifications:

- for heat: *mu dan pi* (Moutan cortex), 6–9 g; *zhi zi* (Gardeniae fructus), 3–5 g
- for fear or depressive mood: *he huan pi* (Albizziae cortex), 4–6 g; *suan zao ren* (Ziziphi spinosi semen), 6–9 g
- for constipation or flatulence: *da fu pi* (Arecae pericarpium), 6–9 g; *bing lang* (Arecae semen), 6–9 g
- for phlegm stagnation in polycystic ovaries (PCO): *ban xia* (Pinelliae rhizoma), 4–6 g; *zao jia ci* (Gleditsiae spina), 4–6 g
- for blood stasis, *qi* or phlegm stagnation in myomas or polycystic ovaries (PCO): *tu bie chong* (Eupolyphaga seu steleophaga), 3–5 g; *e zhu* (Curcumae rhizoma), 4–6 g

- for sperm antibodies, add blood-moving substances: *dan shen* (Salviae miltiorrhizae radix), 6–9 g; *tao ren* (Persicae semen), 6–9 g; *hong hua* (Carthami flos), 3–6 g
- for reduced sperm motility: *wang bu liu xing* (Vaccariae semen), 4–6 g; *lu lu tong* (Liquidambaris fructus), 4–6 g

Pondering and Reflection—Weakness of Spleen *Qi*

Causes and Disease Development

The spleen supplies the kidney—which serves as the reservoir of both congenital and acquired essence *(jing)*—with all those energies that the person can absorb from the environment and digest. This can take place on the material, spiritual, and emotional level. The spleen has the function of absorbing *qi* from the environment in its various forms and transforming it into the body's own substrate. Diet and metabolism: these are the sources of the energy *qi* (in addition to the lung) —on the physical, spiritual, and mental level. By consuming fast food and junk food, we miss paying the necessary attention to what is good for the body and what it truly needs. The results are nutritional deficits, metabolic disorders, states of deficiency, and accumulations of dampness due to non-transformed substances.

Human *qi* is fed from three sources:

- from the inborn potential of the kidney
- from respiration (lung) and
- from the diet (spleen)

The functions of the kidney, spleen, and lung in turn consume *qi*. Chronic diseases or stress lead to excessive strain on these sources of energy and thereby ultimately to the exhaustion of the fundamental reserves and potentials of the person. These elemental potentials are, however, stored in the kidney—the basis for reproduction and sexuality.

Empathy is an essential function of the spleen. If the two partners are unable during sexual intercourse to be responsive to each other or to put themselves in each other's place, sexual satisfaction is impossible.

Confidence, including confidence in oneself, is the Confucian virtue associated with the earth phase. On the one hand, this includes the aspect in interpersonal relationships. It means that we accept our partner the way he or she is, in the entirety of the person. Fear, insecurity, role-playing are no longer necessary—and thus the backdrop is formed for an unforced corporeality. On the other hand, though, this also includes the aspect of confidence in oneself, in one's own body. Introspection with the result that we are content with ourselves the way we are.

The spleen reflects the earth phase in the human body and therefore also our ability to remain in the middle, that is, in our own center. This also concerns the physical level because one of the important functions of the spleen is to lift the or-gans and tissues and keep them in their place. In spleen vacuity, we see sagging of the organs, especially of the pelvic organs. An absence of the spleen's uplifting power can also affect the ability to get an erection.

Symptoms

Soft-liquid stools, possibly containing pieces of undigested food. The abdomen is distended, in conjunction with generalized cold sensations. We can also find a tendency to hernias. Drooping manifests in varicosis, uterine or bladder prolapse, and possibly dribbling after urination.

Tongue: pale, swollen
Pulse: vacuous, fine

Table 18.3 Key symptoms for sexuality and reproduction: weakness of spleen *qi*

	Woman	Man
Sexuality and reproductive organs	Bladder prolapse, uterine prolapse	Feelings of pressure and heaviness; reduced libido
Reproduction and menstruation	Vaginal discharge Early miscarriage (first to third month) Morning sickness from the 12th week on (spleen disorder)	Varicocele

Therapy

Strengthen spleen *qi*, supplement the lung and *yang* in the kidney.

Acupuncture

Table 18.4 Acupuncture points in weakness of spleen *qi*

Points	Name	Indication/Effect
SP-6	San yin jiao	Lifts and holds *qi* especially in the pelvic region, erectile dysfunction
SP-8	Di ji	Especially for feelings of fullness, irregular menstruation, or intermenstrual bleeding
ST-30	Qi chong	Regulates *qi* and blood in the entire pelvis, unites the energies of the kidney, spleen, and stomach
ST-27	Da ju	Especially for impotence and feeling of fullness
CV-8	Shen que	Strengthens the center, moxa
GV-20	Bai hui	Lifts *qi*, especially for anal and uterine prolapse and impotence
CV-6	Qi hai	Strengthens *qi*, combine with *dan zhong*, CV-17

Medicinal Therapy

Rx. Bu Zhong Yi Qi Tang (Center-supplementing Qi-boosting Decoction); Modification for the Treatment of Infertility and Sexual Disorders:

- huang qi (Astragali radix), 9–12 g—supplements and lifts spleen qi, strengthens qi and wei (defense)
- ren shen (Ginseng radix), 4–6 g—strengthens original qi, strengthens the spleen and stomach, quiets the spirit
- bai zhu, 9–12 g—supplements the spleen, strengthens qi, dries dampness, stabilizes wei (defense)
- zhi gan cao (Glycyrrhizae radix cum liquido fricta), 3–6 g—supplements the spleen, strengthens qi, harmonizes the formula
- dang gui, 4–6 g—supplements and quickens blood, quiets the spirit, moistens the intestine
- chen pi (Citri reticulatae pericarpium), 3–5 g—moves and regulates qi, strengthens the spleen, downbears qi, transforms dampness
- sheng ma (Cimicifugae rhizoma), 3–5 g—strongly upbears qi, frees the surface
- chai hu, 3–5 g—strongly upbears qi, soothes liver qi
- du zhong, 6–9 g—supplements liver and kidneys, contains the essence, downbears ascending liver yang
- tu si zi, 6–9 g—supplements kidney yang, contains essence, supplements liver yin

Modifications:

- for leucorrhea: cang zhu (Atractylodis rhizoma), 4–6 g; huang bai (Phellodendri cortex), 2–3 g
- for fullness in the abdomen: zhi ke (Aurantii fructus), 4–6 g; hou po (Magnoliae officinalis cortex), 4–6 g; mu xiang (Aucklandiae radix), 4–6 g; sha ren (Amomi fructus), 3–5 g

Missing Clarity—Dampness and Dampheat

Causes and Disease Development

The spleen transforms the energies absorbed from the diet into bodily substances. This ability (which consumes qi and yang) is strained considerably when we assimilate very solid, heavy, and simply hard to digest or fluid components of the diet. Fluids must be reabsorbed adequately from the intestine and either incorporated into tissue,

flesh, or blood, or eliminated via the intestine and bladder. If the spleen does not receive sufficient qi or requires too much qi for digesting, fluids begin to collect in the body: the tissue becomes edematous, both in the extremities and, for example, in the abdomen. The sweat becomes damp and sticky, and all other fluids eliminated by the person become turbid and possibly malodorous. Unprocessed thoughts, the continuously turning merry-go-round of thoughts, and the tendency to pondering are manifestations of this dampness on the spiritual-mental level.

In **men**, this pattern manifests in prostate disorders, but also in disorders of sexuality as erectile dysfunctions; in **women**, in vaginal discharge or formation of cysts.

Note. The fact that dampness can sink downward always indicates the simultaneous existence of an energetic deficit in this part of the body. The reason is that the kidney—especially kidney yang—is also an uplifting force. When kidney yang is exhausted, an "energetic vacuum" results, into which dampness can sink in accordance with its heavy nature. Furthermore, the warming function of kidney yang is essential for the spleen's metabolic function.

Symptoms

Feelings of heaviness, sluggishness, reluctance to move, frequent and possibly frustrated urge to urinate to the point of incontinence, damp and itchy genitals, vaginal discharge, soft stools, possibly hemorrhoids.

Additional Blockages: Heat and Dampness in the Liver and Gallbladder

Causes and Disease Development

When the liver is unable to distribute qi evenly, becomes congested, and forms heat, this heat can collect together with the dampness in the lower burner. As a result, we see symptoms of damp-heat especially along the course of the liver channel and its network vessels.

Because this syndrome complex (spleen qi vacuity, dampness, and kidney vacuity) is a digestive and metabolic disorder, a balanced diet is very important both to provide relief for the metabolism and to supply sufficient amounts of essences acquired from the diet. Fats and other foods that are difficult to digest strain the digestive process excessively. The consumption of raw foods also uses up a lot of *qi* in its metabolism. This overload results in accumulations of fluid in the lower abdomen. Consequently, damp-heat arises when alcohol, sugar, fried foods, and smoking furthermore add a lot of *yang*. As a result, we see destructive inflammatory changes like prostatitis, herpes, or yellow vaginal discharge.

Symptoms

Feelings of heaviness and drooping in the lower abdomen, continuous frequent and possibly frustrated urge to urinate to the point of incontinence, tendency to damp-inflammatory changes in the penis, vagina, and urethra, also genital herpes, soft unformed stools, sweating and itching in the genital area.

Tongue: thick, white or yellow, with sticky fur, especially on the root of the tongue

Pulse: thin and slippery with internal disorders; replete, stringlike, and slippery with invasion of external factors; in heat patterns, rapid; in cold patterns, slow

Table 18.5 Key symptoms for sexuality and reproduction: heat and dampness in the liver and gallbladder

	Woman	Man
Sexuality and reproductive organs	Bartholinitis, drooping of the uterus, cysts, uterine/anal prolapse, genital itch, eczemas, burning, dark urine, yellow vaginal discharge	Genital itch, eczemas, burning, dark urine, difficulty stopping urinating Acute prostatitis (in younger men) Inability to achieve a complete erection
Reproduction and menstruation	Distention before menstruation, menstruation with hesitant onset and dark blood, yellow vaginal discharge Inconspicuous ovulation, pregnancy is possible, the baby will have rashes	Yellow sticky ejaculate with bacteria (no apparent problems with sperm quality)

Therapy

Transform and eliminate dampness, strengthen the *qi* of the spleen and kidney, clear heat.

Acupuncture

Table 18.6 Acupuncture points in heat and dampness in the liver and gallbladder

Points	Name	Indication/Effect
SP-9	Yin ling quan	Dampness in the lower burner, drooping organs
LR-10	Zu wu li	Kidney wind and dampness lead to itching in the testicles; needle to supplement or apply moxa
BL-34	Xiao liao	Dampness with heat in the lower abdomen
KI-8	Jiao xin	Dampness, *yin* vacuity
GB-8	Shuai gu	Dampness in the head, dazed spirit
ST-40	Feng long	Disperses blockages of dampness and phlegm, especially in the stomach channel

Medicinal Therapy for Spleen *Qi* Vacuity with Dampness

Rx. Xiang Sha Liu Jun Zi Tang *(Costusroot and Amomum Six Gentlemen Decoction); Modification for the Treatment of Infertility and Sexual Disorders:*

- *ren shen*, 4–6 g—strengthens *yuan qi*, strengthens the spleen and stomach, quiets the spirit
- *bai zhu*, 6–9 g—supplements the spleen, strengthens *qi*, dries dampness, stabilizes *wei* (defense)
- *fu ling*, 6–9 g—strengthens the spleen, harmonizes the center, eliminates dampness, quiets the spirit
- *zhi gan cao*, 3–5 g—supplements the spleen, strengthens *qi*, harmonizes the formula
- *ban xia*, 6–9 g—dries dampness, downbears lung and stomach *qi*
- *chen pi*, 4–6 g—moves and regulates *qi*, strengthens the spleen, downbears *qi*, transforms dampness
- *sha ren*, 3–5 g—moves *qi* and supplements the spleen and stomach, transforms dampness
- *mu xiang*, 4–6 g—moves *qi*, regulates *qi* in the intestine, supplements spleen *qi*
- *zhi cang zhu* (Atractylodis rhizoma praeparatum), 4–6 g—dries dampness, strengthens the spleen, clears dampness in the lower burner
- *ai ye* (Artemisiae argyi folium), 3–5 g—warms, supplements, and dries the uterus
- *chao qian shi* (Euryales semen frictum) 6–9 g—absorbs dampness, strengthens the spleen and checks diarrhea, secures the kidney and essence
- *chao shan yao* (Dioscoreae rhizoma frictum), 6–9 g—supplements and supports the spleen, stomach, and lung, nourishes the kidney; when processed, checks vaginal discharge
- *chao lian zi* (Nelumbinis semen frictum), 6–9 g —astringes, strengthens the spleen and checks diarrhea, clears heart heat, nourishes the kidney

or:

Rx. Er Miao San *(Mysterious Two Powder); Modification for the Treatment of Infertility and Sexual Disorders:*

This formula clears damp-heat:

- *zhi cang zhu*, 6–9 g—dries dampness, supplements the spleen
- *huang bai*, 4–6 g—eliminates damp-heat, cools vacuity heat in the kidney

- *che qian zi* (Plantaginis semen), 6–9 g—clears heat, promotes urination
- *shi wei* (Pyrrosiae folium), 4–6 g—clears heat, stanches bleeding
- *fu ling*, 6–9 g—strengthens the spleen, harmonizes the center, eliminates dampness, quiets the spirit
- *shan yao* (Dioscoreae rhizoma), 6–9 g—supplements the spleen and stomach, promotes fluid production, supplements kidney *qi* and *yin*
- *ze xie* (Alismatis rhizoma), 4–6 g—eliminates dampness, cools vacuity heat in the kidney, clears damp-heat
- *bi xie* (Dioscoreae hypoglaucae seu semptemlobae rhizoma), 4–6 g—separates the turbid from the clear, eliminates dampness
- *zhu ling* (Polyporus), 4–6 g—promotes urination, eliminates dampness
- *yi yi ren* (Coicis semen), 9–12 g—eliminates dampness, treats damp-heat
- *tong cao* (Tetrapanacis medulla), 1–2 g—eliminates dampness, clears heat, functions as courier

or:

Rx. Bi Xie Fen Qing Yin *(Fish Poison Yam Clear–Turbid Separation Beverage); Modification for the Treatment of Infertility and Sexual Disorders:*

- *bi xie*, 9–12 g—access to the bladder, liver, and stomach, separates the turbid from the clear, bitter, also clears damp-heat in the skin
- *shi chang pu* (Acori tatarinowii rhizoma), 4–6 g —opens the senses and dissolves phlegm, transforms turbid dampness, harmonizes the center burner, heart, spleen, and liver
- *yi zhi ren* (Alpiniae oxyphyllae fructus), 6–9 g—supplements *yang*, warms the kidney and spleen
- *wu yao* (Linderae radix), 4–9 g—moves the *qi* in the lower burner, warms the kidneys, spleen, stomach, and lung

Modifications:

- for ejaculate with reduced viscosity and prolonged liquefaction time: *huang bai*, 4–6 g; *zhi mu* (Anemarrhenae rhizoma), 6–9 g
- for sperm agglutination: *wang bu liu xing*, 6–9 g; *mu gua* (Chaenomelis fructus), 6–9 g; *wan can sha* (Bombycis feces), 4–6 g

Medicinal Therapy for Damp-heat in the Liver or Gallbladder

Rx. Long Dan Xie Gan Tang *(Gentian Liver-draining Decoction); Modification for the Treatment of Infertility and Sexual Disorders:*

- *chao long dan cao* (Gentianae radix fricta): 4–6 g—drains damp-heat from the liver and gallbladder channels, clears liver-fire
- *jiao shan zhi zi* (Gardeniae fructus ustum), 3–5 g—clears heat and drains damp-heat in the triple burner
- *sheng di huang* (Rehmanniae radix exsiccata seu recens), 4–6 g—nourishes kidney *yin*, cools the blood and *yang*
- *mu tong* (Akebiae trifoliatae caulis), 3–5 g
- *ze xie*, 6–9 g—eliminates dampness, cools vacuity heat in the kidney, clears damp-heat
- *shan yao*, 6–9 g—supplements and supports the spleen, stomach, and lung, and nourishes the kidney
- *chao jing jie* (Schizonepetae flos frictus), 4–6 g —access to the liver, *qi*, and blood levels, relieves itching, when processed, less effective for freeing the surface
- *che qian zi*, 6–9 g—clears heat, promotes urination
- *zhi cang zhu*, 4–6 g—dries dampness, supplements the spleen
- *chao bai zhu* (Atractylodis macrocephalae rhizoma frictum), 3–5 g—supplements the spleen, strengthens *qi*, dries dampness, stabilizes *wei* (defense)
- *chao chai hu* (Bupleuri radix fricta), 3–5 g— strongly upbears *qi*, soothes liver *qi*
- *chao qing pi* (Citri reticulatae pericarpium viride frictum), 3–5 g—regulates liver *qi*, dries and transforms phlegm
- *huang bai*, 3–5 g—eliminates damp-heat, cools vacuity heat in the kidney, diuretic
- *yi yi ren*, 9–12 g—eliminates dampness, treats damp-heat
- *chuan niu xi* (Cyathulae radix), 6–9 g—access to the liver and kidney, moves the blood and drains dampness
- *bi xie*, 4–6 g—separates the turbid from the clear, eliminates dampness

Modifications:

- For prostate hypertrophy after acute inflammation in younger men two to three of the following softening substances: *xia ku cao* (Prunellae spica), 6–9 g; *mu li* (Ostreae concha), 9–12 g;

zhe bei mu (Fritillariae thunbergii bulbus), 6–9 g; *xuan shen* (Scrophulariae radix), 6–9 g

The Source Dries Up—Kidney Vacuity

Causes and Disease Development

According to TCM, the kidney is the central reservoir of the energies that are significant for maintaining life, for reproduction, and therefore also for sexuality. This pool is emptied both by emotional and physical overexertion, but also by chronic tension—that is, due to liver *qi* congestion. The inborn potential of essence inevitably decreases during the course of human life. We can slow down this loss only by leading a moderate life, by avoiding overexertion and excess. In any case, the kidney depends on being refilled by receiving postnatal potential (*jing*). Otherwise, the result is kidney *yin* or *jing* vacuity.

Vacuity of the kidney and hence also of sexuality is often influenced by an insecure future and the resulting existential fear. Unemployment, involuntary mobility, and the loss of professional, biographical identity show that the social safety net has become coarse-meshed and that life security is disappearing. All this can cause profound insecurity. Other mechanisms that "get under the skin" also affect this fundamental level, such as any experience of trauma in the sexual realm, violence, or humiliation.

Physical overexertion—this includes, for example, childbirth, pregnancies, and serious hormonal strain such as after attempted artificial fertilization—most commonly results in an exhaustion of kidney *yang*, but can also result in a weakness of kidney *yin*, which in turn cause disorders in other viscera and bowels. This weakness of kidney *yin* appears mostly in men or in overexertion of the mental capacities (see spleen weakness). In kidney vacuity, we will often find a vicious cycle in men: weakness of kidney *yin* leads to vacuity fire with an increased sex drive, whose expression in excessive sexuality in turn further aggravates the *yin* vacuity.

An exhaustion of kidney *yang* can be rebuilt neither with rest nor with sufficient sleep. One possible source could be diet—it should be easily digestible and warm in its nature. Other elements of the lifestyle should also aim at balancing the physiological exhaustion with moderate movement and appropriate warmth—that is, supplying *yang* from the outside.

The kidney is "the source of *yin* and *yang*," as the *Su Wen* states,[7] and hence we are often dealing with combined symptoms of *qi*, *yin*, and *yang* vacuity in the kidney.

Symptoms

Fear and insecurity, feelings of panic and heat, increased libido, insomnia, disquietude, dizziness, heat symptoms (e. g., a red face, hot palms and soles), pain in the lower back, exhaustion, "steaming bones," tinnitus, "light" feeling in the head, impaired hearing, all symptoms aggravated by lack of sleep or after sexual activity because of the exertion of *yin*, a gaunt appearance, constipation in cases of insufficient fluids.

Tongue: thin, reddish, dry
Pulse: thin to the point of disappearing, rather superficial and rapid

Table 18.7 Key symptoms for sexuality and reproduction: kidney vacuity

	Woman	Man
Sexuality and reproductive organs	Insufficient lubrifaction of the vagina After a few minutes of intercourse, burning, pain, dryness, increased sensitivity	Premature ejaculation Sex makes the person restless and sleepless Night sweating in the lower half of the body
Reproduction and menstruation	Regular cycle is possible During menstruation: disquietude, dark red, thick blood, shortened menstruation After menstruation: pain in the lower back/sacrum/heel/KI-1 No ovulation, high temperature curve, ovulation takes place but eggs are smaller and weaker, as are the babies Possibly miscarriage (sixth to seventh month)	Reduced amount of ejaculate Reduced sperm count Increased number of dead/abnormal sperm cells

Therapy

Strengthen the spleen, stomach, and kidney.

Medicinal Therapy

Rx. Da Bu Yin Wan *(Major Yin-Supplementing Pill); Modification for the Treatment of Infertility and Sexual Disorders:*

- *zhi gui ban* (testudinis carapax et plastrum cum liquido fricti), 9–12 g—nourishes *yin*, anchors *yang*, cools and nourishes blood, supplements the heart
- *zhi mu*, 6–9 g—clears heat, supplements *yin*, and moistens dryness in the lung, stomach, and kidney
- *huang bai*, 3–5 g—eliminates damp-heat, cools vacuity heat in the kidney, has a diuretic effect
- *shu di huang* (Rehmanniae radix praeparata), 6–9 g—supplements blood, nourishes kidney and liver *yin*, strengthens essence

Modifications:

- for vacuity heat or internal heat: *di gu pi* (Lycii cortex), 6–9 g; *mu dan pi*, 4–6 g; *bai wei* (Cynanchi atrati radix), 4–6 g
- for disquietude and insomnia: *long chi* (Mastodi dentis fossilia calcinata), 6–9 g; *suan zao ren*, 9–12 g
- for night sweating: *fu xiao mai* (Tritici fructus levis), 6–9 g; *wu wei zi* (Schisandrae fructus), 4–6 g; *nuo dao gen* (Oryzae glutinosae radix), 6–9 g
- for exaggerated libido to cool the ministerial fire: *ci shi* (Magnetitum), 9–12 g; *zhi mu*, 9–12 g; *huang bai*, 6–9 g
- for reduced sperm count: *gou qi zi* (Lycii fructus), 6–9 g; *nü zhen zi* (Ligustri lucidi fructus), 6–9 g; *tu si zi*, 6–9 g
- for an increased number of abdnormal sperm cells: *dan shen*, 6–9 g; *tao ren*, 6–9 g; *hong hua*, 0.2–0.3 g; added after decocting

Weakness of Kidney *Yang* with Cold and Dampness

Causes and Disease Development

Exhaustion of kidney *yang* also has a lasting effect on the *qi* and *yang* of the spleen. At the same time, dampness accumulates and therefore we see the pattern of "repletion cold-damp"—or in other words, a "damp uterus". Here, pregnancy will rarely be possible, even by means of in vitro fertilization.

Symptoms

In female patients, we see cold sensations in the lower abdomen, legs, and vagina, with greater cold at night (midnight), rising from the uterus so strongly that the patient wakes from her sleep, watery vaginal discharge, aggravation of symptoms by rain and cold, a pale swollen face, edema, lack of appetite but overweight, diarrhea or soft or sticky stools, frequent urination, clear urine, and severe exhaustion. In male patients, watery fluid is discharged from the penis during bowel movements, there is a feeling of cold and dampness at the dam (CV-1), as well as possibly incontinence.

Tongue: swollen, with tooth marks, moist slimy fur that can be white, grey, or even black

Pulse: sunken, slow, and slippery, especially in the spleen position

Table 18.8 Key symptoms for sexuality and reproduction: weakness of kidney *yang* with cold and dampness

	Woman	Man
Sexuality and reproductive organs	Decreased libido	Decreased libido Weak or overly short erections; cold sensations in the penis Spermatorrhea at night (aggravated by fatigue and overwork)
Reproduction and menstruation	Menstruation/ovulation can be normal or irregular, or weak eggs Abortion threatens in the first months (especially in cold or with heavy lifting): bedrest and no cold foods (ice-cream), otherwise abortion threatens, low temperature curve	Fertility: watery ejaculate, reduced sperm count, increased number of dead/inactive sperm

Therapy

Strengthen kidney *yang*, warm, transform dampness.

Medicinal Therapy

Rx. Zan Yu Dan (Procreation Elixir); Modification for the Treatment of Infertility and Sexual Disorders:

- *fu zi* (Aconiti radix lateralis praeparata), 3–5 g—revives collapsed *yang*, warms the fire in the kidney, strengthens spleen and kidney *yang* (**beware: toxic!**)
- *rou gui* (Cinnamomi cortex), 3–5 g—warms the kidney, strengthens *yang*, guides the fire back to the source
- *rou cong rong* (Cistanches herba), 4–6 g—supplements kidney *yang*, moistens the stool

- *ba ji tian* (Morindae officinalis radix), 6–9 g—supplements the kidney, strengthens *yang* and the sinews and bones, expels wind
- *yin yang huo* (Epimedii herba), 6–9 g—supplements the kidney, strengthens *yang* and *yin*, downbears ascending liver *yang*
- *jiu zi* (Allii tuberosi semen), 4–6 g—warms the kidney, supplements *yang*, contains essence
- *xian mao* (Curculiginis rhizoma), 4–6 g—supplements the kidney, strengthens *yang* (**beware: toxic!**)
- *du zhong*, 6–9 g—supplements the liver and kidney, contains essence, downbears ascending liver *yang*
- *shu di huang*, 6–9 g—supplements blood, nourishes kidney and liver *yin*, strengthens essence

243

- *chao dang gui* (Angelicae sinensis radix fricta), 4–6 g—supplements and quickens blood, quiets the spirit, moistens the intestine
- *gou qi zi*, 6–9 g—supplements the liver and kidney, strengthens *yin*, blood, and *jing*, clears the vision
- *bai zhu*, 6–9 g—supplements the spleen, strengthens *qi*, dries dampness, stabilizes *wei* (defense)
- *tu si zi*, 6–9 g—supplements kidney *yang*, contains essence, supplements liver *yin*
- *pao jiang tan* (Zingiberis rhizoma praeparatum), 2–4 g—warms the center, dispels cold, prepared for treating the lower burner
- *chao ai ye* (Artemisiae argyi folium frictum), 4–6 g—warms, supplements, and dries the uterus
- *xiao hui xiang* (Foeniculi fructus), 3–5 g—warms the kidneys, regulates the flow of *qi* in the liver and lower burner
- *yi zhi ren*, 6–9 g—supplements *yang*, warms the kidney and spleen

---

He yin yang (合阴阳 = "**sex**"): in women, *yin* exhaustion causes the source to dry up; in men, a loss of *yin* causes consuming *yang*.

A Limp Lumbus—Weakness of Kidney *Qi*

Causes and Disease Development
In addition to the cold sensation, especially in the feet, which we can observe in kidney *yang* vacuity as a key symptom, the present pattern manifests in more pronounced symptoms of **lack of strength**. The kidney receives its *qi* also from the lung, which downbears it. As a result of weakness in the lung, we subsequently see a weakness of *qi* in the kidneys. Overconsumption of *qi* arises especially in endurance sports and after long-term severe physical strain.

Symptoms
Cold sensations in the lower back, abdomen, hands, and feet, fatigue and exhaustion, lower back pain, fatigue from sexual intercourse, lack of strength with lumbar pain and weakness, dribbling urination, and headache accompanied by feelings of emptiness in the head.

Tongue: thin, strengthless, light-colored
Pulse: sunken, fine

Table 18.9 Key symptoms for sexuality and reproduction: weakness of kidney *qi*

	Woman	Man
Sexuality and reproductive organs	Vaginal discharge Decreased libido	Cold sensations in the penis Decreased libido Decreased strength and duration of erections; nightly seminal emissions without sexual activities or dreams
Reproduction and menstruation	No ovulation Watery pink menses (weakness of *chong mai* and *ren mai*) Stronger cold sensations during menstruation	Lower sperm count, increased count of dead/inactive sperm

Therapy

Strengthen and lift *qi*, supplement the lung and spleen.

Acupuncture

Table 18.10 Acupuncture points in weakness of kidney *yin*, kidney *yang*, or *qi*

Points	Name	Indication/Effect
BL-43	Gao huang shu	Extensive exhaustion of essence, construction, and the spirit
BL-58	Fei yang	Fear, weakness in the lumbus and legs
KI-3	Tai xi	Kidney vacuity with heat
KI-6	Zhao hai	Generalized vacuity, vacuity of the *shen* and restless *gui* (ghosts and demons)
BL-35	Hui yang	Weakness of kidney *yang*
BL-23	Shen shu	Vacuity of kidney *yin* and *yang*
BL-52	Zhi shi	Strengthens the will and consolidates identity
LR-4	Zhong feng	Weakness of kidney *yang*, fear, lack of sensitivity, withdrawal
CV-5	Shi men	For infertility and frigidity **Beware**: moxa is preferable—needles make infertile!
CV-6	Qi hai	Concentration and mobilization of *qi* and *yang*; together with CV-12 and CV-17 for general quickening of *qi*
CV-4	Guan yuan	Moxa for infertility and stagnation of *yin*; cold below, heat above
KI-2	Ran gu	"Dragon Spring"—as fire point, it is most suitable for stimulating kidney *yang*; moxa!
KI-1	Yong quan	Quickens *qi* and *yang*; moxa!
ST-36	Zhu san li	As earth point on the stomach channel for absorbing *qi* and hence supporting *yang*, indirectly also for strengthening *yin*
GV-4	Ming men	To mobilize the *ming men* fire and hence original *qi*, for listlessness
KI-13	Qi xue	Sterility, moxa!
SP-6	San yin jiao	Upbears *qi*, especially in the pelvic region to the center, for erectile dysfunction
KI-7	Fu liu	Moves water, strengthens kidney *yang* and *qi*
ST-30	Qi chong	Moves *qi* in the lower burner and *chong mai*, supplies the lower abdomen with blood and *qi*
GV-20	Bai hui	Strongly upbears *qi*, e.g., for impotence and prolapse
BL-16	Du shu	Hairloss
BL-67	Zhi yin	Seminal emissions, weakness in the legs, hot feet
BL-11	Da zhu	Weak bones, osteoporosis
GB-19	Nao kong	The "gate to the brain," supports the marrow, in combination with GB-39, for headaches after sex and after excesses
GB-39	Xuan zhong	Sea of marrow, i.e., nourishing the bones and brain and enriching essence
LU-3	Tian fu	Mobilizes essence *qi* to the brain, "celestial window" point, for extensive exhaustion
HT-6+ KI-7	Yin xi+fu liu	Kidney *yin* vacuity negatively affecting the heart; exhaustion and disquietude after excesses
LR-8	Qu quan	Loss of essence, liver blood, and *yin* after excesses, nourishes the uterus
LR-9	Yin bao	For preserving *yin*, strengthening the uterus and liver blood

Medicinal Therapy for Weakness of Kidney *Yang* and Kidney *Qi*

Rx. Jin Gui Shen Qi Wan *(Golden Coffer Kidney* Qi *Pill); Modification for the Treatment of Infertility and Sexual Disorders:*

- *shu di huang*, 9–12 g—nourishes kidney *yin*, cools blood and construction
- *shan zhu yu* (Corni fructus), 6–9 g—nourishes liver and kidney *yin*, contains essence, checks sweating
- *shan yao*, 9–12 g—supplements the spleen and stomach, promotes fluid production, supplements kidney *qi* and *yin*
- *fu zi*, 2–3 g—revives collapsed *yang*, warms kidney fire, strengthens spleen and kidney *yang* (**beware: toxic!**)
- *gui zhi* (Cinnamomi ramulus), 3–5 g—warms the kidney, strengthens *yang*, guides the fire back to the source
- *fu ling*, 6–9 g—strengthens the spleen, harmonizes the center, eliminates dampness, quiets the spirit
- *mu dan pi*, 4–6 g—cools and quickens blood, cools vacuity heat, cools liver fire
- *ba ji tian*, 4–6 g—supplements the kidney, strengthens *yang*, strengthens the sinews and bones, extinguishes wind
- *rou cong rong*, 6–9 g—supplements kidney *yang*, moistens the stool
- *suo yang* (Cynomorii herba), 6–9 g—supplements the kidneys, strengthens *yang*, nourishes blood and essence, moistens the intestines
- *gou qi zi*, 6–9 g—supplements the liver and kidney, strengthens *yin*, blood, and essence, clears the vision
- *yin yang huo*, 6–9 g—supplements the kidney, strengthens *yang* and *yin*, downbears ascending liver *yang*

Strengthless—Weakness of Lung *Qi*

Causes and Disease Development

The lung is the source of *qi*—through respiration, we absorb celestial *qi* (*da qi*), the guarantor of life and vigorous activity, also and especially in the area of sexuality and reproduction. The movements of the pelvic muscles, pelvis, and lumbar region are as dependent on this force as are the strength and duration of erections, because the *qi* absorbed by the lung is physiologically directed downward to the kidneys whence it supplies the entire lower burner with tautness and vitality.

Any physical as well as psychological strain can overexert *qi* over time or impede the distribution of *qi* into the lower abdomen, ultimately leading to impaired sexuality. Internal factors like chronic disease, especially lung disorders and also smoking, affect the absorption of *qi* by the lung. Both too much and too little physical activity can exhaust *qi* as well. An additional internal factor is the strain on the lung from separation and mourning processes.

According to TCM, the lung, by means of the corporeal soul *po*, is the agency that guarantees the receptivity for feelings and emotions. The "*entzauberung*" (disenchantment) of sexuality and reproduction that occurs in the course of fertility treatment in the framework of modern biomedicine can then also affect this aspect of the lung and thereby make a satisfying "fiery" sexuality more difficult.

Symptoms

Shortness of breath, quiet strengthless voice, great need for sleep, quiet coughing.
    Pulse: sunken, fine
    Tongue: light-colored, possibly swollen

Table 18.11 Key symptoms for sexuality and reproduction: weakness of lung *qi*

	Woman	Man
Sexuality and reproductive organs	Easily exhausted after sex; lacking sensation of pleasure	Easily exhausted after sex; weak erections; lacking sensation of pleasure
Reproduction and menstruation	Prolonged cycle, intermenstrual bleeding	No changes

Therapy

Strengthen the lung and *qi*.

Acupuncture

Table 18.12 Acupuncture points in weakness of lung *qi*

Points	Name	indication/effect
LR-4	*Zhong feng*	Weakness of kidney *yang*, fear, lack of sensitivity, withdrawal
ST-30	*Qi chong*	Regulates *qi* in the entire pelvis, unites the energies of the kidney, spleen, and stomach
BL-36	*Cheng fu*	Weakness of *yang* and *qi*, lack of strength in the lumbus, impotence

Medicinal Therapy

Rx. Si Jun Zi Tang *(Four Gentlemen Decoction); Modification for the Treatment of Infertility and Sexual Disorders:*
This formula strengthens *qi* and lifts it upward, but also conserves liver and kidney *yin* and supplements and astringes essence:

- *ren shen*, 4 g—strengthens original *qi*, spleen, and stomach, quiets the spirit
- *bai zhu*, 8 g—supplements the spleen, strengthens *qi*, dries dampness, stabilizes defense
- *fu ling*, 8 g—strengthens the spleen, harmonizes the center, eliminates dampness, quiets the spirit
- *zhi gan cao*, 3 g—supplements the spleen, strengthens *qi*, harmonizes the formula
- *ban zia*, 6 g—dries dampness, downbears lung and stomach *qi*
- *huang qi*, 10 g—supplements the spleen, upbears *yang qi*
- *wu wei zi*, 4–6 g—preserves lung *qi*, quiets the spirit, contains essence, checks diarrhea and sweating
- *mai men dong* (Ophiopogonis radix), 4–6 g—moistens the lung and nourishes *yin* in the lung, heart, and stomach
- *shan zhu yu*, 4–6 g—nourishes liver and kidney *yin*, contains essence, checks sweating
- *han lian cao* (Ecliptae herba), 4–6 g—nourishes the liver and kidney
- *nü zhen zi*, 4–6 g—nourishes liver and kidney *yin*

Note. Nowadays, we often substitute a double dose of *dang shen* for *ren shen* because it is cheaper.

Chilled—Weakness of Heart *Yang*

Causes and Disease Development

Heart *yang* sinks downward and thereby promotes, in concert with kidney *yang*, the strength of erections. It is the "ruler of the viscera and bowels," as the eighth chapter of the *Ling Shu* states. As such, it ensures the harmony and smooth functioning of all vital processes in the body. Its connection to heaven is, like the heart in the human body, the agency of union: of *yin* and *yang*, man and woman, love and desire. It is this process, the union of *yin* and *yang* in the fire of love, that produces *qi* and a new life.

Heart *yang* makes it possible for us to communicate; our openness represents the above-mentioned social-communicative dimension of sexuality.

The energy of the heart contributes unconditionality and unintentionality to interpersonal relationships—different from and in addition to the desire and lust that is the manifestation of kidney energy.

Desire and lust then frequently lead to "wanting" and "having to" engage in sexual intercourse, the stormy urge to conquer, as we have described it, for example, under liver *qi* congestion. The heart as the manifestation of the earth phase in the human body introduces the warmth of love to a partnership and to sex—both as explosive consuming outbursts (*yan* 炎) and as life-sustaining slow-glowing warmth (*shuo* 爍):

"This glowing warmth is what holds people together after long-term partnerships, in crises and doubts. This type of fire certainly leads a shadowy existence in the background of contemporary attention—as the tabloid press and Hollywood blockbusters both only reflect that dramatic-explosive variety of the young heart-fire, promoting the illusion of eternally being in love."[10]

Nevertheless, *shuo*, the warmth of the fire, is what builds and sustains life. Furthermore, *shuo* is life-giving because of the fact that the movement of its fire is directed downwards. As a result, it has a lasting strengthening effect on kidney *yang* and its *ming men* fire. The fire from the heart and kidney is the source of warmth in the penis and of the strength of erection and ejaculation. When we notice pronounced fatigue and need for sleep after sex, this is a sign that the life-sustaining fire is exhausted.

Symptoms

Palpitations, general listlessness and fatigue, short-ness of breath, cold sensations, especially in the hands, reluctance to speak, quiet voice, mime-like lack of expressiveness, gloominess, fearfulness and bitterness, and impotence (erections during sleep and with masturbation, on the other hand, are in-conspicuous).

Pulse: fine, weak, sunken

Tongue: light-colored, moist white fur

Table 18.13 Key symptoms for sexuality and repro-duction: weakness of heart *yang*

	Woman	Man
Sexuality and reproductive organs	Decreased libido Pronounced listlessness; gloominess	Decreased libido No or incom-plete erections Unsatisfying sexuality
Reproduction and menstruation	Normal fertility During men-struation, pronounced cold sensations, exhaustion, and shortness of breath	Sperm quality inconspicuous

Therapy

Strengthen the heart, warm the kidney and spleen.

Acupuncture

Table 18.14 Acupuncture points in weakness of heart *yang*

Points	Name	Indication/Effect
LR-4	*Zhong feng*	Weakness of kidney *yang*, fear, lack of sensitivity, with-drawal
BL-52	*Zhi shi*	Lacking self-confidence, identity, and sense of self
GV-11	*Shen dao*	Strengthens heart *yang* by means of the kidney, up-bears kidney *yang*
BL-15	*Xin shu*	Regulates heart *yang* and *qi*
PC-6	*Nei guan*	Protects the heart from hurt feelings
GV-4	*Ming men*	Brings life perspectives to the fore, strengthens the libido

Medicinal Therapy

Rx. Cheng Yang Li Lao Tang *(Yang-supporting Fatigue-controlling Decoction); Modification for the Treatment of Infertility and Sexual Disorders:*

- *gao li shen* (Ginseng radix coreensis), 4–6 g—strengthens original *qi*, warms the lung, spleen, and stomach, warms heart *yang* and *qi*, quiets the spirit
- *huang qi*, 6–9 g—supplements and upbears spleen *qi*, strengthens *qi* and defense
- *wu wei zi*, 4–6 g—supports the heart and quiets the spirit, supplements the kidney and contains essence
- *zhi gan cao*, 4–6 g—supplements the heart, spleen, and stomach, strengthens *qi*, harmo-nizes the formula
- *gui zhi*, 3–5 g—warms and unblocks heart *yang* and the channels and blood vessels
- *sheng jiang*, three slices—warms *yang* in the lung, spleen, and stomach
- *bai zhu*, 6–9 g—supplements the spleen, strengthens *qi*, dries dampness, stabilizes *wei* (defense)
- *chen pi*, 3–5 g—moves and regulates *qi*, strengthens the spleen, downbears *qi*, trans-forms dampness
- *dang gui*, 4–6 g—supplements and quickens blood, quiets the spirit, moistens the intestine
- *da zao*, three pieces—supplements the center, strengthens the spleen and stomach, supple-ments blood, quiets the spirit, harmonizes the formula
- *fu zi*, 3–5 g—revitalizes collapsed *yang*, supple-ments *yang* in the heart, kidney, and spleen, warms the kidney fire, unblocks the channels and blood vessels (**beware: toxic!**)
- *jiu zi*, 4–6 g—supplements *yang* and warms the kidney, secures essence, warms the stomach
- *yi zhi ren*, 6–9 g—supplements *yang*, warms the kidney and spleen

■ Differentiation between Patterns

Table 18.15 presents an overview for additional differentiation between the patterns discussed above.

Table 18.15 Overview of key symptoms in the treatment of infertility and sexual disorders.

Pattern	Tongue	Pulse	Symptoms General	Symptoms Sexuality	Symptoms Reproduction	Etiology
Kidney *qi* vacuity	Thin, strengthless, light-colored	Sunken, fine	Lack of strength with lumbar pain and weakness, dribbling urination, headaches accompanied by feelings of emptiness in the head	Decreased libido, inability to achieve an erection, seminal emissions without sexual activities	Inadequate sperm quality, reduced sperm count, higher number of dead or inactive sperm, no ovulation	Fear, exhaustion
Weakness of kidney *yang* with cold and dampness	Pale swollen tongue body	Sunken, slow, slippery	Cold sensations (feet), large amounts of clear urine, nycturia, weak lumbus and knees, thin white vaginal discharge	Listlessness	Low temperature curve, watery ejaculate, reduced sperm count and quality, no ovulation, bad eggs	Physical overexertion, chronic disease (see above)
Kidney *yin* vacuity	Thin red tongue body	Thin, rapid	Fatigue, dizziness, heat sensations, yellow urine, insomnia, palpitations	Spermatorrhea, hyperactivity, insufficient lubrification, burning sensations in the vagina, weak erections	Low ejaculate volume, bad sperm quality and amount, no ovulation, high temperature curve	Excessive masturbation, excesses, mental overstrain, aphrodisiacs (see above)
Liver *qi* stagnation	Tense	Tight	Frustration, tautness in the costal arch, sighing, pain and dysmenorrhea	Impotence, vaginitis	Insufficient sperm motility, irregular cycle, pain during ovulation and menstruation	Irregular cycle
Damp-heat in the liver and gallbladder	Yellow slimy tongue fur	Slippery, tight, rapid	Itching, yellow vaginal discharge, feeling of heaviness, bitter taste in the mouth, yellow urine	Weak erections, burning sensations	Yellow sperm, bacteria	Chronic liver *qi* congestion, wrong diet
Weakness of spleen *qi*	Pale, swollen	Vacuous, fine	Sloppy stools, drooping, incontinence	Vaginal discharge, varicocele, reduced libido, feeling of heaviness	Early miscarriage, from the 12th week on	
Weakness of heart *yang*	Light-colored, moist white tongue fur	Fine, weak, sunken	Palpitations, general listlessness and fatigue	Pronounced listlessness, gloominess	Sterility	Exhaustion, injury, bitterness

Note: Modified after Noll and Peineke[9].

• **Antibodies against spermatozoa**, both as auto-immune reaction of the man to his own sperm (autoantibodies), for example after a breach of the normally impermeable blood-testis barrier due to injury or inflammation, and also as immune reaction of the woman to the male semen (isoantibodies). Autoantibodies are common, but do not necessarily impair fertility.

TCM Diagnostics and its Most Relevant Diagnoses

A comparative, somewhat mechanistic consideration of male and female anatomy already suggests that it must be far easier to treat male fertility problems.

In addition to comprehensive questioning and tongue and pulse diagnosis within the framework of a **TCM medical history**, we recommend recourse to biomedical findings under all circumstances. An up-to-date spermiogram is required, if necessary with raster electron microscopy to differentiate malformations. This should be checked after several weeks. Spermiograms should always be done by the same specialist to ensure their comparability. It should be determined whether a varicocele is present.

Besides checking for the above-mentioned risks, the medical history should deal in particular detail with the patient's lifestyle. Questions on diet, stress, sports, sex life, clothing, smoking, alcohol, medications, and exposure to chemicals or fine dust are also important for concurrent behavioral recommendations.

A spermiogram can also be translated directly into a **TCM diagnosis**. In simplified terms, we can say that the sperm itself and its motility are associated with *yang*, while seminal fluid, sperm count, and morphology are associated with *yin*, or in the latter case also with *jing*. Exact differentiations and corresponding formulas have been introduced by Clavey[5,6] in particular and are found in Liang.[16]

In the diagnosis of fertility problems, the **kidney** as the root of life and storehouse of essence lies at the center of our therapeutic interest. The kidney determines a person's ability to reproduce. Diagnosis generally does not pose any particular problems and provides a clear approach for therapy. As the mirror image of our Western lifestyle, we find **vacuity patterns** and **repletion patterns**.

Vacuity Patterns

Vacuity patterns, especially weakness of kidney *yang* and weakness of blood, tend to be the result of a consuming lifestyle and great professional demands, especially at an advanced age. Problems with the libido are not always only caused by a lack of *yang*, but are in men, as well as in women, frequently related to a liver *qi* stagnation, due to stress in one's professional and/or personal life, not the least of which can be reproductive stress.

Repletion Patterns

In general, repletion patters are related primarily to damp-heat and to *qi* stagnation and blood stasis. We often find a varicocele.

Due to the lack of research, general statements on the relevance of these TCM diagnoses are difficult. Thus, we are limited to personal therapeutic experiences, which in the present case are based in particular on patients who had already undergone measures of artificial insemination.

■ Treatment of Male Infertility

Biomedical Therapies

The options of biomedicine are in essence limited to the treatment of infections and the surgical removal of varicoceles, as well as the retrieval of sperm from the testicles when the seminal tract is obstructed.

TCM Therapies

In cases with impaired findings in the spermiogram, TCM under all circumstances recommends treatment. Hereby, **Chinese medicinal therapy** offers the most comprehensive options and should form the focus.* Nevertheless, **acupuncture** and **moxibustion** also offer valuable assistance, especially with regard to sperm motility. There is no doubt that we can also achieve positive results by

---

* Below, we only describe formulas that are not found in Bensky.[2]

means of *qi gong, tui na,* and Chinese dietetics (see Chapters 9, 10, and 13).

Medicinal Therapy

Medicinals

The following medicinals can be used in the treatment of male infertility:
- **Kidney *yin* supplements**: *shu di huang* (Rehmanniae radix praeparata) supplements kidney *yin* and nourishes essence and blood; *sang shen* (Mori fructus) mildly strengthens blood, *yin*, and essence; *gou qi zi* (Lycii fructus) supports *yin* and blood; *yu zhu* (Polygonati odorati rhizoma) for pronounced *yin* vacuity and emaciation, moistening.
- **Kidney *yang* supplements**: *du zhong* (Eucommiae cortex), *xu duan* (Dipsaci radix), *tu si zi* (Cuscutae semen), *yin yang huo* (Epimedii herba), *ba ji tian* (Morindae officinalis radix), *lu rong* (Cervi cornu pantotrichum).
- **Astringing medicinals**: *shan zhu yu* (Corni fructus) secures essence and sperm motility; *fu pen zi* (Rubi fructus) strengthens kidney energy.
- **Supplementing medicinals**: *shan yao* (Dioscoreae rhizoma) as *qi* supplement, also supports kidney *yin*; *huang jing* (Polygonati rhizoma) strengthens kidney essence and sperm production.
- **Envoy**: *wang bu liu xing* (Vaccariae semen) is of special significance as envoy for the testicles and thereby increases the effect of the formula.

Guiding Formulas

The following two formulas give an overview of the application of suitable medicinals for the treatment of male infertility.

Rx. Bu Shen Yi Jing Fang (Supplement the Kidneys Benefit the Jing Formula)[17]:
- *he shou wu* (Polygoni multiflori radix)
- *shu di huang*
- *gou qi zi*
- *shan yao*
- *shan zhu yu*
- *tu si zi*
- *fu pen zi*

- *nü zhen zi* (Ligustri lucidi fructus)
- *bai shao yao* (Paeoniae radix alba)
- *mu dan pi* (Moutan cortex)
- *dang shen* (Codonopsis radix)
- *huang qi* (Astragali radix)
- *yin yang huo*
- *rou cong rong* (Cistanches herba)
- *ba ji tian*
- *suo yang* (Cynomorii herba)
- *dan shen* (Salviae miltiorrhizae radix)
- *lu jiao shuang* (Cervi cornu degelatinatum)

Each in high dosages, with a daily dose of 12–15 g.

Modifications for Insufficiency of Kidney Yin *and* Heat:
- *han lian cao* (Ecliptae herba), *tian men dong* (Asparagi radix), *huang bai* (Phellodendri cortex).
- Remove *yin yang huo* and *suo yang* and reduce the dosage of *ba ji tian* and *rou cong rong*.

Bei Tu Tang[*]:
- *bi xie* (Dioscoreae hypoglaucae seu semptemlobae rhizoma), 15 g
- *tu si zi*, 10 g
- *fu ling* (Poria), 15 g
- *che qian zi* (Plantaginis semen), 9 g
- *ze xie* (Alismatis rhizoma), 9 g
- *mu li* (Ostreae concha), 15 g
- *gou qi zi*, 12 g
- *xu duan*, 12 g
- *shan yao*, 20 g
- *sha yuan ji li* (Astragali complanati semen) 20 g
- *dan shen*, 20 g
- *shi chang pu* (Acori tatarinowii rhizoma), 3 g
- *huang bai*, 12 g
- *gan cao* (Glycyrrhizae radix), 3 g

Additions and Modifications
This formula was created for all "male problems," such as impotence, spermatorrhea, bloody semen, low liquefaction, or chronic prostatitis. Handle it flexibly in accordance with the particular diagnosis. In heat patterns, for example, leave out *tu si zi*, and in *yang* insufficiency leave out *huang bai*; for varicocele, on the other hand, add blood-moving medicinals.

---

[*] According to Clavey,[5,6] after Xu Fusong. Designed by Xu Fusong, Journal of Chinese Medicine, 1996: 9. Vol. 37, p. 532.

Acupuncture, Ear Acupuncture, and Moxibustion

Mazin Al Khafaji[1] lists several studies on the efficacy of acupuncture in male infertility. Already in 1984, a German study of 28 men found a statistically relevant improvement of sperm quality after only 10 treatments in 3 weeks. A Brazilian investigation of 19 patients concluded that two treatments a week with acupuncture and moxibustion over 10 weeks resulted in a significant increase of normal findings. A study from Tel-Aviv examined 20 men with azoospermia and severe OAT syndrome. It found a clear increase in sperm count in two-thirds of the men with azoospermia, especially in men with inflammations in the genital tract.

Lewis[15] points to a study by Shanghai University of TCM on electroacupuncture on SP-6 (*san yin jiao*), CV-4 (*guan yuan*), and CV-12 (*zhong wan*). In addition to an improvement in symptoms and sperm in all parameters, the researchers found a normalization of hormone values, especially estrogen (57.1%) and testosterone (65.1%).

Especially when treating insufficiency of kidney *yang*, **moxa therapy** is indicated. To complement treatment, we can also use **ear acupuncture**, for example on the points for the testicles, endocrinium, *shen men*, the antiaggression point, or also specifically to stop smoking.

Combined TCM Therapy in Accordance with TCM Diagnoses

For the various disease patterns of male infertility, treatment with a combination of medicinal therapy and acupuncture and moxibustion can occasionally be suitable. Experience shows, however, that the use of Chinese medicinal therapy alone already offers excellent treatment results. We have dispensed here with presenting any typical symptoms. For this information, the reader should refer to the standard texts by Maciocia[18] and the advanced literature, but also to the case studies below and other contributions in this book.

Insufficiency of Kidney *Yin*

Rx. *Zuo Gui Wan* (Left-restoring [Kidney *Yin*] Pill
Rx. Yang Jing Zhong Zi Fang (*Essence-nourishing Seed-planting formula*):
- *huang jing*
- *shu di huang*
- *shan zhu yu*
- *tu si zi*
- *gou qi zi*
- *shan yao*
- *dan shen*
- *bai shao yao*

Acupuncture
- CV-4 (*guan yuan*), GV-4 (*ming men*), BL-23 (*shen shu*), KI-3 (*tai xi*), KI-7 (*fu liu*), SP-6 (*san yin jiao*)

Insufficiency of Kidney *Yang*

Rx. *You Gui Wan (Right-restoring [Life Gate] Pill)**
Rx. Wu Zi Yan Zong Wan (*Five Seeds Pills for Abundant Descendants*)[19]
- *tu si zi*
- *wu wei zi* (Schisandrae fructus)
- *gou qi zi*
- *fu pen zi*
- *che qian zi*; 6 g each

Acupuncture
CV-4 (*guan yuan*), CV-6 (*qi hai*), GV-4 (*ming men*), BL-23 (*shen shu*), ST-36 (*zu san li*), SI-3 (*hou xi*) plus BL-62 (*shen mai*): to activate the *du mai*.

Moxa
GV-4, BL-23

---

* Also known as Right (Kidney)-restoring Pill.

Damp-heat

Rx. Long Dan Xie Gan Tang *(Gentian Liver-draining Decoction)*

Acupuncture
CV-4 *(guan yuan)*, LR-8 *(qu quan)*, SP-6 *(san yin jiao)*, SP-9 *(yin ling quan)*, LI-11 *(qu chi)*, BL-40 *(wei zhong)*, KI-7 *(fu liu)*

Qi Stagnation

Rx. Xiao Yao San *(Free Wanderer Powder)*

Acupuncture
Yin tang, LR-1 *(da dun)*, LR-3 *(tai chong)*, GB-34 *(yang ling quan)*, SP-6 *(san yin jiao)*

Blood Stasis

Rx. Xue Fu Zhu Yu Tang *(House of Blood Stasis-expelling Decoction)*

Acupuncture
SP-10 *(xue hai)*, LR-8 *(qu quan)*, ST-29 *(gui lai)*, SP-6 *(san yin jiao)*, ST-29 *(gui lai)*, SP-4 *(gong sun)* plus PC-6 *(nei guan)*: to activate the *chong mai*

Lower Jiao Blood Stagnation (Varicocele)

Rx. Gui Zhi Fu Ling Wan *(Cinnamon Twig and Poria Pill)*
Lewis points to a Japanese study that found that after 3 months of taking this formula, the varicocele disappeared in 80% of cases, the sperm count improved in over 70% of cases, and sperm motility in over 60%.[15]

TCM Therapy in Accordance with a Spermiogram

Low Volume

Treatment Principle
Supplement *yin* and blood and support essence, for example with:
- *nü zhen zi*
- *han lian cao*
- *he shou wu*
- *huang jing*

Low Motility

Treatment Principle
Support *yang* and *qi*, for example with:
- *tu si zi*
- *yin yang huo*
- *ba ji tian*
- *xian mao* (Curculiginis rhizoma)
- *du zhong*
- *xu duan*
- *lu rong*

Malformations

Treatment Principle
Move blood, for example with:
- *dan shen*
- *ji xue teng* (Spatholobi caulis)
- *huai niu xi* (Achyranthis bidentatae radix)
- *tao ren* (Persicae semen)

Lower Jiao Blood Stegnation (Varicocele) in Oligospermia

Treatment Principle
Move and disinhibit blood, for example with:

Rx. Tong Jing Jian *(Channel-freeing Brew)*[5]:
- *dan shen*
- *e zhu* (Curcumae rhizoma)
- *chuan niu xi* (Cyathulae radix)
- *chai hu* (Bupleuri radix)
- *huang qi*
- *mu li*

For all men, the partners were also receiving treatment. In only one case the man alone had taken the initiative and his partner had followed him.

In 87% of cases, only medicinal therapy was used; in seven cases, acupuncture and partly moxa as well. Forty-three treatments were carried out to conclusion. Ten men were still in treatment at the time of the deadline. Fifty-one percent of men stopped treatment early or never started in the first place.

Altogether 15 of the partners became pregnant, eight after additional artificial fertilization and seven naturally. In three cases, the pregnancies happened after just a few weeks of treatment. Thirteen healthy children were born, among them two pairs of twins. In two cases, artificial fertilization resulted in miscarriage early on in the pregnancy.

Thirteen of the 15 pregnancies occurred in women whose partner had persevered with the treatment for over 3 months, which means that in this group 62% of partners became pregnant. In an additional four cases, control spermiograms were done, which all showed positive findings. Among the 21 men who had persevered with the treatment, 17 cases showed verifiable effects with the occurrence of pregnancy or a control spermiogram, and only four cases failed to do so. Among these 17, only two results were judged as negative (miscarriage in early pregnancy) but 15 as positive, which corresponds to a success rate of 88%. Even if we take the 51% of prematurely stopped treatments into consideration, the success rate is still 44%. In light of the fact that most patients were cured, this is an acceptable result, which could certainly be improved further with more consistent therapy. The present description does not even take into account any additional positive health effects of the therapy. In addition, we can see a clear tendency for prematurely stopped treatments to drop and for success rates to go up.

Conclusions from the Study

As a rule, fertility treatment should always include **both partners** to optimize chances for a baby. Already in the **patient's history** we can often find valuable information from the partner. While the woman should undergo a biomedical examination of the endometrium, ovaries, fallopian tubes, and luteal phase, the man should absolutely be examined early on in regards to his fertility. The andro-logical findings are essential information for the work of the TCM practitioner. Up-to-date spermiograms by a specialist are therefore indispensable before the beginning of therapy, if possible two spermiograms to eliminate any coincidental results.

If limitations are found, **TCM therapy** should be carried out in all cases. This applies also to artificial fertilization, to increase the chances and reduce the risk of miscarriages and malformations. In this context, the patient should be informed that his health insurance may no longer cover the expenses of artificial fertilization if his medical findings improve.

The **treatment duration** should be set in accordance with the duration of spermiogenesis to a minimum of 3 months. It should be agreed that an additional spermiogram will be done after 3 months to check the effects of the therapy, unless a pregnancy has already occurred. Exact documentation of the treatment is self-explanatory. The use of a database program that can be tailored to the individual requirements of the user is very helpful.

A combined treatment with **Chinese medicinal therapy** and **acupuncture** is optimal. **Medicinal therapy** should be employed in all cases. It offers the greatest opportunities and requires a comparatively small expenditure of time. For practical reasons, granular mixtures are preferred, with a daily dose between 12 g and 18 g. Pressing these into tablets would certainly further improve acceptance, but is unfortunately associated with considerable additional costs. For vacations, it can be appropriate to temporarily fall back on ready-made tablets, for example Seven Forests'[8] Man's Treasure or Gentiana 12, or Golden Flower's[20] *Jing Qi* or *Gui Zhi Fu Ling Wan*.

After determining on the diagnosis, initially prescribe a formula in a low dosage on a trial basis for one week to test the patient's tolerance. Further prescriptions follow. In cases of damp-heat or *qi* stagnation and blood stasis, treat these first and then, after the symptoms have improved accordingly, support the constitution and strengthen the kidney. As a rule, add *wang bu liu xing* as envoy for the testicles.

Consistent **acupuncture treatment** is desirable. At a minimum, you should try to treat the man with acupuncture before the partner's ovulation. Body acupuncture can be complemented with ear acupuncture. In insufficiency of kidney *yang*, **moxa treatments** can under certain circumstances and after appropriate instruction also be performed by the partner.

Sooner or later, the couple's love life is negatively affected by infertility; expert advice should therefore also be given in this respect. The **pelvic floor muscles** are probably the group of muscles that receives the least amount of attention in health clubs. Both men and women should therefore be advised to exercise their pelvic floor as well.

The treatment package is topped off with **recommendations** for a healthy diet, tips for relaxation exercises, moderate physical activity, and if necessary, quitting smoking, which is supported by ear acupuncture. Under all circumstances, avoid overheating the testicles.

In addition to TCM treatment, a targeted **orthomolecular therapy** can be appropriate, especially when there are signs of chronic inflammations, deficiency states, and exhaustion. This often means an existent mitrochondropathy that can no longer be fixed by means of diet alone. It is possible that the oxidative stress damages the sperm as well. With antioxidative therapy, the proportion of sperm with breaks in the DNA strands is significantly reduced after a few weeks of treatment with oral antioxidants.[12] A study by the University of California[13] demonstrated that an increased intake of antioxidants leads to improved sperm quality.

Lewis[15] recommends the intake of vitamin C, B_{12}, E, beta-carotene, selenium, zinc, L-arginine, and L-carnitine to promote sperm motility. Zinc is important for sperm production and testosterone metabolism. Choose an appropriate compound preparation that contains all the necessary dietary supplements. Austrian urologists[10] report a pilot study on the efficacy of one such preparation. The examination of 30 men showed an obvious improvement in sperm quality and quantity as well as an increase in motile sperm cells. Every third man regained normal values. A continuing study is planned from the fall of 2006 on.

In spite of the fact that the treatment of male infertility is basically simple and promising, it often presents problems in clinic because many men have a skeptical attitude towards the treatment of their problem, especially by means of naturopathic medicine.

Very few men refuse treatment, but many allow the treatment to peter out after only a short time. Factual information and clear agreements should therefore be presented at the beginning of the treatment. In general, consistent treatment **for at least 3 months with Chinese medicinal therapy, acupuncture, and dietary supplements** is the key to the greatest possible success. In certain cases, it can be necessary to carry out measures of artificial fertilization, which should then be accompanied by TCM treatment. For this purpose, you should seek cooperation with a center for reproductive medicine.

Notwithstanding all this euphoria, we should always be realistic about the limitations of therapy. Some of the couples will remain childless in spite of all therapeutic efforts.

■ Conclusion

The treatment of male infertility with TCM is a very effective approach in fertility therapy and should be employed consistently. In comparison with measures of artificial fertilization, it is very cost-effective and, if performed by professionals, free of harmful side-effects. On the contrary—many men feel that the treatment is good for them all around. It is often only with the relief over an improved spermiogram or the unexpected pregnancy that we see how much stress the diagnosis of infertility means for men as well. Most importantly, though, this approach can allow many women to avoid artificial fertilization, which they experience as very distressing physically and emotionally, as well as financially. According to the National Institute of Health, male infertility is involved in approximately 40% of the 2.6 million infertile married couples in the United States. These men are a challenge for TCM that practitioners should respond to much more actively. This is a great and wonderful task that is worth working for. TCM practitioners and their associations should do a better job at informing the public on treatment options and should also influence health policy.

Literature

Currently, not much literature on the treatment of male infertility with TCM exists. Only Maciocia[19] includes a small appendix on "male sterility." Dr. Steven Clavey from Sydney devoted more attention to male infertility as well in a seminar in the spring of 2001 and presented a broad range of formulas for the various spermiogram results, differentiated according to TCM diagnoses. Unfortunately, he has not yet published his experiences.[5,6]

1. Al-Khafaji M. *Research into Acupuncture and Abnormality of Sperm.* Clinical Center of Chinese Medicine.
2. Bensky D, Barolet R. *Chinesische Arzneimittelrezepte und Behandlungsstrategien.* Kötzting: VGM Wühr; 1996.
3. U.S. Department of Health & Human Service: U.S. BIRTH RATE REACHES RECORD LOW, News Release, June 25, 2003. http://www.hhs.gov/news/press/2003pres/20030625.html.
4. Cheung CS, Golden RS (translator/editor). *TCM and Male and Female Infertility.* San Francisco: Harmonious Sunshine Cultural Center; 1995. (Includes extensive chapters on male infertility and TCM.)
5. Clavey S. Seminar on Infertility at Offenbach (unpublished); 2001.
6. Clavey S. *Male Infertility.* Sydney (unpublished); 2003.
7. Czichos J. *Überaktives Immunsystem Macht Frauen Unfruchtbar.* Bild der Wissenschaft. January 10, 2002.
8. Dharmananda S, Melleh A. *Beutel mit Perlen.* Hawthorne, Portland: Institute for TCM and Preventive Health Care; 2002.
9. Dunson D. Reproductive functions of the ageing male. *Human Reproduction.* 2002;17(5):1399–1403. http://humrep.oxfordjournals.org/cgi/reprint/17/5/1399.pdf
10. Forum für Wissenschaft, Industrie und Wirtschaft (Austria). Erste Fruchtbarkeitspille für den Mann. Innovationsreport. May 1, 2006.
11. Gminski R, Mersch-Sundermann V. Gesundheitliche Bewertung der Exposition Gegenüber Tonerstäuben und Gegenüber Emissionen aus Laserdruckern und Kopiergeräten—Aktueller Erkenntnisstand. *Umweltmed Forsch Prax.* 2006; 11:269–300.
12. Greco E, Lacobelli M, Rienzi L. Reduction of the Incidence of Sperm DNA Fragmentation by Oral Antioxidant Treatment. *J Androl.* 2005; 26: 349–353.
13. Eskenazi B, et al. Antioxidant intake is associated with semen quality in healthy men. *Human Reproduction.* 2005;20(4):1006–1012. http://humrep.oxfordjournals.org/cgi/reprint/20/4/1006.
14. Jacobi H. Rückgang der Spermienqualität in Deutschland und Europa. WWF 1999: Chemikalienpolitik, http://www.tu-cottbus.de/BTU/Fak4/AllgOeko/Biologie/scripte_deutsch/WWFsperm.pdf.
15. Lewis R. *The Infertility Cure.* Boston: Little, Brown; 2004. (With extensive chapters on male infertility and TCM. See also http://www.easternharmonyclinic.com [accessed May 9, 2009]).
16. Liang L. *Acupuncture & IVF.* Boulder: Blue Poppy Press; 2003. (With extensive chapters on male infertility and TCM.)
17. Lyttleton J. *Treatment of Infertility.* London: Churchill Livingstone; 2004: 255–276. (With extensive chapters on male infertility and TCM.)
18. Maciocia G. *Die Grundlagen der Chinesischen Medizin.* Kötzting: VGM Wühr; 1994. (With extensive chapters on male infertility and TCM.)
19. Maciocia G. *Die Gynäkologie in der Praxis der Chinesischen Medizin. Infertilität.* Appendix: Sterilität des Mannes. Kötzting: VGM Wühr; 2000: 279.
20. Monda L, Scott J, Waltz P (translator). *Golden Flower—Chinese Herbs.* Karlsruhe: Peter Waltz; 1999.
21. Robert-Koch-Institut/Statistisches Bundesamt. *Ungewollte Kinderlosigkeit, Gesundheitsberichterstattung des Bundes.* 2004; 20.
22. Sokol R. *Verminderte Fruchtbarkeit—Ozon Tötet Spermien.* Los Angeles: University of Southern California, Environmental Health Perspectives. http://www.focus.de/gesundheit/ratgeber/sexualitaet/verminderte-fruchtbarkeit_aid_106 599.html (accessed May 9, 2009).
23. Spielmann W. Reproduktionstoxikologie. German Federal Institute for Risk Assessment [Bundesinstitut für Risikobewertung]. Lecture, 12 December, 2005.
24. Statistisches Bundesamt, Bevölkerungsentwicklung Deutschlands bis 2050.
25. Stelting HJ. Krank durch Toner? Erfahrungen mit einer Nanopathologie. *Umweltmed Forsch Prax.* 2006;11:329–337.
26. Stelting HJ. Tonerallergie. *Internistische Praxis.* 2005;45:457–462.
27. Tauber R, Pfeiffer D. *Jungen von heute ... Väter von Morgen? Varikozele testis—Wenn der Kinderwunsch Versagt Bleibt.* Barmbek: AK Barmbek; 2001.
28. TNF-alpha-Informationszentrum, www.tiz-info.de (accessed May 9, 2009).
29. Troge A. President of the Federal Environment Agency [Umweltbundesamt]: Wissenschaft im Dialog. Berlin: BMWF; May, 2003.
30. Verband der Reproduktionsmediziner (BRZ). Offener Brief an Bundeskanzlerin Merkel. Saarbrücken; 2006.
31. Wyrobek AJ, Eskenazi BS, Young S et al. Advancing age has differential effects on DNA damage, chromatin integrity, gene mutations, and aneuploidies in sperm. *PNAS.* 2006:103:9601–9606.

Endometriosis (*nei ji* 内积, "inner accumulation") is a benign disorder that affects approximately 20–30% of women with fertility problems. It occurs exclusively during women's reproductive years and is diagnosed most frequently between the age of 30 and 40. In its development, it is dependent on hormones, occasionally disappears completely during pregnancy, but can recur after childbirth. Endometriosis declines with the onset of menopause.

■ Causes and Pathogenesis from the Biomedical Perspective

In this disorder, dispersed uterine tissue (endometrium) appears in the abdominal cavity and forms so-called **endometriosis lesions**. These lesions cause localized inflammatory lesions that change the surrounding tissue and can trigger the formation of adhesions. With regard to fertility, this is highly problematic since it can lead to occlusion or agglutination of the fallopian tubes, as a result of which neither semen nor egg can pass through. The adhesions caused by endometriosis can lead to impaired mobility of the ovaries and fallopian tubes as well as to a disturbed reception of the ovum. This means that this disorder frequently affects the functions of the fallopian tubes (i. e., reception of the ovum, ovum transport, fertilization, and embryo transport). Nevertheless, the fallopian tubes are not affected in all women who suffer from endometriosis. Endometriosis lesions often occur on one or both ovaries, in which case cysts can develop, most notably chocolate cysts. When these cysts are removed and analyzed, a brown viscous substance (old menstrual blood) is found that looks like chocolate. In addition to the uterus and peritoneum, endometriosis can also spread to the intestines and the bladder. Depending on the severity of endometriosis, the affected

organs can even adhere to each other. This can lead to symptoms that are not subjectively linked to the menstrual cycle, such as pain during defecation or urination.

Parallel to the mechanical problems triggered by endometriosis, around 45% of affected women show a luteal corpus insufficiency (functional weakness of the corpus luteum) and around 20% show an anovulatory cycle, which likewise limits fertility.

Until now, biomedicine has failed to provide a conclusive theory for the origin of endometriosis. There are many theories, however, that explain the mechanism by which it spreads. The so-called displacement theory states that menstrual blood enters the fallopian tubes and is displaced from there into the abdominal cavity. Endometrial cells also spread through the lymph drainage paths and the vessels. Whenever these cells get stuck in one place, an endometriosis lesion can form there. Because numerous lymphatic and vascular connections exist between the uterus, ovaries, fallopian tubes, and the lesser pelvis, lesions can occur in the entire lower abdomen.

The theory of direct expansion states that endometriosis is caused by the direct penetration of endometrial tissue from the outside of the uterus into the bladder, ureter, and intestine. We also find descriptions of immunological changes that lead to localized inflammations around the endometriosis lesions. This reaction is partly responsible for the pain associated with endometriosis. Thus, we find considerably more macrophages in women with endometriosis than in women without this condition, while the activity of the natural killer cells is reduced.

Symptoms

It must be noted here that this condition can run its course without detectable complaints by the patient, as a result of which she will frequently only learn about an existing endometriosis from a laparoscopic diagnosis in the context of testing fallopian tube patency.

The following medicinals can be used:

- *da huang* (Rhei radix et rhizoma), 5–10 g
- *tao ren*, 10 g
- *san leng*, 10 g
- *e zhu*, 10 g

■ Important Disease Patterns

The following section covers important disease patterns and their treatment in TCM:

- liver *qi* congestion and blood stasis
- stasis due to external cold
- insufficiency of kidney *yang* with internal cold (blood stasis)
- damp-heat in the lower burner with blood stasis
- damp-heat in the lower burner with blood heat

Liver *Qi* Congestion and Blood Stasis

Liver *qi* congestion can lead to liver blood stasis. With regard to menstruation, liver *qi* moves the blood before and during the menstrual period. If blocked, the blood fails to move sufficiently, as a result of which we see menstrual pain and dark clotted menstrual blood. The stronger the pain, the more severe is the blood stasis.

Causes and Disease Development
Long-lasting emotional problems, unprocessed anger, disappointment.

Symptoms
Premenstrual irritability, tension in the breasts, delayed onset of menstruation, dark clotted blood, sharp stabbing pain before and during the period, internal disquietude. The tongue is pale red, also bluish, with congested sublingual veins; the pulse is stringlike.

Acupuncture
- For opening the chong mai, SP-4 (*gong sun*) and PC-6 (*nei guan*)
- LI-4 (*he gu*) and SP-8 (*di ji*), particularly effective for relieving pain 3–7 days before the onset of menstruation
- SP-8 (*di ji*): regulates the blood in the uterus and relieves pain
- LR-3 (*tai chong*): moves blood and *qi*, regulates the chong mai
- CV-6 (*qi hai*): moves *qi* in the lower abdomen
- KI-14 (*si mian*): moves blood in the lower abdomen and eliminates blood stasis in the *chong mai*

Medicinal Therapy
Numerous formulas exist for this pathology. A large number of these is related to the basic formula *Tao Hong Si Wu Tang* with *hong hua* and *tao ren* plus *qi*-regulating medicinals.

Rx. Tao Hong Si Wu Tang (*Peach Kernel and Carthamus Four Agents Decoction*):
- *shu di huang* (Rehmanniae radix praeparata), 9–12 g
- *bai shao yao* (Paeoniae radix alba), 9–15 g
- *dang gui* (Angelicae sinensis radix), 9–12 g
- *chuan xiong* (Chuanxiong rhizoma), 3–6 g
- *tao ren*, 6 g
- *hong hua*, 3 g

In severe pain, the formula *Ge Xia Zhu Yu Tang* can achieve good results. This formula is not only effective for relieving pain due to blood stasis; it also contributes to the elimination of abdominal masses like cysts or myomas.

Rx. Ge Xia Zhu Yu Tang (*Infradiaphragmatic Stasis-expelling Decoction*):
- *wu ling zhi*, 9 g
- *dang gui*, 6 g
- *chuan xiong*, 9 g
- *tao ren*, 6 g
- *mu dan pi* (Moutan cortex), 6 g
- *chi shao yao* (Paeoniae radix rubra), 6 g
- *wu yao* (Linderae radix), 6–12 g
- *yan hu suo*, 3 g
- *gan cao* (Glycyrrhizae radix), 9 g
- *xiang fu* (Cyperi rhizoma), 4.5 g
- *hong hua*, 9 g
- *zhi ke* (Aurantii fructus), 4.5 g

Stasis due to External Cold

Cold slows down the blood flow and thereby causes blood stasis in the channels and in the uterus.

Causes and Disease Development
External cold, often in combination with external dampness, can penetrate into the channels and uterus. A special risk factor is inappropriate clothing in climate zones that are dominated by cold and dampness, such as wearing nylon stockings on cold days. In women who practice a lot of water sports and go swimming during or shortly after their menstrual period, cold and dampness can easily enter the uterus. In particular, young girls and younger women tend to suffer from this pathology.

Symptoms
Sharp stabbing pain before and during menstruation that is relieved by application of warmth, clotted, sparsely flowing, shiny red menstrual blood, back pain, shivering. The tongue is pale bluish with congested sublingual veins, the pulse slowed down, sunken, and rough, or sunken and stringlike.

Acupuncture
- CV-4 (*guan yuan*): use fire needle to warm the uterus.
- CV-6 (*qi hai*): use fire needle to move qi and eliminate cold from the lower abdomen.
- ST-28 (*shui dao*): apply direct moxibustion, to eliminate cold from the uterus.
- LI-4 (*he gu*) and SP-8 (*di ji*) are particularly effective for relieving pain 3–7 days before the onset of menstruation.

Medicinal Therapy
In clinical practice, three formulas with the appropriate additions have proven very effective:

Rx. Gui Zhi Fu Ling Wan (*Cinnamon Twig and Poria Pill*):
- *gui zhi* (Cinnamomi ramulus), 9–12 g
- *fu ling* (Poria), 9–12 g
- *bai shao yao*, 9–15 g
- *mu dan pi*, 9–12 g
- *tao ren*, 9–12 g

This formula is often employed with good results. The main medicinal *gui zhi* is a very effective herb for opening and warming the channels and network vessels. It warms *yang* especially in the *chong mai* and *ren mai* and contributes to the regulation of the *qi* and blood flow in these channels. In combination with *fu ling*, it eliminates dampness and phlegm, which is highly significant in the treatment of endometriosis.

If the cold is very pronounced, *xiao hui xiang* (Foeniculi fructus), 3–8 g, is suitable for warming the kidney and liver channels and for increasing the effect of the formula in the lower burner.

This prescription is used in many gynecology departments of Chinese hospitals for the purpose of reducing uterine myomas.

Rx. Shao Fu Zhu Yu Tang (*Lesser Abdomen Stasis-expelling Decoction*):
- *xiao hui xiang*, 1.5 g
- *gan jiang* (Zingiberis rhizoma;), 0.6 g
- *yan hu suo*, 3 g
- *chuan xiong*, 3 g
- *dang gui*, 9 g
- *mo yao*, 3 g
- *guan gui* (Cinnamomi cortex tubiformis), 3 g
- *chi shao yao*, 6 g
- *pu huang*, 9 g
- *wu ling zhi*, 6 g

Rx. Sheng Hua Tang (*Engendering Transformation Decoction*):
- *dang gui*, 24 g
- *chuan xiong*, 9 g
- *tao ren*, 6–9 g
- *pao jiang* (Zingiberis rhizoma praeparatum), 1.5 g
- *zhi gan cao* (Glycyrrhizae radix cum liquido fricta), 1.5 g

Insufficiency of Kidney *Yang* with Internal Cold (Blood Stasis)

Causes and Disease Development
Physical overexertion, chronic disease, long-lasting insufficiency of spleen *yang*.

Symptoms

Deep dull pain before and during menstruation, relieved by a hot bath or hot water bottle, shivering, aversion to cold, **weak menstrual period with black clots**, sensation of pain and cold in the area of the lumbar vertebrae, menstruation weakens the patient. The tongue is pale blue, swollen, and moist; the pulse is sunken, tight, or fine.

Acupuncture

- SP-6 (*san yin jiao*): use fire needle
- CV-4 (*guan yuan*): use fire needle to warm the uterus
- CV-6 (*qi hai*): use fire needle to move *qi* and eliminate cold from the lower abdomen
- BL-23 (*shen qu*): use fire needle to strengthen kidney *yang*
- GV-4 (*ming men*): for insufficiency of kidney *yang* with pronounced symptoms of internal cold

Medicinal Therapy

Rx. Wen Jing Tang *(Menses-warming Decoction):*
- *wu zhu yu* (Evodiae fructus), 9 g
- *gui zhi*, 6 g
- *dang gui*, 9 g
- *chuan xiong*, 6 g
- *shao yao* (Paeonia radix), 6 g
- *e jiao* (Asini corii colla), 6 g
- *mai men dong* (Ophiopogonis radix), 9 g
- *mu dan pi*, 6 g
- *ren shen* (Ginseng radix), 6 g
- *gan cao*, 6 g
- *sheng jiang* (Zingiberis rhizoma recens), 6 g
- *ban xia* (Pinelliae rhizoma), 6 g

Rx. Dang Gui Jian Zhong Tang *(Chinese Angelica Center-fortifying Decoction):*
- *yi tang* (Maltosum), 18–30 g
- *gui zhi*, 9 g
- *shao yao*, 18 g
- *gan cao*, mix-fried in honey, 6 g
- *sheng jiang*, 9 g
- *da zao* (Jujubae fructus), 12 pieces
- *dang gui*, 9 g

Rx. Gui Zhi Fu Ling Wan *(Cinnamon Twig and Poria Pill):*
- *gui zhi*, 9–12 g
- *fu ling*, 9–12 g
- *shao yao*, 9–15 g
- *mu dan pi*, 9–12 g
- *tao ren*, 9–12 g

Damp-heat in the Lower Burner (with Blood Stasis)

Causes and Disease Development

Dampness can enter from the outside, but also often arises internally from an underlying weakness of spleen *qi*. Dampness is heavy, sticky, and tends to sink into the lower burner. There, it obstructs the flow of *qi* and blood on the one hand, while at the same time engendering heat or combining with pre-existing heat.

Damp-heat blocks the flow of *qi* especially in the liver/gallbladder channel, which can then also lead to disturbance in the *dai mai* and manifest in vaginal discharge. Because the *dai mai* encircles the leg channels, any disharmony in this extraordinary vessel can result in lower abdominal pain that radiates into the back, or in an irregular menstrual cycle or tendency to miscarriage.

In general, damp-heat does not cause pain but can, in patients with endometriosis, lead to occlusions, especially in the fallopian tubes. Damp-heat in the lower burner blocks the circulation of *qi* and blood, as a result of which menstrual pain can arise. If damp-heat encounters pre-existing blood stasis in the abdomen, the problem of stagnation is further aggravated.

Treatment Principle

The treatment principle corresponds to that of damp-heat in the lower burner (with blood heat).

Damp-heat in the Lower Burner (with Blood Heat)

Heat in the blood arises among other factors from deep-lying liver *qi* congestion that transforms into liver fire. Because the liver stores the blood, liver fire can heat up the blood, which manifests in a very heavy menstrual period. Heat in the blood frequently coincides with damp-heat. The heat can damage the bodily fluids, which leads to impaired fluidity of the blood and causes stagnation in the blood flow. As a result, we also see pain in relation to the menstrual cycle.

Causes and Disease Development

Living or working in damp surroundings as well as inappropriate clothing allow dampness to penetrate into the body. Excessive consumption of uncooked foods and/or cow's milk products harm the functions of spleen *qi*. As a result, the impaired transformation of this food causes dampness to form, which can then sink into the lower burner. This dampness can combine with heat, which arises from factors like spicy foods or alcohol.

Symptoms

Yellow, occasionally malodorous, vaginal discharge, vaginal itching, pain before and during menstruation with a downward-pulling sensation, reddish sticky menstrual blood with small clots, cyclically occurring urinary tract infections, sloppy stools. The tongue has a thick and oily yellow fur, especially in the back third of the tongue. The pulse is slippery and also stringlike.

Any further differentiation is not helpful because these acupuncture points treat both damp-heat with blood stasis and with blood heat.

Acupuncture

- to open the dai mai, GB-41 (*zu lin qi*) and TB-5 (*wai guan*)[4]
- GB-26 (*dai mai*): regulates menstruation, eliminates dampness, stabilizes the dai mai
- GB-27 (*wu shu*): regulates menstruation, stabilizes the dai mai, relieves pain
- SP-9 (*yin ling quan*): eliminates dampness in the lower burner
- GB-34 (*yang ling quan*): clears the liver and eliminates damp-heat from the liver and gallbladder
- CV-3 (*zhong ji*): eliminates dampness from the lower burner
- ST-28 (*shui dao*): regulates the lower burner and eliminates stagnation
- acupuncture points that move the blood (see above)
- SP-10 (*xue hai*) and LI-11 (*qu chi*): cool the blood

Medicinal Therapy

The recommended basic formula for eliminating damp-heat is *Er Miao San*, which is composed of only two ingredients. This formula must therefore be supplemented in light of the differentiated disease pattern.

Rx. Er Miao San (Mysterious Two Powder):
- *cang zhu* (Atractylodis rhizoma)
- *huang bai* (Phellodendri cortex)

If pain during menstruation is in the foreground, you can additionally employ the formula *Shi Xiao San*.

Rx. Shi Xiao San (Sudden Smile Powder):
- *wu ling zhi*
- *pu huang*

Grind both substances into a fine powder. The daily dose is 6 g, mixed into warm white wine or vinegar. Can also be given as a decoction.

Modifications for Blocked Fallopian Tubes:
- *hong teng*
- *zao jia ci*
- *bai jiang cao*
- *lu lu tong*
- *chuan lian zi*

Modifications for Ovarian Cysts:
- *ban xia*
- *fu ling*
- *kun bu*
- *hai zao*
- *san leng*
- *e zhu*

Modifications for Heat in the Blood with Heavy Periods:
- *chi shao yao*
- *mu dan pi*
- *dan shen* (Salviae miltiorrhizae radix)

Modifications for Recurrent Urinary Tract Infections:
- *che qian zi* (Plantaginis semen)
- *tu fu ling* (Smilacis glabrae rhizoma)
- *tong cao* (Tetrapanacis medulla)

The remaining patterns, which refer to states of energetic insufficiency, are insufficiency of *qi* and blood, insufficiency of *yang* and blood, and insufficiency of kidney and liver *yin*. They are not covered here because they generally do not cause severe, but rather dull pain during or after menstruation. In cases with acute symptoms caused by endometriosis, they are not of primary importance.[5] In contrast to other practitioners, the author has achieved excellent results with an initial treatment of the repletion state. Once the symptoms are alleviated, treatment should then possibly address the underlying vacuity state.

■ Treatment during Menstruation

In this phase, that is, on the first to third days of the period, we can treat as long as the woman's vitality permits it. In extremely severe pain, we recommend regulating the *qi* and quickening and moving the blood. It is especially important to move the blood downward, which allows the remaining heat to be discharged to the outside. This generally occurs by voiding the intestines. It is therefore useful in this treatment phase to use *da huang*. For this purpose, we should decoct it at least as long as the other medicinals. In spite of the fact that this herb partly loses its purging effect due to the longer decocting time, its strong downward-draining effect remains; this applies particularly to its ability to clear residual damp-heat as well as to eliminate blood stasis. Many women report clearly reduced menstrual pain if they fast or take a laxative on the day before the onset of menstruation.

The basic formulas *Tao He Cheng Qi Tang* or *Ge Xia Zhu Yu Tang* are indicated here, to resolve blood stasis and thereby relieve pain.

Rx. Tao He Cheng Qi Tang (*Peach Kernel* Qi-coordinating Decoction):
- *tao ren*, 12–15 g
- *da huang*, 12 g
- *gui zhi*, 6 g
- *mang xiao* (Natrii sulfas), 6 g
- *gan cao*, mix-fried in honey, 6 g

Rx. Ge Xia Zhu Yu Tang (*see above*)
In this phase, you can also prescribe anal enemas (see above).

Here, we must emphasize once again that the treatment strategies discussed above **apply only to the preparation for pregnancy** and can only be employed for the appropriate symptoms. The severity of endometriosis can vary from mild to severe. In spite of a diagnosis confirmed by laparoscopy, many women show no symptoms at all, nor is their fertility automatically disturbed by small endometriosis lesions.

As soon as symptoms have been relieved by treatment with acupuncture and Chinese medicinals, you can begin with the true treatment: to create the ideal energetic conditions for conception. This is done by:
- strengthening kidney *yin* and *yang*
- regulating liver *qi*
- harmonizing the *ren mai* and *chong mai*

Subsequently, you should no longer prescribe blood-moving substances that were necessary for the treatment of the endometriosis.

■ Case Study

Infertility due to Endometriosis

This case study illustrates the methodology of TCM in the treatment of infertility due to endometriosis. For this purpose, it explains the different treatment strategies in rhythm with the menstrual cycle.

Medical History
The patient, Ms. Andrea G., had been trying to get pregnant for 2 years. A laparoscopy, which had been done 3 months previously, confirmed the suspected diagnosis of endometriosis in the 30-year-old patient. Two chocolate cysts with a diameter of 6 cm were removed on both ovaries. In addition, many adhesions in the pouch of Douglas were removed. The right fallopian tube had been blocked. After surgery, the pain in the vaginal canal during sexual intercourse and urination disappeared. Nevertheless, the menstrual pain, which was particularly severe and spasmodic on the first and second day of the period, continued to occur. The period was frequently accompanied by a feeling of nausea. It was relatively weak but prolonged (up to 8 days). The menstrual blood was red and contained small clots.

Symptoms
The patient complained of pronounced premenstrual symptoms. Irritability and tense and painful breasts stood in the foreground. The menstrual cycle was 29 days long and regular. The patient's

general state of health was good. She appeared emotionally very stable.

The tongue was pale red, with a slightly reddened tip, the fur was oily and yellow on the root of the tongue. The sublingual veins were slightly congested. The pulses were strong and tight.

Diagnosis

Liver *qi* stagnation with blood stasis and blockage of *qi* and blood in the *chong mai*.

The inadequate movement of liver *qi*, which manifested in the pronounced premenstrual symptoms, had caused blood stasis. In spite of the fact that the pain was severe during menstruation, the other signs of blood stasis were not yet extreme. The blood contained small clots, the sublingual veins were not very conspicuous. The tongue, however, indicated an accumulation of dampness and heat in the lower burner, which might have been a contributing factor to the adhesions in the lower abdomen. The damp-heat aggravated the existing stagnation problem in the lower abdomen. The pulses highlighted the repletion state.

Treatment Principle

Regulate liver *qi,* eliminate blood stasis, draw out damp-heat.

Medicinal Therapy

Two formulas were combined with each other and prescribed from the 14th day of the cycle on in the form of a decoction:

Rx. Chuan Lian Zi San *(Toosendan Powder) and* Xiao Yao San *(Free Wanderer Powder):*
* *chuan lian zi*, 5 g
* *yan hu suo*, 10 g
* *chai hu* (Bupleuri radix), 5 g
* *dang gui*, 5 g
* *bai shao yao*, 7 g
* *bai zhu* (Atractylodis macrocephalae rhizoma), 5 g

* *fu ling*, 5 g
* *qing pi* (Citri reticulatae pericarpium viride frictum), 7 g
* *wu ling zhi*, 10 g
* *zao jia ci*, 5 g
* *gan cao*, 3 g

From the first to the third day of menstruation, *Chuan Lian Zi San* was prescribed with additions:
* *chuan lian zi*, 3 g
* *yan hu suo*, 10 g
* *wu ling zhi*, 10 g
* *san leng*, 7 g
* *bai shao yao*, 7 g
* *zhi gan cao*, 5 g
* *zhi da huang* (Rhei radix et rhizoma praeparata), 3 g

Result

After two cycles, menstruation became painless. Treatment was therefore stopped during menstruation. All in all, treatment was continued for another 3 months. Then, the patient decided on artificial fertilization. She became pregnant in the first attempt and 9 months later gave birth to a healthy girl.

Bibliography

1. Chen J. *Chinese Medical Herbology and Pharmacology.* City of Industry, CA: Art of Medicine Press; 2001.
2. Clavey S. *Fluid Physiology and Pathology in Traditional Chinese Medicine.* London: Churchill Livingstone; 2003.
3. Feige A. *Frauenheilkunde.* Munich: Urban & Fischer; 2006.
4. Kirschbaum B. *Die 8 Außerordentlichen Gefäße in der Traditionellen Chinesischen Medizin.* Uelzen: ML; 2000.
5. Maciocia G. *Obstetrics and Gynecology in Chinese Medicine.* London: Churchill Livingstone; 1998.

21 PCO Syndrome and Fertility

Jacqueline Peineke

The term polycystic—or better: polyfollicular—ovaries refers to ovaries that contain 10 or more immature follicles with a maximum 9 mm diameter and whose central connective tissue is increased.

Under ultrasound, multiple antral follicles—without a dominant follicle—and, as a whole, clearly enlarged ovaries are detected. The follicles fail to mature into a tertiary follicle ready for ovulation. Ovulation fails to take place and menstrual periods are accordingly irregular or absent.

The so-called **PCO syndrome (PCOS)** includes several symptoms, among which **hyperandrogenism** (increase of male sex hormones) is the obligatory key symptom. The source of the androgens can be the ovaries themselves or the adrenal cortex. The consecutive disturbance in follicular maturation is an important cause of unwanted childlessness and absent menstruation.

Potential findings in PCOS:

- menstrual disorders (absent or rare menstrual periods)
- increased body hair in a typical male pattern (hirsutism)
- obesity
- sterility
- changes in the fat and carbohydrate metabolism (insulin resistance)
- acne
- hair loss

What appear to be polycystically changed ovaries are encountered in many young women (20–25%). Among these, however, only a relatively small percentage develops a true PCO syndrome. Nevertheless, the practitioner will often be confronted with this syndrome in fertility treatment. Elevated levels of androgen—the key symptom of PCOS—are found in almost all patients.

■ How Does PCOS Arise?

Different hormonal (obesity) and cellular regulatory disturbances (androgen receptor polymorphism), which we are unable to discuses in detail here, form the basis of PCOS. To summarize, we can state that the proper cooperation of hypothalamus, hypophysis, and ovaries—as the so-called axis of reproduction—is disturbed. **Follicular maturation is impaired**, which is due to insulin resistance in the follicle and increased production of androgens.

Especially in obesity (i.e., in an increase of visceral fat tissue), elevated ovarian, as well as more rarely adrenal, production of androgen can result—discernible by an obvious "masculinization" with regard to the distribution of body fat and hair; this can be compounded by a diabetic metabolism.

■ Treatment with Biomedicine

As the first step, the pituitary gland and ovarian functions are temporarily suppressed by means of oral ovulatory inhibitors, that is, the "pill." In this context, antiandrogen progestagens are preferred. The excess weight must be reduced in order to lower the elevated estrogen levels and therefore also the rise in LH secretion that was caused by the increase in fat tissue. In patients with a diabetic metabolism, oral anti-diabetic drugs can be prescribed as well, to lower insulin resistance. This covers the treatment of PCOS; to additionally assist in the promotion of fertility, the following are indicated:

- as a rule, gonadotropins in low dosage after so-called down regulation
- in appropriate cases, ovarian stimulation with clomifen (e.g., indication: ovulatory disturbances)

- surgical drilling and thereby destruction of excess antral follicles (exception)
- in ovarian overreaction to the stimulation: in vitro fertilization (IVF)

Ovarian overstimulation syndrome and an undesired multiple pregnancy are a risk of these therapies, which should only be employed by experienced professionals.

The ovarian stimulation desired in the framework of these biomedical concepts must be distinguished from an **overstimulation syndrome**. This rare but serious complication can vary in its manifestation—from mildly affected well-being to a life-threatening clinical picture. The pathogenesis of overstimulation syndrome is still unclear; it involves a massive increase in vessel permeability. This leads to the formation of edemas, ascites, and pleural and pericardial effusions. We can also see a thickening of the blood with an increased hematocrit and the risk of thromboembolic complications.

For basic information on complementary treatment with TCM in the framework of reproductive medicine in accordance with the different stages (preparation, down-regulation, menstruation, stimulated follicle maturation, extraction, transfer), refer to Chapter 6.

Treatment with TCM

From the perspective of TCM, we can describe PCOS in terms of **root vacuity** (*ben xu*) and **tip repletion** (*biao shi*).

The kidneys are responsible for reproductivity. Most patients with infertility suffer from kidney vacuity. According to TCM, the kidneys store essence (*jing*); essence and blood (*xue*) share the same source. A lack of essence and blood impairs the functions of the extraordinary vessels *chong mai* and *ren mai*; under these conditions, it is difficult to become pregnant. Kidney vacuity hence forms the basis, whence phlegm-dampness repletion, fire resulting from liver *qi* stagnation, or *qi* stagnation with blood stasis follow and facilitate each other.

Affected organs are the **liver, spleen**, and **kidneys**; the disturbance manifests in the *chong mai* and *ren mai*. We differentiate the following four **patterns**:

- kidney vacuity
- phlegm-damp
- liver fire
- *qi* stagnation with blood stasis

Treatment focuses primarily on replenishing kidney vacuity. To complement this, we can choose to:

- strengthen the function of the spleen, to regulate *qi* and transform phlegm
- soothe liver *qi*, to resolve stagnation and reduce fire
- quicken the blood, to resolve the stasis and regulate menstruation

Both the treatment principle and the choice of medicinals follow this pattern differentiation in accordance with the presenting pathology.

The goal of treatment is always to regulate menstruation and thereby harmonize the interplay of **kidneys—*tian gui*—*chong mai*** and ***ren mai*—uterus**. In this way, we can effectively treat an existing infertility.

Expressed in biomedical terms, a regular menstrual cycle stems from the correct cooperation of hypothalamus, hypophysis, and the ovaries. To regulate menstruation means here to regulate this connection (axis of reproduction).

Differential Diagnosis

The following section describes the four above-mentioned patterns in more detail, including their symptoms and the corresponding treatment principles. Basic formulas and modifications follow. Complementing this, we give acupuncture points that can accompany treatment with Chinese medicinals. Treatment with the Chinese patent medicines that are also listed here should be regarded as an alternative to the recommended formulas. Because in this case the practitioner has no way of influencing the dosage of individual ingredients in relation to each other, the possibilities for tailoring treatment to the particular condition of individual patients are limited.

Kidney Vacuity

Symptoms
- delayed menstruation, brightly colored blood, or amenorrhea
- infertility
- tinnitus
- pain in the lower back
- cold sensations
- polyuria
- soft stools
- reduced libido
- overweight

Tongue: pale, with a thin white fur
Pulse: fine, sunken

Therapy

Nourish the kidney, replenish essence, regulate the *chong mai* and *ren mai*.

Medicinal Therapy
Rx. You Gui Wan *(Right-restoring [Life Gate] Pill)*—*Modification for the Treatment of Infertility in PCOS:*
- *shu di huang* (Rehmanniae radix praeparata), 10 g
- *shan yao* (Dioscoreae rhizoma), 20 g
- *shan zhu yu* (Corni fructus), 10 g
- *gou qi zi* (Lycii fructus), 10 g
- *lu jiao jiao* (Cervi cornus gelatinum), 10 g
- *tu si zi* (Cuscutae semen), 12 g
- *du zhong* (Eucommiae cortex), 10 g
- *dang gui* (Angelicae sinensis radix), 10 g
- *rou gui* (Cinnamomi cortex), 6 g
- *fu zi* (Aconiti radix lateralis praeparata), 6 g **(beware: toxic!)**

Additional Modifications:
- for delayed menstruation or amenorrhea:
  - *ze lan* (Lycopi herba), 12 g
  - *chuan niu xi* (Cyathulae radix), 12 g
  - *ji xue teng* (Spatholobi caulis), 20 g
- For very young patients or patients with malformation of the uterus:
  - *zi he che* (Hominis placenta, pre-cooked), 10 g
  - *he shou wu* (Polygoni multiflori radix), 10 g

---

* Also called Right (Kidney)-restoring Pill.

- *rou cong rong* (Cistanches herba), 10 g
- *yin yang huo* (Epimedii herba), 10 g

Patent Medicine
You Gui Wan: three times daily one pill.

Acupuncture
- BL-23 (*shen shu*): supplements the kidney, *yang*, essence and *yin*, warms the uterus
- GV-4 (*ming men*): supplements kidney *yang* and the *ming men* fire
- CV-6 (*qi hai*): supplements the kidney, *yang*, and *qi*, regulates *qi* and harmonizes the blood
- SP-6 (*san yin jiao*): supplements the kidney and harmonizes the liver, regulates menstruation, quickens blood, and stimulates the channels

Phlegm-damp

Symptoms
- scant or delayed menstruation
- amenorrhea
- infertility
- leukorrhea
- dizziness, feeling of heaviness in the head
- feeling of pressure in the thorax
- nausea
- feeling of heaviness in the extremities
- soft stools
- obesity

Tongue: enlarged, white slimy fur
Pulse: slippery

Therapy

Dissolve phlegm, transform dampness, regulate *qi* and menstruation.

Medicinal Therapy
Rx. Cang Fu Dao Tan Wan *(Atractylodes and Cyperus Phlegm-abducting Pill):*
- *cang zhu* (Atractylodis rhizoma), 10 g
- *xiang fu* (Cyperi rhizoma), 10 g
- *fu ling* (Poria), 12 g
- *ban xia* (Pinelliae rhizoma), 10 g
- *chen pi* (Citri reticulatae pericarpium), 10 g
- *gan cao* (Glycyrrhizae radix), 3 g
- *dan xing* (Arisaema cum bile), 10 g
- *zhi ke* (Aurantii fructus), 10 g
- *shen qu* (Massa fermentata medicata), 10 g

- *sheng jiang* (Zingiberis rhizoma recens), three slices

Modifications:
- For obesity and change in body hair (to dissolve phlegm and activate the network vessels):
  - *shan ci gu* (Cremastrae seu pleiones pseudobulbus), 10 g (**beware: toxic!**)
  - *xia ku cao* (Prunellae spica), 10 g
  - *zao jia ci* (Gleditsiae spina), 15 g
  - *shi chang pu* (Acori tatarinowii rhizoma), 10 g
- For masses in the lower abdomen (to soften hardenings and disperse accumulations):
  - *kun bu* (Laminariae/Eckloniae thallus), 15 g
  - *hai zao* (Sargassum), 15 g
  - *xia ku cao*, 10 g
  - *e zhu* (Curcumae rhizoma), 12 g

Patent Medicine
Qi Zhi Xiang Fu Wan (Sevenfold Processed Cyperus Pill): 6 g daily.

Acupuncture
- CV-6 (*qi hai*): supplements the kidney, *yang*, and *qi*, regulates *qi* and harmonizes the blood
- SP-8 (*di ji*): regulates menstruation and quickens the blood
- ST-30 (*qi chong*): regulates the *chong mai* and *qi* in the lower burner
- SP-6 (*san yin jiao*): supplements the kidney and harmonizes the liver, regulates menstruation, quickens the blood, and stimulates the channels

Liver Fire

Symptoms
- amenorrhea
- scant or irregular menstruation
- infertility
- muscle growth
- increased or thick hair
- facial acne
- feeling of tension or pain in the thorax, hypochondrium, or breasts
- galactorrhea
- dry mouth, desire to drink water
- constipation

Tongue: yellow, thin fur
Pulse: rapid and tight

Therapy

Soothe liver *qi* and clear heat, to reduce fire.

Medicinal Therapy
Rx. Dan Zhi Xiao Yao San *(Moutan and Gardenia Free Wanderer Powder)—Modification for the Treatment of Infertility in PCOS:*
- *mu dan pi* (Moutan cortex), 10 g
- *zhi zi* (Gardeniae fructus), 10 g
- *dang gui*, 10 g
- *bai shao yao* (Paeoniae radix alba), 15 g
- *chai hu* (Bupleuri radix), 6 g
- *bai zhu* (Atractylodis macrocephalae rhizoma), 10 g
- *gan cao*, roasted, 5 g
- *chuan niu xi*, 10 g

Additional Modifications:
- for constipation:
  - *da huang* (Rhei radix et rhizome), 6 g, to clear heat, reduce fire, and support bowel movement
  - *mai ya* (Hordei fructus germinatus), roasted, 60 g
  - *ku ding cha* (Ilicis folium), 10 g
- For tension pain in the thorax, hypochondrium, or breasts (to soothe liver *qi* and free the network vessels):
  - *yu jin* (Curcumae radix), 15 g
  - *wang bu liu xing* (Vaccariae semen), 15 g
  - *lu lu tong* (Liquidambaris fructus), 10 g

Patent Medicine
Xiao Yao Wan (Free Wanderer Pill): 10 g, three times a day.

Acupuncture
- LR-3 (*tai chong*): soothes liver *qi*, regulates menstruation, regulates the lower burner, nourishes liver blood and *yin*
- LI-4 (*he gu*): activates the channels, relaxes in combination with LR-3
- LR-2 (*xing jian*): clears liver fire, soothes liver *qi*, regulates the lower burner

Qi Stagnation with Blood Stasis

Symptoms
- delayed, scant, or interrupted menstruation
- abdominal pain that is aggravated by pressure
- menstrual period with clots, pain that is relieved by discharge of clots
- amenorrhea
- infertility
- depression
- feeling of fullness in the thorax and hypochondrium

Tongue: crimson, with dark spots on the margin and tip
Pulse: sunken and tight

Therapy

Regulate *qi*, quicken the blood, resolve stasis, regulate menstruation.

Medicinal Therapy
Rx. Ge Xia Zhu Yu Tang *(Infradiaphragmatic Stasis-expelling Decoction)—Modification for the Treatment of Infertility in PCOS:*
- *dang gui*, 10 g
- *chuan xiong* (Chuanxiong rhizom), 5 g
- *chi shao yao* (Paeoniae radix rubra), 10 g
- *tao ren* (Persicae semen), 10 g
- *hong hua* (Carthami flos), 6 g
- *zhi ke*, 10 g
- *yan hu suo* (Corydalis rhizoma), 10 g
- *wu ling zhi* (Trogopteri feces), 10 g
- *mu dan pi*, 10 g
- *bai shao yao*, 10 g
- *xiang fu*, 10 g
- *gan cao*, 5 g

Additional Modifications:
- For feeling of tension in the thorax or breasts, tension pain in the lower abdomen, depression, and PMS, to soothe liver *qi*, resolve stagnation, and activate *qi*, for pain relief:
  - *qing pi* (Citri reticulatae pericarpium viride), 10 g
  - *mu xiang* (Aucklandiae radix), 9 g
  - *chai hu*, 6 g
- for masses in the abdomen, to quicken blood, resolve stasis, and disperse masses:
  - *san leng* (Sparganii rhizoma), 10 g
  - *e zhu*, 10 g
  - *mo yao* (Myrrha), 10 g
  - *lu lu tong*, 10 g

Patent Medicine
Da Huang Zhe Chong Wan (Rhubarb and Ground Beetle Pill): one pill, two to three times a day in hot water or ginger decoction.

Acupuncture
- LR-3 (*tai chong*): soothes liver *qi*, regulates menstruation, regulates the lower burner, nourishes liver blood and *yin*
- LI-4 (*he gu*): activates the channels, relaxes in combination with LR-3
- ST-30 (*qi chong*): regulates the *chong mai* and *qi* in the lower burner
- ST-29 (*gui lai*): regulates menstruation
- SP-10 (*xue hai*): moves blood and resolves stasis

Bibliography
1. Feige A, Rempen A, Würfel W, Caffier H, Jawny J. *Frauenheilkunde.* Munich: Urban & Schwarzenberg; 1997.
2. Lyttleton J. *Treatment of Infertility with Chinese Medicine.* London: Churchill Livingstone; 2004.
3. Zuo Y. *Gynecology of Traditional Chinese Medicine.* Shanghai: University of TCM Publishing House of Shanghai; 2002.

In vitro fertilization/embryo transfer (IVF/ET) is a technique of reproductive medicine. Following controlled ovarian stimulation (COS), eggs are retrieved from the ovaries. After these eggs are cultivated and fertilized and have developed into embryos of a certain size, they are transferred to the uterus for implantation and growth.

Children "created" by means of IVF/ET treatment are referred to in China as "test-tube babies." Since the first test-tube baby was born in Great Britain in 1978, IVF/ET procedures have experienced rapid growth and development, for example with the following techniques:

- intracytoplasmic sperm injection (ICSI)
- cryoconservation and transfer
- co-cultivation
- assisted hatching
- blastocyst transfer
- in vitro maturation (IVM)
- pre-implantation diagnosis (PID)

These techniques are common all over the world. With their assistance, reproductive medicine has been able to help many infertile couples so far.

The IVF/ET procedure is a milestone in the treatment of infertility. But even with this method there are difficulties, such as the low success rate (live birth rate 8–30%), low responders (9–20%), high drop-out rate (15–24%), long treatment duration, and high costs, to name just the most important ones.

For these reasons, more and more couples are turning to TCM for support. Apart from this fact, many open-minded IVF/ET specialists have begun referring their difficult patients to TCM practitioners whom they trust, to receive further assistance

■ History of Fertility Treatment in TCM

TCM has a history of treating infertility that goes back more than a thousand years. It has therefore gathered a wealth of experience with resulting opinions and scientific foundations. Already in the 11th century BCE, the famous physician Zhou Yi stated: "Infertility refers to the state when women are not pregnant after 3 years." This is the first mention of this disorder with reference to a time frame.

The *Bei Ji Qian Jin Yao Fang (Essential 1000-Gold Formulary for Emergencies*; see Chapter 8), composed in 652 CE by Sun Simiao, mentions *quan bu chan* ("primary infertility"), *duan xu* ("secondary infertility"), and their causes and treatment.

The *Su Wen* chapter "*Shang Gu Tian Zhen Lun*" ("Treatise of Heavenly Truth from Remote Antiquity"), written around the first century CE, is the first text to describe the physiological processes of fertility: "At the age of 7, kidney *qi* becomes stronger, ... at the age of 14, the *tian gui* arrives, the *ren mai* opens, the *chong mai* becomes strong, and the menses begin to flow regularly, ... then a woman can get pregnant."

The *Su Wen* chapter "*Gu Kong Lun*" ("Treatise on Bone Hollow") states that "in disease of the *du mai*, the woman will be infertile." This is the first reference to the pathology by which an insufficiency of *yang* causes infertility.

The section on women's formulas in the *Jin Gui Yao Lüe (Essential Prescriptions of the Golden Coffer)* from the Han period (206 BCE– 220 CE) states: "Women who have cold in the abdomen will not be pregnant for a long time." The same text also refers to the formula *Wen Jing Tang* (Menses-warming Decoction), the first formula for regulating menstruation and hence the production of progesterone. The section on women in the *Zhen Jiu Jia Yi Jing (Systematic Classic of Acupuncture and Moxibustion)* from the Western *Jin* period (265–316 CE) states: "Women with blood stasis will be infertile and can be treated at *guan yuan* (CV-4)." This is the first time that the pathology of blood stasis and its treatment with acupuncture are mentioned.

The chapter on "childlessness" (*wu zi*) in the classic *Zhu Bing Yuan Hou Lun (On the Origins and Symptoms of the Various Diseases),* which was composed in the Sui period (581–618 CE), elaborates: "Disharmony in the *chong mai* and *ren mai* is the main cause of women's diseases."

Since then, TCM has developed a complete scientific system for the physiology, pathology, and treatment of infertility, with excellent results. Like Western reproductive medicine, TCM has also grown step by step in this area and continues to achieve better and better results.

■ Preliminary Results

From October 2000 to February 2006, I have supported IVF/ET treatments with TCM in China and abroad (Israel and Swizerland) and gathered detailed data on 86 cases. The average age of the patients was 34.4 ± 3.6 years (the range was 27–44 years). The mean duration of infertility was 7.3 ± 3.2 years (the range was 2–20 years). There were 51 cases of primary infertility (59.3%) and 35 cases of secondary infertility (40.7%).

Among these patients, the following **causes** of infertility were found:
- PCOS (polycystic ovary syndrome, n = 5)
- PCOS/fallopian tube-based infertility (n = 6)
- PCOS/infertility of the partner (n = 3)
- infertility of the partner (n = 15)
- fallopian tube-based infertility (n = 18)
- infertility of the partner/fallopian tube-based infertility (n = 10)
- latent ovarian insufficiency (FSH-level > 15mIU/mL^4, n = 6)
- endometriosis and/or adenomyosis (n = 8)
- thin endometrium (<7 mm during implantation, n = 4)
- thin endometrium/infertility of the partner (n = 2)

- other factors (hyperprolactinemia, intrauterine myomas, hypogonadotropic hypogonadism, n = 2)
- infertility of unknown causes (n = 7)

All partners had already received treatment with reproductive medicine. The average of received IVF/ET or ICSI/ET treatments was 3.6 ± 1.5 (the range was 1–9 times). Seventy-nine cases were treated with TCM for 1–4 months before the start of the IVF/ET treatment. Seven cases started both therapies in the same month. All patients were treated with TCM at least until hCG proof (pregnancy); pregnant women continued to receive treatment at least until the 10th week of pregnancy; pregnant women with miscarriage history were treated until the month of their previous miscarriage.

Among these 86 cases, 48 resulted in pregnancies, 33 patients (38.4%) became pregnant in the first round of treatment, 15 (17.1%) in the second round.

Four patients lost the child in the first trimester; 39 children were delivered (among these three pairs of twins).

The remaining eight cases were pregnancies that went past the 12th week, with good fetal development. The clinical pregnancy rate (pregnancies/total number of patients treated with TCM) was 51.2%, the miscarriage rate (miscarriages/pregnancies) was 8.3%.

Most patients in this group had a prehistory of infertility. Multiple failures had both exhausted them mentally and aggravated their endocrinologic disturbances. Treatment with TCM to support IVF/ET therapy was able not only to alleviate the symptoms and strengthen the confidence and starting condition of the patients; it was also able to increase the number of pregnancies and reduce the number of miscarriages.

I work as a gynecologist for integrated TCM and Western medicine at the Beijing Hospital of TCM, Capital University of Medical Science, which does not have a department of reproductive medicine. The starting situation of individual patients tends to vary greatly, for example by age, BMI, menstrual period, length of infertility, cause of infertility, or type of previous treatments (medications or invasive). This complicates the comparability of the study.

In addition, it is difficult to suggest participation in a control group without TCM treatment to patients whose concern it is to support their IVF/ET treatment with TCM. For this reason, we do not have comparative data for IVF/ET treatments with TCM support and without support. What we need, though, are clearly designed, foresighted, and randomized studies. More and more studies on supporting IVF/ET or ICSI/ET therapy with TCM show results that sound optimistic.

When and For Which Patients is IVF/ET or ICSI/ET Treatment Appropriate?

In spite of the fact that the question might seem superfluous and that we could argue that IVF/ET treatments are appropriate for all types of infertility, opinions differ on this topic.

Complications in IVF/ET or ICSI/ET Treatments

Complications that can arise in the course of IVF/ET or ICSI/ET procedures include for example:

- The miscarriage rate (18.4–30%) is higher than in natural pregnancies (10–18%).
- Abdominal pregnancies occur more frequently (3.8–5%) than in natural conception (2%).
- The number of multiple pregnancies is high (30%).
- The rate of ovarian hyperstimulation syndrome (OHSS), a critical iatrogenic complication, lies around 23.3%.
- Micromanipulation of gametes has raised the question of the safety of ICSI; we must consider the fact that a slight rise in chromosomal deviations in 1082 caryotypes has been noticed in ICSI children, without defects.

In addition, the low success rate, high costs, and other factors that we have already mentioned at the beginning of this chapter discourage many couples from deciding on these methods.

Which Method for an Infertile Couple?

We have a few suggestions on this topic:

Principle of Differentiation

Treatment with TCM should be initiated in accordance with the principle of pattern identification as the basis for determining treatment (*bian zheng lun zhi*). At the same time, we should look for the cause of the infertility. TCM offers a rich treasure trove of experience. If no serious circumstances are found, the couple will get pregnant after a short time. We can achieve even better results by combining Chinese pattern identification with biomedical pathology. For example, a female patient whose infertility is accompanied by problems such as endometriosis, PCO syndrome, luteal phase defect (LPD), or dysfunctional uterine bleeding can become pregnant when treated with TCM.

According to my experience, some patients who had previously received various IVF/ET or ICSI/ET treatments with no success were able to have children after treatment only with Chinese medicinals.

Combination with Biomedicine

If no pregnancy has occurred after 3–6 months of TCM therapy, it should be combined with biomedicine. A patient with PCOS, for example, can supplement TCM treatment with Clomifen/hCG or Metformin, to profit from the advantages of both methods.

If endometriosis patients are still not pregnant after several months of TCM treatment, a laparoscopy is advised. Afterwards, we should continue treatment with TCM because the pregnancy rate 6 months after laparoscopy is high. This results either from the stimulation of ovulation or from the additional softening of adhesions and tissue growths, as a result of which the function of the ovaries and fallopian tubes is supported.

Patients after a laparoscopy should not go without additional treatment. This would reduce the possibility of a pregnancy because these patients often suffer also from lack of ovulation, LPD, luteinized unruptured follicle syndrome (LUFS), or immune problems. Moreover, endometriosis relapses are common.

In infertility due to occluded fallopian tubes, it has proven effective to treat patients internally and externally for 2 months with TCM and then to repeat a patency test with fluid instillation (introduction). If at this point we find signs of an opening such as reduced pressure or less fluid backflow, treatment should be continued. In the author's opinion, an opening of the fallopian tubes occurs within 2–6 months in nearly half of the patients receiving this combined therapy.

Good results can also be achieved with TCM in the treatment of male infertility patients in whom sperm density is less than 20 million/mL and sperm activity is reduced.

Most problems can be solved with TCM or in combination with biomedicine without requiring IVF treatment. In these cases, we spare patients the massive side-effects of medications that are otherwise given in high dosages, such as hot flashes, localized reactions at the puncture sites, mood swings, headache, or menstrual problems. Most importantly, TCM does not carry any risks comparable to those of IVF/ET or ICSI/ET treatment. In addition, the costs are much lower.

Who is an Appropriate Candidate for IVF/ET or ICSI/ET Treatments?

In the following cases, it is advisable for patients to immediately undergo IVF/ET or ICSI/ET treatment, for the sake of saving time:

- For women in whom both fallopian tubes are occluded, especially when the obstruction is found in the proximal part of the tubes, or for women whose fallopian tubes were removed in a fallopian tube removal; for women who have a prehistory of pelvic tuberculosis because this disorder increases the likelihood of an abdominal pregnancy since the TB has destroyed the inside of the ovaries. Even if treatment with TCM would result in patency, it would still be difficult to restore peristalsis and the walls of the tubes. Regardless of this fact, women above the age of 38 should directly undergo IVF/ET treatment in view of the quality and number of their eggs.

- For women whose partner suffers from severe oligo-astheno-teratozoospermia syndrome (OATS), because here it is impossible to produce a child naturally or via intrauterine insemination (IUI).

How Can We Support IVF/ET Treatment?

Depending on the case, there are different protocols for controlled ovarian stimulation and fertilization methods. Nevertheless, the principle of IVF/ET treatment is always the same: in general, we find the stages of **down-regulation, retrieval of the ovum**, and **embryo transfer**. The treatment principle of TCM changes in accordance with the different steps. In our experience, there are six stages that we can accompany with TCM:

1. Preparatory
2. Down-regulation
3. Menstrual
4. Oocyte maturation
5. Follicle punction
6. Embryo transfer

Preparatory Phase—Regulation (*Tiao* 调)

In order to successfully carry out an IVF/ET or ICSI/ET treatment, it is important to balance the patient's *yin* and *yang*, *qi* and blood, the viscera and bowels (*zang* and *fu*) for 2–3 months by means of TCM.

Why is the Preparation Phase Necessary?

- According to the TCM theory that "the kidneys are responsible for the ability to reproduce (*shen zhu sheng zhi* 肾主生殖)," most infertility patients suffer from kidney vacuity. In TCM, "the kidneys store the essence (*shen cang jing* 肾藏精, and "essence and blood share the same source (*jing xue tong yuan* 精血同源)". An insufficiency of essence and blood negatively affects the function of the *chong mai* and *ren mai*. Under these circumstances, it is difficult to become pregnant. On the other hand, though, controlled ovarian stimulation (COS) induced the development of a larger amount of follicles within a very short time, which consumes a lot of essence and blood. This in turn causes additional damage to kidney essence and liver blood. The chapter on "Principles of Women's Problems" in the text *Jing Yue Quan Shu (Complete Works of Jing Yue)* describes it this way: "The only cause of infertility is insufficiency of essence in men and insufficiency of blood in women." Now we know that the man's essence and the woman's blood form the material foundation of pregnancy. In this case, how could we expect good results with a precondition of insufficient liver blood and kidney essence?

- Shortly after failed IVF/ET treatments, women often describe menstrual disorders such as a delayed or shortened cycle, increased menstrual bleeding, or amenorrhea. In such cases, we must first regulate menstruation before a new IVF/ET treatment is initiated. In the "Principle of Gynecological Diseases in Pregnancy" chapter we find the following statement: "The method for achieving pregnancy is to regulate menstruation to plant seeds" (*tiao jing zhong zi* 调经种子). It is certainly easier to become pregnant when menstruation is regular. From the biomedical perspective, a regular menstrual cycle is the result of the proper interplay of hypothalamus, hypophysis, and the ovaries. To regulate menstruation means to regulate this connection (the reproductive axis).

- Large amounts of hormones that have collected in the body after a failed IVF/ET treatment can affect the interplay of the body's own hormones and disrupt the maturation of the ovum and the construction of the endometrium and development of the embryo. In this case, it is good to regulate the imbalances in the body for 2–3 months with TCM and to disburden it of the leftovers from previous hormone treatments.

- Many patients suffer from liver *qi* stagnation. The causes of this can consist of: long-lasting infertility, failed IVF/ET treatments, excessive expectations, but also the increasing pressure and psychological strain from family, society, and the patient's professional and economic situation. Liver *qi* stagnation leads to disturbance in the *qi* and blood, which in turn affects the function of the liver and kidney because "the liver and kidney share the same source" (*gan shen tong yuan* 肝肾同源). According to TCM theory, this leads to a corresponding disturbance of the axis "kidney–*tian gui*–*chong mai*

and *ren mai*–*bao gong* (uterus)." If such women continue biomedical treatment immediately after a failed IVF/ET attempt, an additional failure will further aggravate the stagnation, which causes a vicious circle. Therefore, more and more failures result. This is called "infertility due to liver depression" (*gan yu bu yun* 肝郁不孕). Some patients suffer from depression or nervous agitation, which gives rise to or aggravates additional symptoms like exhaustion, insomnia, or changes in appetite and weight. After a failed IVF/ET treatment, we recommend treating the patient for 2–3 months with TCM to regulate and harmonize.

Common **patterns** during the preparatory and regulatory phases are:
- kidney vacuity with liver *qi* stagnation
- liver fire due to liver *qi* stagnation
- vacuity heat due to liver and kidney *yin* vacuity
- *yang* vacuity in the kidney and spleen, in combination with dampness and phlegm
- damp-heat accumulation in the lower burner

The treatment principle for prescribing medicinals and/or selecting acupuncture points depends on a **differential diagnosis**.

The ideal condition for an IVF/ET treatment includes:
- a comparatively abundant amount of blood and essence to support the pregnancy
- relaxation, to allow the axis "kidney–*chong mai* and *ren mai*–*bao gong*" to function
- correct pulse and tongue findings that express the balance of *yin* and *yang*, *qi*, blood, and the organs, as well as the absence of pathogenic factors that could impact the treatment, for example:
  – a red tongue body with no fur indicates severe *yin* vacuity with vacuity heat, which could lead to agitation, reduced quality of oocytes and endometrium, and hence potentially to a miscarriage
  – a thick tongue fur that indicates dampness and phlegm, which could lead to shifting of the uterus and its network vessels and hence to infertility
  – a dark tongue body with stasis macules or bleeding that suggests blood stasis, which could lead to an impaired microcirculation in the reproductive organs

– a very fine and weak pulse, especially at the cubit (*chi mai*, i.e., kidney position), which indicates that liver blood and kidney essence are too weak to support the oocytes

These deviations from the ideal state provide the explanation for a continued lack of pregnancy in spite of the fact that the biomedical preconditions, for example, an endometrial thickness of 10 mm, good embryo morphology, and an optimal hormonal state, are fulfilled. TCM always treats the whole person. A healthy appetite and sleep, balanced emotional state, and regular digestion are good and important signs for the patient.

Down-regulation Phase—Supplementing (*Bu* 补)

In this phase, the patient receives high doses of GnRH-a (gonadotropin-releasing hormone agonist), often for a "long protocol" of COS, to inhibit the activity of the reproductive axis and the body's own hormones. This is called down-regulation and often begins in the luteal phase of the previous cycle. Patients with endometriosis and adenomyosis are treated for 2–3 months to control the endometriosis lesions. Patients with an irregular cycle or FSH (follicle-stimulating hormone) levels of more than 15 U/L are often given the "pill," for example Marvelon, for 1–3 months prior to the start of IVF/ET treatment.

Therapy

Replenish and supplement blood and essence to regulate and strengthen the *chong mai* and *ren mai*.

Medicinal Therapy

Rx. Yang Xue Tian Jing Fang (养血填精方, *Blood-nourishing Essence-replenishing Formula*) *with modifications:*
- *dang gui* (Angelicae sinensis radix)
- *chuan xiong* (Chuanxiong rhizoma)
- *bai shao yao* (Paeoniae radix alba)
- *e jiao zhu* (Asini corii gelatini pilula)
- *shu di huang* (Rehmanniae radix praeparata)

- *he shou wu* (Polygoni multiflori radix)
- *gou qi zi* (Lycii fructus)
- *tu si zi* (Cuscutae semen)
- *chai hu* (Bupleuri radix)
- *shan zhu yu* (Corni fructus)
- *fu ling* (Poria)

Note: It is necessary to select one of these groups for the main formula.

Necessary Additions:
- For kidney *yang* vacuity, add *rou cong rong* (Cistanches herba) and *fu pen zi* (Rubi fructus).
- For kidney *yin* vacuity, add *nü zhen zi* (Ligustri lucidi fructus) and *han lian cao* (Ecliptae herba).
- For excessive heat, replace *chuan xiong* with *dan shen* (Salviae miltiorrhizae radix) or *chi shao* (Paeoniae radix rubra).

Modifications:
- liver *qi* stagnation: add *yu jin* (Curcumae radix) and *xiang fu* (Cyperi rhizoma)
- insufficiency of *qi*: add *dang shen* (Codonopsis radix) or *tai zi shen* (Pseudostellariae radix)
- *yin* vacuity: add *sha shen* (Adenophorae seu glehniae radix), *yu zhu* (Polygonati odorati rhizoma), or *huang jing* (Polygonati rhizoma)
- insomnia: add *suan zao ren* (Ziziphi spinosi semen), *bai zi ren* (Platycladi semen), *zhen zhu mu* (Concha margaritifera), or *yuan zhi* (Polygalae radix)

Beware!
It is important to avoid medicinals that stimulate or heat kidney *yang* too strongly, such as *rou gui* (Cinnamomi cortex), *huang qi* (Astragali radix), *lu rong* (Cervi cornu pantotrichum), *yin yang huo* (Epimedii herba), *xian mao* (Curculiginis rhizome), or *suo yang* (Cynomorii herba). The same rule applies to substances that move the blood too strongly, such as *su mu* (Sappan lignum), *e zhu* (Curcumae rhizome), and *san leng* (Sparganii Rhizoma), unless their function is necessary.

The "down-regulation phase" or "supplementing phase" serves to replenish and supplement blood and essence without stimulating the reproductive function, which would run counter to the down-regulation by GnRH-a.

Acupuncture

- CV-12, CV-6, CV-4, ST-36, SP-6, KI-3, GV-20, HT-7, LR-3

Menstrual Phase—Gently Free the Blood (*Tong* 通)

During this phase, the menstrual blood is flowing. Menstruation is the beginning of a new cycle. During this time, it is important to "drain instead of storing" (*xie er bu cang* 泻而不藏) and to "create a smooth passage by freeing the flow" (*yi tong wei shun* 以通为顺). The blood should be freed and purged gently to cause the old endometrium to be eliminated completely and thereby ensure that the new endometrium can grow in a renewed environment. Treatment begins 2–3 days before the onset of menstruation and continues for another 3–4 days afterwards.

Therapy

Nourish blood and support the flow of blood to regulate menstruation.

Medicinal Therapy

Rx. Tiao Jing Fang (调经方, *Menses-regulating Formula*), with modifications:

- *dang gui*
- *chuan xiong*
- *shu di huang*
- *bai shao yao*
- *pu huang* (Typhae pollen)
- *xiang fu*
- *yi mu cao* (Leonuri herba)
- *he shou wu*
- *gan cao* (Glycyrrhizae radix)

Modifications:

- heavy menstrual periods or periods with clots: add *chai hu, qian cao* (Rubiae radix), powdered *san qi* (Notoginseng radix), or *pu huang tan* (Typhae pollen carbonisatum)
- scant and dark periods: add *ze lan* (Lycopi herba), *dan shen, hong hua* (Carthami flos), or *tao ren* (Persicae semen)
- dysmenorrhea: add *yan hu suo* (Corydalis rhizoma), *chuan lian zi* (Toosendan fructus), *wu yao* (Linderae radix), or *li zhi he* (Litchi semen); for cold pain, add *wu zhu yu* (Evodiae fructus) and *gao liang jiang* (Alpiniae officinarum rhizoma)

Acupuncture

- CV-6, CV-3 SP-6, SP-10, SP-8, LR-3

It is possible that the menstrual period will fail to arrive after 2–3 months of taking GnRH-a. Be this as it may, as soon as stimulation of the oocyte development is initiated in the course of the IVF treatment, continue with phase 4 (oocyte maturation phase), under certain circumstances also by-passing the menstruation phase.

Oocyte Maturation Phase—Promoting (*Cu* 促)

This phase corresponds to the length of time that the patient is taking gonadotropin-FSH or hMG (human menopausal gonadotropin) to stimulate the maturation of the oocyte.

Therapy

Warm and supplement the kidneys, quicken the blood, and regulate the *chong mai* and *ren mai*, to promote oocyte maturation.

Medicinal Therapy

Rx. Zi Shen Tiao Chong Fang (滋肾调冲方, *Kidney-enriching Thoroughfare-regulating Formula*), with modifications:

- *dang gui*
- *chuan xiong*
- *dan shen*
- *tu si zi*
- *qou qi zi*
- *ba ji tian* (Morindae officinalis radix)
- *xu duan* (Dipsaci radix)
- *zi he che* (Hominis placenta)
- *su mu*

Note: It is necessary to select one of these groups for the main formula.

Necessary Additions:

- kidney *yang* vacuity: add *lu rong, yin yang huo, ji xue teng* (Spatholobi caulis), and *rou gui*
- kidney *yin* vacuity: add *gui ban* (Testudinis plastrum), *nü zhen zi, han lian cao, chi shao*, or *mu dan pi* (Moutan cortex)

Modifications:

- liver *qi* stagnation: add *yu jin* and *mei gui hua* (Rosae rugosae flos)

285

- blood stasis: add *san leng* and *e zhu*
- constipation: add *rou cong rong* and *tao ren*
- vacuity heat in the heart, leading to nervousness and disquietude: add *bai he* (Lilii bulbus) and *lian zi xin* (Nelumbinis plumula)

For vacuity of *qi* and *yin* and insomnia, add the same medicinals as in the down-regulation phase.

Beware!
The principle "warm the kidney and supplement essence, quicken the blood and regulate the *chong mai*" has the effect that the ovaries bring a large number of follicles into the development stage, by replenishing essence and blood. Nevertheless, it is wrong to think "the more follicles the better." Apparently, if the number of mature follicles is higher than 13, the likelihood of OHSS (ovarian hyperstimulation syndrome) increases.[5] In addition, from the perspective of TCM, follicular development requires the support of essence and blood. Maturing an excessive number of follicles consumes too much essence and blood and negatively affects egg quality.

The analysis of 104 cases of IVF/ET treatments at the Beijing Third Hospital of Beijing Medical University revealed that the pregnancy rate in "high responders" (more than 13 mature follicles) was 0%; "low responders" (less than three mature follicles) had a pregnancy rate of 25%, and "middle responders" (3–13 mature follicles) had a rate of 30.6%.[5]

For patients who did not show elevated levels of FSH in the first COS and had more than 13 mature follicles to begin with, it is therefore better to select the formula *Yang Xue Tian Jing Fang*, to preserve and improve the quality of the oocytes. For patients who developed only few follicles during COS, we recommend the use of acupuncture in addition to *Zi Shen Tiao Chong Fang*.

Acupuncture—Main Points
- CV-4 (*zi gong*), ST-29, ST-36, SP-6 (*yin tang*)
- BL-13, BL-15, BL-17, BL-18, BL-20, BL-23 (*wu zang shu + ge shu*), GV-20

Use points from both groups in alternation.

Modifications:
- kidney *yang* vacuity: add GV-4 and BL-20
- kidney *yin* vacuity: add KI-3 and KI-6
- liver *qi* stagnation or liver fire: add LR-3 and LR-2
- disharmony of heart and kidney: add *si shen xue* (*si shen cong*, HT-7, GV-24, GB-13)
- ear acupuncture: endocrinium, liver, kidney, spleen, *shen men*

Follicle Punction Phase—Relax (*Song* 松)

This phase begins at the point in time when the follicles are almost fully matured and lasts until 1 day before the embryo transfer (ET). During this time span, patients undergo a variety of tests (blood tests, ultrasound, etc.) and surgeries; they are therefore often very tense.

Therapy

Regulate liver *qi* and quiet the spirit, strengthen the kidney and move the blood.

Medicinal Therapy
Rx. Zi Shen Tiao Chong Fang (滋肾调冲方, *Kidney-enriching Thoroughfare-regulating Formula*) plus:
- *yu jin*
- *he huan pi* (Albizziae cortex)
- *bai he* or *lian zi xin*

Acupuncture
- *si shen cong*, HT-7, GV-24, LR-3, SP-6, SP-10, *wu zang shu + ge shu*
- ear acupuncture: endocrinium, liver, *shen men*, uterus

Beware!
Avoid acupuncture points in the area of the ovaries, such as *zi gong* and ST-29, to avoid injuring the swollen ovaries.

Embryo Transfer Phase—Securing and Astringing (*Gu* 固)

This phase comprises the time span from the embryo transfer to the serum hCG test (pregnancy test) after 12–14 days.

Therapy

Replenish the kidneys and spleen to secure the *chong mai* and *ren mai*.

Medicinal Therapy

Rx. Yi Shen Gu Chong Fang (益肾固冲方, *Kidney-boosting Thoroughfare-securing Formula*):
* *tu si zi*
* *fu pen zi*
* *gou qi zi*
* *xu duan*
* *shan zhu yu*
* *shu di huang*
* *shan yao* (Dioscoreae rhizoma)
* *dang gui*
* *bai shao yao*
* *chai hu*

Necessary Additions:
* kidney *yang* vacuity: add *bu gu zhi* (Psoraleae fructus) or *rou cong rong, dang shen* or *huang qi*
* kidney *yin* vacuity: add *nü zhen zi, han lian cao, sha shen*, or *yu zhu*

Modifications:
* spleen vacuity with diarrhea: add *bai zhu* (Atractylodis macrocephalae rhizoma), *fu ling*, or *bian dou* (Lablab semen album)
* blood heat: add *huang qin* (Scutellariae radix) and *chun gen pi* (Toonae radicis cortex)

Beware!

In this phase, *yin* has already turned into *yang*. By stimulating *yang qi*, *yin* essence is continuously transformed into *yin* and blood. *Yin* and *yang* support each other and give rise to each other, reach the uterus and uterine vessel, and thereby create the ideal circumstances for the embryo transfer. The balance of *yin* and *yang* is the key to maintaining a functioning corpus luteum.

Treatment in accordance with Chinese pattern identification can here lead to success. It is not always appropriate to stimulate kidney *yang* to support the luteal function. You should particularly avoid medicinals that precipitate. It is important to both support the kidney and spleen and secure the *chong mai* and *ren mai*. It is said in TCM that "pregnancy can easily give rise to fire (*tai qian san ba huo* 胎前三把火)." For this reason, we treat patients suffering from blood heat with medicinals that nourish kidney *yin* and clear heat, to avoid a disturbance of the *chong mai* and *ren mai* and hence a potential miscarriage.

Acupuncture

In this phase, it is important to needle gently, to use thin needles, to needle superficially, and not to apply any manipulation. Otherwise, we run the risk of moving the patient's *qi* and blood too strongly and hence triggering uterine contractions and thereby affecting the implantation of the embryo.

Avoid LR-14 and SP-6 in particular, a pair of points that—according to classical literature as well as modern research—induces miscarriage and also labor.[8]

Any contraction from the cervix to the fundus could possibly move the implanted embryo into the fallopian tubes and cause an extrauterine pregnancy, especially since the function of the fallopian tubes is impaired in most patients to begin with. Any contraction from the fundus to the cervix, on the other hand, could propel the implanted embryo to the outside of the uterus. It therefore makes sense to avoid both of these points during the embryo transfer phase until additional research results are available on the effects of these points on the uterus. The positive results of a German study on the use of these two points is only a beginning.

Instead, we can strengthen kidney essence and liver blood in this phase with *wu zang shu* plus *ge shu*. Thereby we support the endometrium and consequently promote the development of the embryo. In patients with stress, you can add GV-20 (*yin tang*) and GV-24.

Case Studies

In the following pages, Dr. Wu Yuning illustrates the complexity of IVF/ET therapy and complementary treatment with TCM by means of several case studies from her practice. These examples clearly show where the quality and potential of TCM is found: in the individualized treatment of each patient beyond biomedical therapy.

Case Study 1: Thin Endometrium

Medical History

Ms. B. R., 32 years old, primary infertility for 2 years, two spontaneous miscarriages, IVF/ET and FET treatment (frozen embryo transfer). Each time, the endometrium was only 4–5 mm thick at the time of implantation, in spite of the fact that the patient was taking aspirin and Progynova. Treatment with TCM began on October 31, 2001, the third ET was planned for November. At the time of this implantation, the endometrium was 6 mm thick but irregular. The treatment proceeded without success. On December 7, 2001, she complained of listlessness, weakness in the lower back and legs, apprehension, disquietude, and great irritability. The tongue was dark with a thin dry white fur; the pulse was fine and string-like with a weak *chi* pulse.

Differential Diagnosis

Kidney vacuity with liver *qi* stagnation and blood stasis.

Treatment Principle

Strengthen kidney essence, soothe liver *qi*, and quicken blood, to resolve the blood stasis.

Medicinal Therapy

- *huang jing*
- *dang gui*
- *bai shao yao*
- *he shou wu*
- *zi he che*
- *sheng di huang* (Rehmanniae radix exsiccata seu recens)
- *tu si zi*
- *yin yang huo*
- *nü zhen zi*
- *ze lan*
- *mu dan pi*
- *yu jin*
- *bai he*
- *wang bu liu xing* (Vaccariae semen)

Result

After treatment, the apprehension, disquietude, and pain in the lower back disappeared. The patient started another IVF treatment with a long protocol as before and concomitantly took a modification of the formula *Yang Xue Tian Jing Fang*. The COS that was initiated after the subsequent menstruation was complemented with a modification of *Zi Shen Tiao Chong Fang*. On February 27, 2002, the embryo transfer took place, at which time the endometrium had a thickness of 6 mm and a good morphology. The formula was changed to *Yi Shen Gu Chong Fang*. On March 11, the hCG test came back positive. Later, the patient had scant bleeding for 1 week and continued treatment with TCM up to the 14th week of pregnancy. Delivery took place according to plan.

Commentary

Research has demonstrated the connection between endometrial thickness and successful implantation. In this case, a thin endometrium was the cause of two spontaneous miscarriages and a third failed treatment with IVF/ET or FET with aspirin and Progynova. An additional IVF/ET treatment, this time accompanied by TCM, resulted in pregnancy. Continuing treatment with TCM later prevented a threatened miscarriage that had announced itself by bleeding.

Case Study 2: Thin Endometrium, PCOS, OATS in the Partner

Medical History

Ms. Li, 33 years old; her husband's spermiogram showed a sperm density of 8.62 million/mL and a motility of 6.18% (a. 1.72%. b. 1.73%, c. 3.09%, d. 93.82%).

COS treatment began in May of 2005 (ultra-short protocol with Decapeptyl). Because of the reduced thickness of the endometrium, the patient additionally took Progynova, 4 mg daily. On June 6, at the time of the embryo transfer, the endometrium was 7 mm thick and grade C. She received two embryos with seven cells and received Progynova and progesterone. On June 22, menstruation began. As a result, the couple decided to request treatment with TCM. In July, the basal temperature (BT) rose for 16 days, which unfortunately turned out to be an ectopic pregnancy. The patient was treated with a laparoscopy and continued treatment with TCM. On September 22, the patient reported a delayed menstrual period, sticky vaginal discharge, soft stools, and white sticky phlegm in the throat. She had a dark tongue body with white fur and a fine slippery pulse.

Differential Diagnosis
Kidney and spleen vacuity with phlegm-damp as well as blood stasis.

Treatment Principle
Strengthen the kidney and spleen, eliminate phlegm-damp, and nourish and move blood.

Medicinal Therapy
- *tai zi shen*
- *fu ling*
- *cang zhu* (Atractylodis rhizoma)
- *dang gui*
- *chuan xiong*
- *ji xue teng*
- *san leng*
- *bei mu* (Fritillariae thunbergii bulbus)
- *tu si zi*
- *yin yang huo*
- *du zhong* (Eucommiae cortex)
- *xu duan*

During treatment, she felt better and prepared herself for the FET. After the last period on December 20, 2005, she started taking a modification of the formula *Zi Shen Tiao Chong Fang*.

Result
On January 4, 2006, the endometrium was 8 mm thick and grade A; the ultrasound examination showed a follicular diameter of 2.1 cm.

The FET took place on January 8. At this time, the endometrium had a thickness of 9 mm, grade A, and the patient began taking a modification of *Yi Shen Gu Chong Fang*. On January 22, the serum-hCG was 1400 mIU/mL; on February 17, the ultrasound examination detected heart beats. The pa-

tient continued treatment with TCM until the 12th week of pregnancy.

Commentary
The endometrium doubtlessly plays an important role in this process. There are no immediate criteria for evaluating the endometrium; its thickness and echogenicity, made visible by means of ultrasound, are merely able to provide information on its development. It is clear that the endometrium changed in the course of treatment with TCM from 7 mm grade C to 9 mm grade A. Likewise, the PCOS was treated and ovulation promoted, which even lead to a natural pregnancy—although this unfortunately developed into an ectopic pregnancy.

Case Study 3: Weak Ovarian Reaction

Medical History
Ms. K. L., 36 years old, secondary infertility and delayed menstrual periods for 3 years. Her FSH value was around 21–28 IU/L. She had received hMG/hCG (human chorionic gonadotropin)/IUI twice, as well as three IVF/ET treatments. The last IVF had been called off due to insufficient follicle size. On January 4, 2002, she started treatment with TCM. At this time, she was preparing for another IVF (long protocol with Decapeptyl). On the third day of her menstrual period, she began with Gonal F (FSH), seven ampoules daily for 5 days, then switched to Menogon (FSH + LH), seven ampoules daily for 15 days. In the fourth IVF/ET treatment, nine eggs were removed, seven were fertilized, only four developed into five cells with weak morphology and were implanted. The treatment failed.

On March 20, she reported pain in the lower back, insomnia, stress, and nervousness. The tongue was swollen and dark, the fur yellow and slimy, the pulse sunken and fine with a weak *chi* pulse.

Differential Diagnosis
Kidney and spleen vacuity with damp-heat.

Treatment Principle
Clear heat and eliminate dampness, strengthen the kidney and spleen.

Medicinal Therapy

Rx. Yang Xue Tian Jing Fang *(Blood-nourishing Essence-replenishing Formula), modified:*

- *yu zhu*
- *huang lian* (Coptidis rhizoma)
- *che qian zi* (Plantaginis semen)
- *zhi ke* (Aurantii fructus)
- *ze lan*
- *chi shao*
- *ye jiao teng* (Polygoni multiflori caulis)
- *e jiao zhu*
- *tu si zi*
- *gou qi zi*
- *shan zhu yu*
- *fu ling*
- *bai he*
- *yuan zhi*

Analysis of the Formula:

- *Huang lian, che qian zi,* and *zhi ke* clear heat and eliminate dampness.
- *Ze lan* moves the blood and promotes urination to eliminate additional dampness.
- *Ye jiao teng* is a replacement for *he shou wu,* which is used in the original formula; *bai he* and *yuan zhi* supplement this medicinal to nourish the heart, quiet the spirit, and relax.
- Because of the yellow sticky tongue fur, *dang gui, chuan xiong,* and *di huang* were removed from the formula, and *bai shao yao* was replaced with *chi shao.*

Acupuncture

The acupuncture points of choice were CV-12, ST-40, ST-36, SP-6, KI-3, LR-2, and HT-7.

COS started on April 1, and she returned for treatment on April 5. Her stress symptoms had decreased, but she reported pronounced lower back pain that increased at night and no bowel movements for the past 2 days. The tongue was swollen and dark with a thin white fur; the pulse was unchanged.

Medicinal Therapy

The patient received a modification of the formula *Zi Shen Tiao Chong Fang* in combination with acupuncture:

Rx. Zi Shen Tiao Chong Fang *(Kidney-enriching Thoroughfare-regulating Formula), modified:*

- *huang jing*
- *dang gui*

- *dan shen*
- *tu si zi*
- *gou qi zi*
- *zi he che*
- *xu duan*
- *ba ji tian*
- *su mu*
- *rou cong rong*
- *yin yang huo*
- *ji xue teng*
- *tao ren*

Acupuncture

The following points were used:

- CV-4, CV-12, ST-29, *zi gong,* SP-10, ST-36, LR-3, KI-3
- BL-13, BL-15, BL-17, BL-18, BL-20, BL-23

Points from both of these groups were needled in alternation, two to three times a week. From April 12 on, the points on the lower abdomen were omitted.

Result

On April 17, five oocytes were removed, three fertilized, two embryos developed well and were implanted. At this time, the endometrium was 11 mm thick. The formula was *Yi Shen Gu Chong Fang,* with the addition of *yu zhu, huang qin,* and *rou cong rong.* This was supplemented with acupuncture treatment on BL-13, BL-15, BL-17, BL-18, BL-20, BL-23, GV-20, ST-36, and *yin tang.* On May 5, the serum β-hCG was 194 U/L, and treatment was continued with TCM until the 10th week of pregnancy. The birth took place as planned.

Commentary

Prescribing high doses of hMG (human menopausal gonadotropin, including FSH and LH) in low responders does not necessarily improve the process;[9] instead, it negatively affects the receptivity of the endometrium (and increases costs). Individualized treatment with Chinese medicinals and acupuncture improved both the responsiveness of the ovaries and the quality of the follicles.

Case Study 4: Advanced Age and Infertility

Medical History

Ms. Y. G., 41 years old, secondary infertility for 4 years. Her FSH level was 15.52 IU/L; the right fallopian tube was occluded. She had already gone through two failed CC/hCG/IUI treatments and three equally unsuccessful Gonal F/hCG/IUI treatments.

During the first IVF/ET treatment (ultrashort protocol), she received Gonal F, five ampoules daily for five days, then Menogon, five ampoules daily for 15 days (75 ampoules total). Four egg cells were removed, one was fertilized and implanted. Implantation was unsuccessful. Treatment with TCM started in December 2001.

Treatment Principle

Strengthen kidney *jing*, nourish and move blood.

Medicinal Therapy and Acupuncture

During the second ICSI/ET treatment, she took Gonal F as before, 25 ampoules, then Menogon, five ampoules daily for 10 days (50 ampoules total). Meanwhile, she received the formula *Zi Shen Tiao Chong Fang* and acupuncture. Six egg cells were removed, two fertilized and implanted, unfortunately unsuccessfully.

In her third ICSI/ET treatment, she received the same protocol as in the second attempt and continued treatment with TCM accordingly.

Result

Five egg cells were removed, three fertilized; two well-developed embryos were implanted, and in June 2002 the patient was pregnant. She continued treatment with a modification of *Yi Shen Gu Chong Fang* until the 10th week of pregnancy.

Commentary

At an advanced age, the quality of the follicles is often lower, or we see a weak ovarian reaction. During treatment with TCM, the dosage of Menogon was reduced by 25 ampoules; in the second accompanied treatment course, two embryos developed and the patient became pregnant.

Case Study 5: Endometriosis and Adenomyomatosis

Medical History

Ms. Qian, 36 years old, primary infertility for 10 years, reduced sperm motility in the husband. She had already undergone one long and one short COS protocol and three failed ICSI/ET attempts. She began treatment with TCM in March 2005. On the fourth embryo transfer, the endometrium had a thickness of 11 mm, three frozen embryos (of six cells) were thawed and implanted. The menstrual period started on May 22. On May 25, she reported disquietude, stress, and insomnia. Because she lived far away from Beijing and only six frozen embryos were available, she requested another FET soon. The tongue was swollen and dark, the fur yellow and white; the pulse was fine, stringlike, and rapid.

Differential Diagnosis

Damp-heat with blood stasis, with kidney vacuity and liver *qi* stagnation.

Treatment Principle

Clear heat, eliminate dampness, and resolve the blood stasis; at the same time, strengthen the kidneys and harmonize liver *qi*.

Medicinal Therapy

- *sha shen*
- *dan shen*
- *san leng*
- *e zhu*
- *yin chen hao* (Artemisiae scopariae herba)
- *huang bai* (Phellodendri cortex)
- *xia ku cao* (Prunellae spica)
- *tu fu ling* (Smilacis glabrae rhizoma)
- *bie jia* (Trionycis carapax)
- *nü zhen zi*
- *gou qi zi*
- *yuan zhi*
- *bai he*

Result

On June 17, a follicle was detected that was 2.6 × 1.9 cm in size, the endometrium was 10 mm thick.

The fifth ET (with an embryo with five to six cells and two embryos with four cells) took place on June 18. To supplement this biomedical ther-

291

apy, the patient took *Yi Shen Gu Chong Fang* plus *huang qin* and *chun pi* (Toonae cortex). On June 30, her serum-hCG was 339 U/L, 7 days later it rose to 7370 U/L and the ultrasound exam revealed heart beats. She took Chinese medicinals up to the 14th week of pregnancy.

Commentary

Bleeding due to an ectopic endometrium in endometriosis or adenomyomatosis corresponds to blood that has left the channels and turned into so-called "vanquished blood." This is described as blood stasis in the pelvis and uterus.

The differential diagnosis was damp-heat with blood stasis, in combination with kidney vacuity and liver *qi* stagnation. After taking Chinese medicinals, the patient became pregnant. Because women with endometriosis and adenomyomatosis are more likely to suffer from miscarriages, it is important to continue treatment until at least the 12th week of pregnancy.

Case Study 6: Five Failed IVF/ET Treatments, OHSS

Medical History

Ms. G. D., 27 years old, secondary infertility for 2 years, G1 P0, removal of the fallopian tubes due to ectopic pregnancy. In addition, she was diagnosed with polycystic ovaries and PMS. The patient received three CC/hCG, three hMG/hCG/IUI, and five IVF/ET treatments (with three COS).

On October 1, 2001, she began with TCM treatment and reported thirst, apprehension, and insomnia, lots of phlegm, cold sensations, a delayed cycle with spotting 5–6 days before the onset of menstruation, tension in the breasts 14 days before menstruation, and scant dry stools with bowel movements every 1–2 days. She was overweight. The tongue was dark and red, the fur grey and dry, the pulse fine, stringlike, and slippery.

Differential Diagnosis

Yin vacuity with vacuity heat, liver *qi* stagnation in combination with phlegm.

Treatment Principle

Nourish kidney *yin* and clear vacuity heat, soothe liver *qi*, and eliminate phlegm.

Medicinal Therapy

- *sha shen*
- *chi shao*
- *sheng di huang*
- *dan shen*
- *tao ren*
- *yu jin*
- *chai hu*
- *han lian cao*
- *nü zhen zi*
- *tu si zi*
- *bei mu*
- *bai he*
- *yuan zhi*

Continued Treatment

On October 21, the phlegm and cold had disappeared, and the thirst, apprehension, insomnia, and dry stools had improved. She began a long protocol with Decapeptyl and a modification of *Yang Xue Tian Jing Fang*. On October 29, her menstrual period arrived, and she took *Tiao Jing Fang* for 5 days before switching to *Zi Shen Tiao Chong Fang*. On November 12, she reported depression, frequent crying, and dry stools. The tongue was slightly swollen and crimson, the fur thin and yellow and partly peeled off at the root of the tongue; the pulse was fine and stringlike. The endometrium had a thickness of 11 mm and there were eight good follicles on each side.

Differential Diagnosis

Yin vacuity with vacuity heat, disharmony of the heart and kidney.

Treatment Principle

Nourish kidney *yin* and clear vacuity heat, nourish the heart and quiet the spirit.

Medicinal Therapy

Rx. Zi Shen Tiao Chong Fang *(Kidney-enriching Thoroughfare-regulating Formula), modified:*

- *sha shen*
- *chi shao*
- *sheng di huang*
- *dan shen*
- *tao ren*
- *yu jin*
- *tu si zi*
- *gou qi zi*
- *han lian cao*
- *nü zhen zi*

- *tian men dong* (asparagi radix)
- *bai he*
- *yuan zhi*
- *lian zi xin*
- *bai zi ren*

Subsequent Treatment

On November 14, 2001, 14 oocytes were removed, seven of which were fertilized. On November 17, three embryos were transferred. On November 20, the patient was in a much better mood, but she reported abdominal tension, lower back pain, a swollen face, and reduced amounts of urine. The tongue was enlarged and red, the fur grayish yellow and partly peeled off at the tongue root, the pulse was fine, stringlike, rapid, and weak at the *chi* position. Ultrasound examination showed an accumulation of fluid in the pelvis.

Differential Diagnosis

Spleen and kidney vacuity with heat and dampness.

Treatment Principle

Strengthen spleen and kidney, eliminate dampness, clear heat.

Medicinal Therapy

Rx. Yi Shen Gu Chong Fang *(Kidney-boosting Thoroughfare-securing Formula), modified:*

- *sha shen*
- *bai shao*
- *tu si zi*
- *gou qi zi*
- *shan zhu yu*
- *xu duan*
- *bai zhu*
- *shan yao*
- *lian zi xin*
- *chai hu*
- *fu ling pi* (Poriae cutis)
- *da fu pi* (Arecae pericarpium)
- *huang qin*

Subsequent Treatment

On November 25, the patient went into the hospital for 4 days because of OHSS. On November 27 (11 days after the embryo transfer), her serum-hCG was 274 U/L. From November 30 on, the amount of urine increased while her body weight decreased. On December 14, *sha ren* (Amomi fructus), *zhu ru* (Bumbusae culis in taenia), and *huo*

xiang (Agastaches herba) were added to the formula because she was suffering from nausea and vomiting. On January 3, 2002, the ultrasound examination showed three yolk sacs and strong heartbeats. The fluid in the pelvis had disappeared. Nevertheless, she suffered from severe pregnancy-related vomiting.

Medicinal Therapy

The formula was changed:

- *sha shen*
- *bai shao*
- *tu si zi*
- *gou qi zi*
- *shan zhu yu*
- *xu duan*
- *bai zhu*
- *shan yao*
- *huang qin*
- *chai hu*
- *sha ren*
- *zhu ru*
- *huo xiang*
- *su geng* (Perillae caulis)
- with 20 drops of fresh ginger juice added daily to the decoction.

Acupuncture

The patient received gentle acupuncture on CV-12, PC-6, ST-44, SP-4, ST-36, and KI-3.

Subsequent Treatment

On February 2, the nausea and vomiting were greatly relieved and the patient reported dryness in the mouth. Reduction of the embryos was planned for February 5. The tongue was tender and red, the fur partly peeled off; the pulse was fine, slippery, and rapid. The diagnosis was *yin* vacuity with vacuity heat. The formula was supplemented with *sheng di huang, lian zi xin, han lian cao,* and *fu pen zi,* while *bai zhu, zhu ru, huo xiang,* and *su geng* were taken out.

Result

The procedure was successful. The patient continued treatment with TCM until the 22nd week of pregnancy and subsequently gave birth to two healthy girls.

Commentary

Following five failed IVF/ET treatments, this patient was suffering from stress with a variety of symptoms. After treatment in accordance with the criteria of differential diagnosis, most of her symptoms improved. Three embryos were implanted. The treatment principles to strengthen the spleen, promote urination, and strengthen the kidneys, relieved the OHSS. During embryo reduction, *yin* was replenished, the heat in the heart was cleared, and the kidneys were strengthened to support the fetuses and prevent a miscarriage. This helped the twins in their healthy development.

Case Study 7: Six Unresolved, Failed IVF/ET Treatments

Medical History
Ms. Duan, 34 years old, G3 P1, secondary infertility for 8 years. Hydrosalpinx and two ectopic pregnancies led to salpingectomy on both sides. The husband's sperm was sufficient for an IVF.

On March 22, she had the sixth FET, the endometrium had a thickness of 12 mm, grade A, three embryos (two with eight cells, one with seven cells) with good morphology. In spite of this, the treatment was unsuccessful, and the patient began treatment with TCM. On May 17, she reported a delayed menstrual cycle with scant dark menses, dry mouth, palpitations, numbness in the hands and arms, headache, and constipation. The tongue was dark with a scant dry fur, the pulse was fine and stringlike.

Differential Diagnosis
Kidney *yin* vacuity with ascending *yang*, blood vacuity combined with liver *qi* stagnation and blood stasis.

Treatment Principle
Strengthen kidney *yin*, regulate ascending *yang*, nourish and move blood, regulate liver *qi*.

Medicinal Therapy
- *yu zhu*
- *dan shen*
- *yu jin*
- *ji xue teng*
- *tao ren*
- *ye jiao teng*
- *e jiao zhu*
- *nü zhen zi*
- *tu si zi*

- *gou qi zi*
- *sheng di huang*
- *lian zi xin*
- *gua lou* (Trichosanthis fructus)
- *gou teng* (Uncariae ramulus cum uncis)

Continued Treatment
After four treatments with TCM, most of the symptoms, such as the palpitations, numbness in the hands and arms, and headache, had disappeared, the patient had one bowel movement a day, and her menstrual period began on July 26 (day 31 of her cycle) with more red blood and less clots. On July 29, she prepared herself for the next FET and received the following prescription:

Rx. Zi Shen Tiao Chong Fang (Kidney-enriching Thoroughfare-regulating Formula), modified:
- *dang gui*
- *chuan xiong*
- *dan shen*
- *tu si zi*
- *gou qi zi*
- *zi he che*
- *xu duan*
- *ba ji tian*
- *su mu*
- *tao ren*
- *nü zhen zi*
- *bie jia*
- *rou cong rong*

On August 12, the endometrium had a thickness of 10 mm, grade A, and three embryos (one with eight cells, one with five to six cells, one with five cells) were transferred. The formula was replaced with a modification of *Yi Shen Gu Chong Fang*.

Result
On April 25, 14 days after the ET, the patient's serum-hCG was 392 U/L; on September 2, the ultrasound showed heart beats. She returned to her home town and continued treatment with TCM until the 12th week of pregnancy.

Commentary
In this patient, six IVF/ET treatments remained unsuccessful—without known cause. How could this happen, given that all attendant circumstances were positive? While in vitro and gene technology are informative, we still do not know

enough about potential defects in fertilization, implantation, and early embryonal development to produce sophisticated diagnoses about infertility and special treatments.

The complexity of this process cannot be evaluated with the standards of normal diagnostic assessments of infertility. Ultrasound, hormone level, and morphology of the embryo are not sufficient to indicate the cause of infertility. Nevertheless, from the perspective of TCM, this patient definitely suffered from kidney *yin* vacuity with ascending *yang* as well as blood vacuity combined with liver *qi* stagnation and blood stasis. Over the course of 2 months, TCM treatment strengthened kidney *yin*, regulated ascending *yang*, nourished and moved blood, and harmonized liver *qi*. As a result, her symptoms disappeared and she undertook another attempt. The FET was successful due to the support with TCM.

Case Study 8: Pronounced Endometriosis

Medical History

Ms. Zhou, 34 years old, primary infertility for 6 years. In 2002, severe endometriosis was detected during a laparoscopy, with adhesions and lesions in the pelvis.

The fallopian tubes were patent. She received GnRH-a three times. Shortly after stopping the injections, severe menstrual complaints returned. The patient then took gestrinone for 2 months. But because she suffered from severe side-effects, she stopped this treatment as well. Subsequently, she attempted for 2 years to become pregnant. All three of the subsequent IVF/ET treatments remained unsuccessful. On June 3, 2004, she began treatment with TCM and prepared for another IVF. She reported frequent stabbing pain in the lower abdomen, thirst, lower back pain, a 30-day menstrual cycle with heavy menstrual periods that lasted for 6 days, and severe symptoms beginning 1 day before the period and lasting until several days after its end. The blood was dark red and mixed with clots. The pain lessened with discharge of the clots. After the IVF, both the pain and the amount of blood and clots increased. The tongue was tender, dark, and red with macules, the fur was thin, yellow, and dry; the pulse was fine and slippery.

Differential Diagnosis

Blood stasis combined with kidney *yin* vacuity and vacuity heat.

Treatment Principle

Move blood to resolve the blood stasis, soften masses, replenish kidney *yin*, and eliminate vacuity heat.

Medicinal Therapy

- *dang gui*
- *dan shen*
- *tu si zi*
- *gou qi zi*
- *bie jia*
- *xu duan*
- *nü zhen zi*
- *san leng*
- *e zhu*
- *zhe chong* (Eupolyphaga seu steleophaga)
- *xia ku cao*
- *lian qiao* (Forsythia fructus)
- *e jiao zhu*
- *sheng di huang*

Result

Because her BBT (basal body temperature) showed two phases, the patient attempted to become pregnant naturally. Her last menstrual period occurred on July 9, 2002, and she received a modification of *Tiao Jing Fang*. Both the menstrual pain and the amount of clots were reduced. She continued taking the formula, which had first been prescribed on May 3, until her BTC (body temperature curve) rose. After that, she switched to *Yi Shen Gu Chong Fang*. On July 29, her urine-hCG was positive; on August 19, her serum-hCG was more than 5000 U/L and the ultrasound showed heart beats. The patient continued treatment with TCM until the 14th week of pregnancy and subsequently gave birth to a healthy son.

Commentary

The patient had attempted to become pregnant for 6 years, including three IVF treatments. In the end, she received treatment with TCM for 2 months and became pregnant. Patients whose infertility is accompanied by endometriosis, even of a severe grade, have a good chance of becoming pregnant when receiving treatment with TCM, especially within 1 year after a laparoscopy. TCM not only improves the blood circulation and thereby softens growths and adhesions, but it also reduces the endometriosis and supports ovulation. If this patient had begun treatment with TCM immediately after the laparoscopy, her treatment would most likely have been considerably easier.

Why Can TCM Support In Vitro Fertilization?

The Gonads are Supported to Improve the Number and Quality of Egg and Sperm Cells

- For thousands of years, replenishing the kidney and liver and nourishing blood and essence have been the basic methods for treating infertility and preparing the material foundation for the egg and sperm.
- Soothing liver *qi*, which causes the patient to relax, can lead to an improvement of the reproductive axis, regulate the hormonal interplay, and increase the responsiveness of the gonads.
- By nourishing and moving blood while replenishing kidney essence, TCM improves microcirculation in the pelvis and the ability of the ovaries to ovulate. Zhang Shucheng's research on young hamsters that were treated with low and high doses of *Bu Shen Sheng Xue Fang*—the formula includes *sheng di huang, shu di huang, shan zhu yu*, and *gui ban jiao* (Testudinis plastri gelatinum), among other ingredients—showed that the number of follicles in a COS increased by 40% or 76% in comparison with the control group, which received water instead (P <0.01[10]). These results proved that the formula is able to improve the ability to ovulate in young hamsters.
- Improvement in the quality of oocytes and in the insemination rate.[1,12] Lian Fang's experimental research on the effect of *Er Zhi Tian Gui*—the formula includes *nü zhen zi, han lian cao, gou qi zi, tu si zi, dang gui*, and *chuan xiong*, among other ingredients—on mice showed that the number of abnormal follicles clearly rose when the total amount of follicles in the group with hMG-intake rose, while follicle quality improved without a simultaneous de-

crease in ovulations in the group in which TCM and hMG were combined (insignificant difference in the rate of ovulation in both groups). Morphology, fertilization rate, and cell division rate were significantly higher in the group with combined TCM/hMG treatment than in the hMG group (P <0.05).

- Improvement of the number and quality of sperm. The success of IVF/ET treatment is intimately linked to the quality and number of sperm cells. Dai Jingcheng's research on malfunctions in the spermatogenesis of mice showed that both the density and motility rate of spermatozoa as well as the weight of the testes and epididymis in the group treated with *Bao Cheng* decoction—the formula includes, among other ingredients, *zi he che, gou qi zi, yin yang huo, tu si zi*, and *huang qi*—were increased significantly compared to the control group (P <0.05, P <0.01[13]). A histopathological preparation of a testicle section showed an obvious recovery of a diseased testicle. This indicates that *Bao Cheng* decoction has a stimulating effect on spermatogenesis and a medicative influence on diseases of the testicles. Yang Ming's research on sperm DNA in patients with kidney *yang* vacuity and infertility after 12 weeks of treatment with *Wu Zi Yan Zong Wan* (Five Seeds Pills for Abundant Descendants) and *Jia Wei Shen Qi Wan* (Supplemented Kidney *Qi* Pill) revealed that the number of haploids rose significantly, shown by means of a quantity analysis of haploids, diploids, and polyploids in the DNA with flow cytometry.[14] The number of sperm with normal morphology increased by 8%. Peng Shoujing's research compared human sperm cells cultivated in a modified tyrode solution (MTS) in vitro with sperms cultivated in a combination of *tu si zi* decoction and MTS in vitro.[15] Sperm motility of the *tu si zi* group was assessed with a sperm capillary penetration test, velocity test, and a sperm activity index calculation. The result was a clear improvement of motility. In addition, the function of the sperm's cell membrane was evaluated by means of a hypo-osmatic swelling test in combination with an eosin test. Thereby, a higher stability after incubation could be proven. Zeng Jingxiong's research has shown that in human sperm that had been co-cultivated in a solution of *huang jing*, the sperm acrosome rate rose significantly compared with the control group (P < 0.05) and the group without medication (P < 0001[16]). This indicates that *huang jing* solution increases the fertilizing ability of human sperm.

- Improvement of fertilizability in older patients. Si Fuchun's systematic research on the reproductive axis and structure in older mice has demonstrated that *Er Xian Tang* (Two Immortals Decoction) with its two partial formulas apparently increased the level of sexual hormones in the blood as well as the gonatropin values, the amount of testosterone receptors in the nucleus and in the cytoplasma of the protate, as well as the number of estradiol receptors in the uterus.[17] Furthermore, it improved age-related cellular changes in the hypothalamus, hypophysis, testicles, ovaries, prostate, and uterus. Zhang Shucheng's study of old hamsters who received low or high doses of *Bu Shen Sheng Xue Fang* showed that the follicle count was significantly higher with COS than in the control group (P < 0.01) and reached 43 % or 70 % of that of young hamsters.[10] This demonstrates that *Bu Shen Sheng Xue Fang* caused a recovery in ovarian function and an improved ability to ovulate in the old hamsters.

The Receptiveness of the Endometrium and the Embryo Implantation Rate are Improved

A careful preparation of the endometrium is of greatest significance in IVF/ET and IVF/ICSI treatment, to balance the asynchrony between the endometrium and the developing embryo.

- TCM states: "The uterine vessel is linked to the kidneys." Hence we know that the physiological functions of the uterine vessel and uterus are closely connected to the state of the kidney. Because replenishing kidney essence is the most important treatment method in TCM and because essence and blood share the same source, this approach guarantees that the uterus is full of blood and essence, like a thick pillow filled with nutrients, to give the sperm a fertile ground.
- By nourishing and moving blood, TCM improves the blood flow and microcirculation in

the uterus and ovaries. Zhang Mingming's research on 23 female patients who after several failed treatments with reproductive medicine received *Bu Shen Huo Xue Tang* (Kidney-supplementing Blood-quickening Decoction)—the formula includes *dan shen, huang qi, dang gui, chuan xiong,* and *sang ji sheng*—for 2 months prior to the next IVF/ET or ICSI/ET treatment, revealed that the endometrium was clearly thicker than before (P < 0.05) and that both the pulsatility index (PI) and the resistence index (RI) were clearly improved (P < 0.05, P < 0.01). These reduced PIs and RIs meant improved circulation in the tissues and increased blood flow and hence promoted not only endometrial thickness but also the microcirculation in the uterine walls. This change increased the receptiveness of the endometrium. Zhang Shucheng's research on the mechanism of *Bu Shen Tiao Jing Fang* (Kidney-supplementing Menses-regulating Formula)—the formula contains *zi he che, dang gui, gou qi zi, tu si zi, ba ji tian,* and *wu ling zhi,* among other ingredients—demonstrated that in old hamsters with kidney vacuity the number of blood vessels in the uterus clearly increased after taking the formula.[19] This result indicates that TCM is able to promote the formation of new blood vessels. Additional studies to compare immune-histological chemically marked growth factors (vascular endothelial growth factor [VEGF] etc.) before and after taking the prescribed medication show a significant rise in the five factors (P < 0.05–0.01[20]). VEGF is a substance that is able to trigger strong growth of the endothel cells, pronounced angiogenesis, as well as an increased permeability of the blood vessels. This suggests that Chinese medicinals have a considerable influence on angiogenesis and on follicular and uterine vascularization, and thereby also on follicular maturation, oocyte quality, fertilizability and development of the embryo, and the synchronicity of the endometrium, as a result of which the establishment and preservation of pregnancy is ensured by means of TCM.

- The rate of pregnancy is increased by an improvement in luteal function.[21,22] In Zhu Wenjie's research on embryo transfer, 104 female patients were divided into two groups. All received hCG to improve luteal function; the members of group A additionally received *Zi*

Shen Yu Tai pills—the formula among other ingredients includes *dang shen*, *xu duan*, *bai zhu*, *ba ji tian*, and *du zhong*—for 14 days. In group A, the serum progesterone, embryo implantation rate, and clinical pregnancy rate (15.42 ± 1.91µg/L, 24.12%, and 51.52%, respectively) were significantly higher than in group B (13.92 ± 1.96µg/L, 16.67% and 34.78%; P < 0.01).

- Medicinals that replenish the kidneys can improve the responsiveness of the hypophysis and ovaries and can regulate the interplay of the hypothalamus-hypophysis-ovaries-uterus axis.[23] They coordinate LH and FSH levels, and the ratio of estradiol (E2) and progesterone, increase the estrogen and progesterone receptors (ER and PR), regulate the synchronization between the endometrium and the developing embryo, and thereby improve the embryo implantation rate.

Embryonal Development is Promoted

The kidneys tie the fetus (*shen yi xi tai* 肾以系胎), the *qi* holds the fetus (*qi yi zai tai* 气以载胎), and the blood nourishes the fetus (*xue yi yang tai* 血以养胎). The formula *Yi Shen Gu Chong Fang* replenishes the kidneys and spleen. The kidneys are responsible for the reproductive processes and conserve essence, the spleen is the source of blood and *qi*. As such, *Yi Shen Gu Chong Fang* provides both kidney essence and blood and *qi* for embryonal development. In this way, it reduces the number of miscarriages and increases the number of live births.

Yang Guiyun investigated the effect of the formula *Bu Shen Huo Xue Tang* (hMG, BSHX) by means of BSHX-containing serum of rabbits as supplement.[12] This was used to co-cultivate sperm and egg cells of unmated mice, and separately the two-cell embryos of mated female mice. Under co-cultivation, the IVF rate increased clearly (P < 0.01), and subsequent embryonal development was promoted in the various phases, especially in that of four- and eight-cell embryos (P < 0.05). The development of eight-cell embryos, morula, blastocysts, and "hatching" were clearly improved. Accordingly, the conclusion was drawn that *Bu Shen Huo Xue Tang* can improve both the fertilization rate and early embryonal development (P < 0.05 or P < 0.01).

Cooperation with Biomedicine Reduces the Side-effects of IVF/ET Treatment

- The TCM treatment principle to nourish and activate the blood improves blood circulation, which increases sensitivity and responsiveness to biomedical treatments.
- TCM affects the emotions of patients. It can relieve tension and fear, stabilize, and restore the function of the reproductive axis even after longer-term infertility or failed IVF/ET treatment. The text *Jing Yue Quan Shu (Complete Works of Jing Yue)* states: "Pregnancy is based on blood and *qi*. Blood and *qi* are based on the emotions. Suppressed emotions will lead to disharmony in the *chong mai* and *ren mai*. This is the cause of infertility."
- Individualized treatment with TCM in accordance with pattern differentiation can reduce the side-effects of treatment with hormones in high doses, such as headache, dizziness, disquietude, exhaustion, abdominal fullness, mood swings, or menstrual disturbances.
- Prevention or reduction of OHSS. OHSS is a serious complication that can arise as the result of taking high doses of hormones. In TCM, this condition corresponds to *zi man* (子满) and is based on an excess of water and dampness (*shui shi fan lan* 水湿泛滥). Causes can include *yang* vacuity in the spleen and kidney, liver *qi* stagnation with spleen *qi* vacuity, collection of damp-heat, or liver and kidney *yin* vacuity. In acute cases, the (superficial) symptoms are treated first, and only afterwards the cause is addressed, to prevent any additional formation of dampness.

Miscarriages are Avoided and Pregnancy Rates Improved

The development of implanted embryos can come to a standstill at any point in their early developmental stages. Miscarriages greatly reduce the success rate and efficacy of reproductive medicine.

TCM can fall back on a history of treating miscarriage that spans many millennia. Threatening miscarriage is referred to as *tai lou* (fetal spotting) or *tai dong bu an* (stirring fetus); habitual miscarriage as *hua tai* (slippery fetus). According to TCM theory, the "reproductive axis" is equated with the connection "kidneys—*tian gui*—*chong mai* and *ren mai*—uterus." This means that "if kidney *qi* is sufficient, the *chong mai* is abundant and the *ren mai* opens up." Furthermore, it is said: "The *chong mai* is the sea of blood and the *ren mai* is responsible for pregnancy" (*chong wei xue hai, ren zhu bao tai*). If the kidneys are weak, the fetus lacks essence and blood, which will lead to a miscarriage. It is therefore extremely important to strengthen the kidney and spleen and to secure the *chong mai* and *ren mai* up to the 10th week of pregnancy. This treatment approach can coincide with an increased luteal function, an improved supply to the uterine walls, and a promotion of embryonal development.

■ Conclusion

TCM as a form of support for IVF/ET treatments constitutes a combination of macrocosm and microcosm, and of traditional and modern techniques. During the different stages of IVF/ET treatment, a number of treatment principles apply; the key to success, however, is found in individualized treatment in accordance with pattern identification (*bian zheng lun zhi*) and the regulation of the entire body (*zheng ti tiao jie* 整体调节). This is the essence of TCM. In addition, it is important to pay attention to the integration of TCM pattern identification into the biomedical differentiation of diseases. We cannot hope for a single formula that is suitable for all patients. The key is the regulation of *yin* and *yang*, *qi* and blood, and viscera and bowels, in order to allow both female and male patients to unfold their full potential. In the future, more and more randomized and controlled clinical studies and research are certain to be carried out, in order to explain the microcosmic changes in TCM and the mechanisms involved.

Acknowledgment
I would like to express my gratitude to my teacher, the nationally famous gynecologist and TCM expert Chai Songyan, and to Zhou Dean, professor of acupuncture, for their long-standing supervision and support. Thanks also to Simon Becker, who edited my original English text.
Wu Yuning

Bibliography
1. Nandedkar TD, Kelkar RL. Potential Researchable Areas in ARTs-oocyte Maturation and Embryo Development. *J Exp Bool.* 2001; 39:1 – 10.
2. Ingrid HL, Shing-Kai Y, Lai PC et al. Adjuvant Low-dose Aspirin Therapy in Poor Responders Undergoing In Vitro Fertilization: A Prospective, Randomized, Double-blind, Placebo-controlled trial. *Fertil. Steril.* 2004;81:557 – 561.
3. Ben-Rafael Z, Bider D et al. Combined Gonadotropin Releasing Hormone Agonist/Human Menopausal Gonadotropin Therapy (GnRHa/hMG) in Normal, High, and Pool Responder to hMG. *J In Vitro Fert Embryo Transf.* 1991;8:33 – 36.
4. Levi AJ, Raynault MF, Bergh PA et al. Reproductive Outcome in Patients with Diminished Ovarian Reserve. *Fertil Steril.* 2001;6:666 – 669.
5. Cao ZY. *Chinese Obstetrics and Gynecology.* 2nd ed. Beijing People's Publication of Health. 2002; 2354 – 2358.
6. Bonduelle M, Ponjaert I, Steirteghem AV et al. Developmental Outcome at 2 Years of Age for Children Born after ICSI Compared with Children Born after IVF. *Hum Reprod.* 2003;18:342 – 350.
7. Lai Y, Duan L. TCM Treatment for Menstrual Disorder after Failure of IVF/ET. *J Sichuan of TCM.* 2003;21:49 – 50.
8. Wang M, Zhu J, Zhang L et al. Study of Mechanism of Promoting Child-birth by Electrical Acupuncture of LI4 and SP6. *J Chin Acupuncture.* 2003;23: 593 – 596.
9. Land JA, Yarmolinskaya MI, Dumoulin JC, et al. High-dose Human Menopausal Gonadotropin Stimulation in Poor Responders Does Not Improve In Vitro Fertilization Outcome. *Fertil. Steril.* 1996;65:961 – 965.
10. Zhang Shucheng, Guo Haizhou, Wu Zhikui. Effect of Prescription of Tonifying the Kidney and Nourishing Blood on Reproductive Cycles and Superovulation of Female GH. *Chin. J Basic Med in TCM.* 1997;5: 24 – 25.
11. Lian Fang, Sun Zhengao, Zhang Jianwei et al. Experimental Study on Effect of *Erzhi Tiangui* Recipe on Quality of Oocytes in Mice. *Chin J Integr Trad and West Med.* 2004;24: 625 – 627.

12. Yang Guiyun, Wang Peijuan, Jiao Xiaobin et al. Effect of *Bushen Huoxue* decoction In Vitro Fertilization and Early Embryonic Development in Mice. *Chin J Integr Trad and West Med.* 2001;21: 522 – 524.
13. Dai Jincheng, Zhou Xiaoping. Influence of *Bao Cheng* Decoction on Testes and Spermatozoon in Mice of Spermatogenesis Dysfunction. *J Fujian College of TCM*, 2002;12:34 – 36.
14. Yang Ming, Wang Shusheng, Chen Zhiqiang. Effects of *Wuziyanzong* Pill and *Jiaweishenqi* Pill on Sperm DNA of Patients with Kidney-*yang* Deficiency and Male Infertility. *Modern J Integr Tradi Chin and West Med.* 2002;11: 889 – 891.
15. Peng Shoujing, Lu Renkang, Yu Lihua et al. Effects of *Tu Si Zi, Xian Mao, Ba Ji Tian* on Human Spermatozoon's Motility and Membrane Function in Vitro. *Chin J Integr Trad and West Med.* 1997;11: 145 – 147.
16. Zeng Jinxiong, Dai Xihu, Liu Jianhua et al. Effects of *Huan Jing* Recipe on Human Spermatazoal Acrosome Reaction. *Chin J TCM Information.* 2002;9: 25 – 26.
17. Si Fuchun. Actuality and Countermeasure of Study on Kidney of TCM from Hypothalomus-Pituitory Reproductive Axis. *Study on TCM.* 1994;7: 2 – 5.
18. Zhang Mingming, Huang GuangYing, Lu Fuer et al. Influence of *Bushenhuo Xuetang* on Patients. *J Microcirculation.* 2002;12: 10 – 13.
19. Zhang Shucheng, Wu Zhikui. *Shen Mingxiu*: Study on Morphologic Observation of Promoting Angiogenesis of Uterine Tissue by Prescriptions of Tonifying the Kidney to Regulate Menstruation and Tonifying the Kidney and Nourishing Blood. *Chin. J Basic Med in TCM.* 1998;4:37.
20. Zhang Shucheng, Liu Xiaoqun, Zhang Zhizhou et al. Effect of Prescription of Tonifying the Kidney to Regulate Menstruation on Angiogenic Factors and their Receptors of Human Endometrium during Implantation. *Chin. J Basic Med in TCM.* 2002;8: 384 – 386.
21. Zhu Wenjie, Li Xuemei, Chen Xiumin et al. Effect of *Zishen Yutai* Pill on Embryo Implantation Rate in Patients Undergoing IVF/ET. *Chin J Integr Trad and West Med.* 2002;22: 729 – 737.
22. Xi Ming. Clinical Research and Development of TCM on Improving Luteal Function. *Modern Diag and Treat.* 1995;6: 6 – 7.
23. Gui Suiqi, Yu Jin, Wei Meijuan et al. Experimental Study on Pituitary, Ovary and Adrenal Gland of Mice with Hyperandrogenic Infertility by Replenishing the Kidney. *Chin J Integr Trad and West. Med.* 1997;17: 735 – 738.

Patient Support 6

23 Inviting the "Heavenly Spark"—*Shen* in the Support of Couples in Fertility Treatment

Ruthild Schulze, Gudrun Kotte

Couples turn to fertility treatment when their intention to conceive and create a child naturally fails. This fact is tied to a number of different internal and external conflicts.

On the level of physical requirements for creation and conception, which we refer to in this chapter as the **jing level**, medicine offers a multitude of possible interventions. In the present chapter, however, we do not want to focus on the *jing* level, or in other words the physical constitution, but on the **shen level**. For this purpose, we present a variety of Chinese medical texts that discuss the necessary preconditions for successful fertility treatment and conception in terms of the "subtle essences," or in other words, the requirements that are found on the *shen* level instead.

Shen (神) is one of those terms in Chinese culture that are open to many possible interpretations, depending on the context. One of the most comprehensive definitions comes from the German sinologist Gudula Linck:

"[...] a person's shen is an active and initiating power, tied to individuation, that is bestowed by Heaven shortly before birth, ... enters the person as he or she comes into being, resides there throughout the entire life—as the person's individual physical disposition, temperament, personality, consciousness, and mental power... Seen from this perspective, shen is a cosmic power that envelops the person, but simultaneously constitutes a particularly subtle form of qi within the person and gives him or her individuality for the duration of life."[9]

Shen has at least as many different meanings as the English term "spirit." *Shen* can be understood as divine power, as individual personality, as life force, as consciousness, and also as divine-cosmic efficacy. In this chapter, we address those aspects of *shen* that are particularly relevant to the practical support of a couple during fertility treatment. This includes, in particular, the following levels of meaning:

- *shen* as consciousness and mindfulness of the practitioner
- *shen* as power of the heart and spiritual connection of the couple

- *shen* as heavenly spark during conception of the child

While this chapter focuses on statements about *shen* in Chinese medical literature, we will depart from the theoretical level in some instances, to show what kind of living and practical help the concept of *shen* can offer to contemporary TCM practitioners. These practical tips can only be approximations and recommendations, not a guideline for standard therapy, because in that case we would miss the immediate potential of the present moment and therefore *shen*. Which competences, emotions, and experiences we include in a therapeutic approach that is oriented towards *shen* depends, above all, on one thing: on our own *shen*!

■ *Shen* as Consciousness and Mindfulness of the Practitioner

The ancient Chinese medical texts provided clear notions on the ethics and personality of an excellent physician. Thus, for example, the gist of statements in the first and 55th chapters of the *Ling Shu* (灵枢 *Magic Pivot*) in the *Huang Di Nei Jing* (黄帝内经 *The Yellow Emperor's Inner Classic** is that a physician with a good *shen* should be able to diagnose a beginning disharmony on the basis

---

* The *Huang Di Nei Jing* is regarded as the oldest and most commonly quoted medical text in China's medicine of systematic correspondences. It consists of a systematic collection of treatises by unknown authors that were compiled around the 1st to 3rd centuries CE. The currently known division of the text into two parts of 81 chapters each, called the *Su Wen* (*Elementary Questions*) and *Ling Shu* (*Magic Pivot*), did not always exist as such. Originally, there appear to have been two additional parts in the *Nei Jing* corpus, namely the *Tai Su* and the *Ming Tang*. Both were supposedly lost in the later Song period. Compare Unschuld 2003[14].

of small changes before it has manifested in symptoms. A practitioner's *shen* is expressed not only in his or her professional skills, but also in the presence, attentiveness, and intuition, in the consciousness, warm heart, and clarity and intelligence. *Shen* resides in the heart and inspires all highly developed **mental functions** that make us human:

* sensitivity
* inspiration
* spiritual aspirations
* the ability to express thoughts, feelings, and emotions

A strong *shen* radiates outward from the forehead and eyes.

Shen as Self-knowledge

As with any other treatment, the success of fertility treatment depends first and foremost on the therapist's clarity within him- or herself. A good *shen* reveals itself here in a critical and honest self-image. To facilitate the patient's reflection, the following questions are helpful:

* Do I have my own personal problems around the issue of wanting children? What are my preconceptions regarding the topics of infertility, miscarriage, adoption, or abortion? Have I addressed and overcome my own affinities or "blind spots"?
* What is my secret opinion about this couple's desire for children?
* How does this attitude influence my diagnosis?
* How precise and consistent is my treatment? Where do I unwillingly get pulled into the dynamics of this couple or of the subject?

Self-reflection, not only at this point, gives the treatment clarity and therefore *shen*. Thus, it is said in Chapter 13 of the *Su Wen* (素问):

"You would then very easily realize that those who carry shen *and energy within them awaken to a flow-ering life and lead a good life compared to those whose* shen *and energy have been lost." ***

Under certain circumstances, a good *shen* can involve the insight that you personally may not be the ideal provider of fertility treatment right at that moment due to your personal concerns. In most cases, though, just the realization of your own sensitivities will already clear up unconscious blockages. Because *shen* stands for consciousness and mindfulness, it is subject to change depending on the situation and must be acquired anew again and again. Regarding this topic, Chapter 73 of the *Ling Shu* states:

"It is absolutely necessary to model yourself after the physicians of antiquity, to learn from them and to show the validity of their teachings also in the present, to pay attention to the most subtle and also the most insignificant conditions of any prevailing state of qi *within the body, and to also transmit this again and again to future generations. A physician with only minor qualifications will pay no heed to such subtleties; the highly-qualified physician, however, will greatly value these details. The reason for this is that the states of* qi *inside the body are so inconspicuous and formless that they are really as mysterious as the spirits."*

It is therefore advisable to foster our concentration and presence and thereby cultivate our *shen* by means of personal reflection, mindfulness exercises, and self-questioning.

Shen as Clarity between Practitioner and Patient

As the second step, the relationship between the practitioner and the couple who want a child must be clarified. The following questions have hereby proven helpful for orientation:

* Do I know both partners?
* How is the contact between myself and the woman and between myself and the man?
* How do I rate the mental state of the couple?

---

* The quotations from the *Huang Di Nei Jing Su Wen* and *Ling Shu* are based in particular on Schmidt[12], but have been slightly modified in some places, following Henry C. Lu[10] and Fu Baotai[2].

- What is my attitude towards them as a couple? Am I moved by certain thoughts or feelings? With whom? When?
- What do I expect from them? What do they expect from me?

If the relationship between the practitioner and the couple is disturbed, this also affects the *shen* of both sides negatively, which will have consequences for the quality and success of the treatment.

General signs of a *shen* **disturbance** include:
- diffuse or lacking eye contact
- vague or unclear language
- incoherent talking, as well as disconnected thoughts and speech

In this context, it is also indicative if a person repeatedly evades questions or contradicts him- or herself in their statements. If you are unable to achieve free-flowing communication even after repeated attempts at clarification, a fundamental requirement for any successful treatment is lacking. The Chinese classics also describe treatment circumstances that make success impossible. A clear *shen* allows us to recognize such cases and to let go without judgment. Thus, for example, Chapter 9 of the *Ling Shu* lists a number of circumstances or patient characteristics under which an experienced physician refuses to treat. Every treatment and every patient is an individual case and requires new sensitivity, as is summarized, for example, in the 29th chapter of the *Ling Shu*:

"When coming to an unfamiliar land, you first have to familiarize yourself with its customs and habits; when visiting the households of unfamiliar families, you have to familiarize yourself with their likes and dislikes; when participating in a celebration, you have to concern yourself with its basic meaning and ritual configuration; and when visiting a patient, you have to grapple with the therapeutic approach that is appropriate in each particular case."

The process of clarification at the beginning of treatment must also always include the general framework such as treatment place, time, and costs, as well as information on the particular situation on the basis of which the couple has entered into TCM treatment. For the treatment to succeed, it is important to know what the couple has experienced and learned in the time since at-tempting to conceive a child. The effects of an unfulfilled wish for a child on the couple's lifestyle and sexual intercourse are part of this initial clarification process as well.

Shen in the Treatment Situation

To integrate the *shen* level into the treatment, the initial contact in particular should be designed very openly. **To give space** and to **take time** are qualities associated with the metal phase. Hence, we express respect and facilitate access to the essential—to water. By this, we are referring to the relationship between the different phases in accordance with the *sheng* (production) cycle. Because metal "produces" water, the clarity, time, and attention associated with metal are requirements for truly embarking on the innermost aspect, which represents the quality of water (see Chapter 70 in the *Su Wen*). It is not uncommon that the couple has already experienced a long search for causes. People visit practitioners for the sake of new impulses. The *shen* level as the level of the heart and spirit can easily be reached by questioning, observation, and open exchange. Our *shen*, which is associated with the phase of fire, contains the ability to speak with warmth and ease and without pressure. With intuition and gentleness, the essential questions can be felt out and asked. Questions for the beginning are:
- What could happen here today that would be beneficial?
- What are your hopes?
- What are your greatest fears?
- What if this treatment does not bring the desired success either?
- Which changes in lifestyle and diet are you as a couple willing to make?

Translated into modern clinical practice, this means a consistent discussion of the couple's positive as well as negative beliefs. Fixations like "We will never succeed in this," "We do not deserve this," or "This is the punishment for previous abortions" present obstacles for treatment. A clear *shen* in the practitioner includes the ability to clearly and consistently press ahead with the investigation of obstacles. The practitioner does not share the couple's "blind spots," but uncovers them with kindness. The following principle applies: you may address anything, including lack of connectedness and hopelessness. Opening up to reality with all its consequences strengthens the *shen* of the couple and of the practitioner and is an ideal starting point for successful patient care. You should turn to any physical treatment only after these essential questions have been resolved. Chapter 25 of the *Su Wen* also stresses that acupuncture cannot have much effect if the *shen* level is not cleared:

"To obtain full efficacy in the treatment with acupuncture, you must first heal the shen. *Afterwards, you must determine the state of the five viscera by taking the pulse ... Only then can you apply the needle."*

According to the "Yellow Emperor," every practitioner should pay special attention to the *shen*. With regard to acupuncture, striving for the *shen* means the greatest possible attentiveness and concentration. Additionally, we can invite the *shen* by selecting special acupuncture points and by the method of needle manipulation. In the framework of this chapter, it is impossible to discuss *shen* in relation to needling techniques in more detail. As an example, let me briefly introduce the supplementing needling technique as it is explained in Chapter 73 of the *Ling Shu*:

"[...] for this purpose, the physician's attitude must be sincere, calm, persistent, and confidence-building; the needle must not be removed immediately after introducing it ... and the hole of the puncture site on the skin must be closed afterwards ... All in all, we can thus say that you must never disregard the importance of restoring the balance of shen *when needling."*

Both during conversation and during needle contact, it is essential to be completely present and to devote your undivided attention to the event. In this way, the unclear background situation of the couple's childlessness can reveal itself more easily.

Similar to *shen* in the contact with oneself and in communication with others, the *shen* aspect in a treatment situation also facilitates a **sharpened perception** of irritations or confusions. By this, we mean disturbances in the clinical process that are normally ignored or appear to be inconspicuous or accidental. This can include, for example, recurring problems with scheduling a visit for the couple, but also "accidents" during a session such as dropping a tea cup. An irritated contact or a *shen* disturbance can express itself in a needle

that cannot be inserted by means of the usual routine or a mix-up of acupuncture points during needling. If irritations or conflicts in the contact with the couple persist in spite of the greatest possible openness and presence of the practitioner, you should reconsider the continuation of treatment.

■ *Shen* as Power of the Heart and Spiritual Connection of the Couple

Once you have established contact with your *shen* and resolved the basic questions, you are solidly grounded, and can now turn to the couple's *shen* level. This refers to the quality of the mental-emotional contact between the two partners, which involves the respective psychological state of each of them as individuals. In this context, it is irrelevant for our consideration of the *shen* here whether the couple could become pregnant naturally or if they are already undergoing fertility treatment at this time. For all couples with the desire to have children, reflecting on the *shen* offers an elemental chance.

Shen as Expression of a Shared Will

When discussing the topic of descendants, the old Chinese texts already devoted special attention to the mental attitude and heart quality between the man and the woman. Anyone who is observing the phenomena of the human body as diligently as we know the early Chinese did cannot ignore the *shen*. In spite of the institutionalized selection of the partner in early China, or perhaps because of this very reason, they checked extensively before linking two people for what was supposed to be eternity. Already the *Fo Shuo Bao Tai Jing* (佛说保胎经 *Sutra on Safeguarding the Fetus*) from the *Jin* period (265–323 CE) found an explanation for infertility in the fact that the couple's *shen* did not resonate in harmony:

"In couples with identical changes, identical thinking, identical magnanimity, identical humbleness, with complete likeness of heart, a fruit will arrive in the mother's womb ... With the same convictions and activities, the same loftiness and lowliness, a child is bound to spring forth, the parents encounter the spirit shen, and a child must come into being."[5]

Here, *shen* contains the meaning of expressing a corresponding mental attitude and individual personality. According to the *Fo Shuo Bao Tai Jing*, to invite the heavenly spark, the couple's mode of thinking must be identical. The question of identical conviction means in this context to inquire about the couple's shared efforts to produce a child. Couples who have a clear *shen* level will also tend to be congruent in their efforts to invite the child. The likeness of heart, the identical magnanimity manifests here as the expression of a shared wish, a shared sense of purpose. It is only under these conditions that the *shen* of the child will meet the parents, the *Sutra* states. It is therefore advantageous to get to know both partners personally in at least one appointment. This also applies when it is a lesbian or gay couple who are undergoing fertility treatment, in which case only the fertility of *one* partner appears to be relevant.

The *Shen* Contact between the Partners during Treatment

When setting the first appointment, the reaction of the conversation partner on the telephone to the offer of a joint first meeting often already reveals a lot of information about the couple's relationship. Typical answers like "I'd prefer to come alone at first" and objections like "But there is something wrong only with *me*, he is perfectly alright" indicate avoidance and can be understood as an expression of possible partner conflicts. Checking this issue in a joint appointment ensures that the treatment with acupuncture or Chinese medicinals is able to fall on "fertile relationship ground." To assess the couple's *shen* level, the first meeting should take place in a situation in which the arrival in the treatment room can be determined by the couple itself. For this purpose, it is helpful if the chairs are not yet placed as needed, because in this way the chosen distance and angle might reveal how the couple stands or

rather "sits" in relationship to each other. Initial silence by the practitioner also creates space for detecting the *shen* level. Illuminating observations in this context are:

- Who starts speaking?
- What is the eye contact and body language like between the two?
- Are they both equally knowledgeable?
- Are they both equally talkative?
- What is the true desire of the man and of the woman?
- What commonalities do we find?

The couple's *shen* reveals itself in the quality of their interaction, in the flow of *qi* from eye to eye and heart to heart. If one of the partners is visibly surprised or touched uncomfortably by the other partner's words, if there is something unclear or unexpressed in the room, or if the contact between the two is full of breaks, such facts can reveal fundamental differences. Likewise, the following principle applies: the more the expressed desire for a child and reality of life diverge, the more necessary it becomes to clear the *shen*. If we find an injured or irritated *shen* in one of the partners or between the two, it is only with difficulty that the heavenly spark can be invited. This aspect of *shen* again involves observations that are easily overlooked if we do not consciously direct our attention there, because the *shen* reveals itself on a subtle, immaterial level. In this context, it is occasionally advisable to work together with psychologically trained experts because an unfulfilled wish for a child should be seen in the context of relationship dynamics and childhood experiences. A complementary network of competences is a blessing in the support of the couple.

To address detected patterns of communication and interaction can mean that whatever could be standing in the way of a child will have the chance to reveal itself. Conception has been unsuccessful so far. Questioning both partners on their contact to the child can be illuminating in this context. Is the child present in dreams or visualizations? Has the couple addressed it? Direct contact with and addressing the desired child are signs of a good *shen* level and are recommended in guidebooks as effective. Thus, in order to support the *shen*, a modern Chinese manual recommends:

"To invite the child enthusiastically to come to this world, the mother is allowed to express the deepest

and most heartfelt love. You should tell the little being: Your mother and your father love you more than anything; they wish that you grow soundly and arrive at your parents' side by a good birth."[17]

Shen as Heavenly Spark during Conception

Up to now, we have discussed *shen* as the expression of a clear spirit and individual personality, as well as the contact and spiritual connection between two hearts. When we speak of the heavenly spark during conception in the following section, this refers to the meaning of *shen* as a divine power that must descend for successful creation and conception. In Chapter 26 of the *Su Wen* in the *Huang Di Nei Jing*, we find a comment that describes *shen* as such a heavenly-spiritual power:

"The Yellow Emperor asked: 'And what does shen mean?'
Qi Bo explained: 'Now regarding shen, what is it? Shen cannot be detected with the ears. You must have excellent eyesight and an open and sensitive heart; in that case, shen, the spirit, reveals itself in your own consciousness. The spirit cannot communicate through the mouth, but only through the heart. To understand shen, you must look very closely, and then you suddenly find what you need to understand. But you can just as quickly lose [such an] understanding again. Shen expresses itself to humans in the same way in which the wind suddenly disperses all clouds. And this is the reason why we speak of shen in this case.'"

In this quotation, *shen* stands for a cosmic or even divine power that is both within us and surrounding us and that we can only realize if we "look very closely" and "have an open and sensitive heart." *Shen* is communicated via the consciousness and the heart. *Shen* works as if the sky were cloudless, as if the world were bathed in radiating brightness as a result. This cosmic side of *shen* is what we mean when we speak of the heavenly spark. The heavenly spark *shen* must be present in the woman's body before a child can be created. The place where *shen* is active, the place of change, lies inside the woman, in her *yin*. The waiting period when we are uncertain about the success of

conception invites us to feel into the invisible, but also allows just as much room for negative projections, pessimistic expectations, or fears. Even where early ultrasound examinations facilitate the visualization at an early point in time, the couple is never spared this phase of waiting. As a result, even artificially supported conceptions are accompanied by a certain small period of introspection. Directing confident hope and visionary power to this time span are creative inspirations on the basis of the wood phase. Because wood gives rise to fire, we can hereby invite the heavenly spark. Thus Zita West and Birgit Zart, for example, as Western authors promote visualizing cellular processes during conception in this phase of fertility treatment.[16,18]

In the following paragraphs, we use selections from the Chinese medical literature of different periods to investigate which additional constellations are most favorable for the arrival of *shen*. For this purpose, we quote primarily texts from the Han, Ming, and Song periods, without being able to discuss the particularities and background of each dynasty in more detail here (see Riegel[11]).

Correct Timing

On the topic of the most favorable time, we find an impressive wealth of recommendations, taboos, tables, and rules. In ancient China, this moment was interpreted primarily in terms of *yin* and *yang* cycles. In the *Fu Ren Da Quan Liang Fang* (妇人大全良方 *Comprehensive Good Formulas for Women*) from the year 1237 by Chen Ziming, which summarizes information from gynecological texts up to the Song period, the male cycle is associated with the progression of the day, while the female cycle is associated with the progression of the month. According to this text, the time of the woman's fertility occurs shortly after her menstrual period while the most fertile time for the man is from midnight to dawn, in accordance with the rise of *yang qi*. In addition, there are astrological rules for lucky and unlucky days and numerous warnings regarding climatic influences. Already the *Li Ji* (禮記 *Record of Rites*), which was created long before the Common Era, warned of the negative influence of thunder:

"Thunder will quickly raise its voice if there is somebody who acts carelessly because such a person will engender children who are imperfect."[11]

While the climatic rules are interesting, they are less relevant to the question of the *shen* aspect than the following popular recommendations. As necessary preconditions for the fertile encounter of man and woman, Chinese texts emphasize mainly the self-cultivation of both the man and the woman, the observance of natural cycles and laws, and erotic passion, depending on the predominant philosophical-religious influence. Among these, the last one is most important from the Western perspective for inviting the *shen*.

Internal Self-cultivation

Texts with a more Confucian or Buddhist orientation focus on perfecting the heart by accumulating hidden merits, on the harmonious interplay of body and spirit (*shen*), and on cultivating piety and virtue, as for example in the *Guang Si Xu Zhi* (广嗣须知 *Essential Knowledge on Increasing Descendants*) from the year 1592 by Hu Wenhuan (胡文煥):

"it is necessary to [preserve] a heart that is free from the desire to harm others. Reverence towards the elderly, concern for children, compassion for orphans, sympathy for widows, help for others in distress, rescuing others from danger ... to the point where my heart becomes one with the heart of heaven, one with its principle. In this way, how could one end up in the miserable position of being unable to engender children?"[11]

In this ancient Chinese text, the **benevolence of the heart** is described as a guarantee for conception. Numerous texts regard virtue and harmony in the parents' nature as an important requirement for inviting the heavenly spark. Even though fertility treatment cannot concern itself with calling on the man and woman to engage in charity, cultivating mindfulness as a quality of the heart is certainly linked to a considerable strengthening of the *shen* and therefore a helpful support of fertility treatment.

Acceptance of Natural Cycles and Laws

In contrast to Confucian self-cultivation, Daoist texts emphasize letting go of all wishes and dedicating oneself to natural laws and cycles as the necessary condition for conception. The Daoist Yuan Mofu (元默甫) wrote in his work *Zhong Si Mi Jue (螽斯秘诀 Secrets to Descendants as Numerous as Grasshoppers)*, 1583, that persons blessed with an abundance of children are mainly those who act without intention and conform to the laws of nature:

"There is in fact no need to employ artificial methods or prescribe supplementing medicinals ... The success of farmers and simple folk who act with no intention lies in the fact that they conform to the rules of nature. They have internalized the laws of nature."[11]

These texts are written with the basic assumption that it is simply the way of nature to produce descendants. They say that if people succeed in cultivating themselves in such a way that their actions are unintentional, impartial, and wasteful like nature herself, they are bound to produce a child. In the Chinese worldview, humans cannot be perceived as separate from cosmic and natural rhythms. Inviting the heavenly spark thus depends on the quality of the heart and on the human approximation to the characteristics and cycles of heaven and earth. A convincing proponent of this view was the pharmacologist Yuan Huang (袁黄) from the Ming period (1533–1606). From a Daoist priest, he had received the prophecy that he would die young and without descendants. His Zen master recommended that he should follow the Buddhist path of accumulating merits. Yuan Huang took this advice to heart. As a result, he not only became a father but also a resolute advocate of believing in the human ability to change one's predestined fate by striving for harmony with nature and cultivating compassion and love in the heart. His work *Qi Si Zhen Quan (祈嗣真诠 True Notes on Praying for Descendants)* therefore is directly addressed to men who—like himself in the past—were hoping for descendants in vain.[11]

The significance of this approach to fertility treatment lies in the space for personal assessment and in the respective openness of the participants. The faith in a kind of predestiny or a deeper justification for "unjust strokes of fate" can imply relief and acceptance for both sides. For the patient and the practitioner, this attitude facilitates strength and confidence in spite of adverse starting conditions, holding out in treatment periods without visible success, or under certain circumstances, dealing with frustration and defeat.

Erotic Passion

Another essential aspect of inviting the heavenly spark is joyful passion. The very early literature on childbirth, but especially texts on the topic of *guang si* (increasing descendants) from the 15th and 16th centuries on devote much attention to the relationship between fertility and the emotional state of the woman.[4] Daoist texts in particular stress the need for mutual pleasure and passion during the act of conception. In this context, the Daoists were not necessarily only concerned with creating descendants. Joyful, conscious sexual intercourse was also seen as a guarantee for longevity and health, in the *nei dan* school even as an alchemistic path to initiation. The Daoists not only teach an "art of the bedchamber" that is entertaining and satisfying for both sides, but even assume that conception cannot succeed without the woman's orgasm. Sexual passion in man and woman is seen as the manifestation of heaven and earth, as universal and individual erotic pleasure, in the words of a Daoist master:

"Of all the things that benefit humans, none can be compared to sexual intercourse. It is fashioned in the image of heaven and receives its form from the earth, it balances yin and rules over yang ... In this way, the seasons follow each other, the man gives, the woman receives; above is action, below receptivity."[1]

According to the above-mentioned Yuan Huang, conception occurs when the sexual union is joyful, spontaneous, and without knowledge or thoughts. Neither *yin* nor *yang* are able to conceive a child on their own, therefore the sexes have to meet in harmony:

"[...] when wives are happy and in harmony, children will come—just as the manifestations of springtime are the result of harmony between heaven and earth."[3]

This is the moment when the heavenly spark (literally: the heavenly *qi*) descends and *jing* begins to lead the new vital processes.

With regard to fertility treatment, this information means most importantly that we should encourage the couple to show more **equanimity and pleasure in their sexuality**. The following questions are illuminating here:

- When do you feel attracted to your partner?
- Do you act on and express your erotic feelings in these situations?
- How much value do you place on the stimulation and fulfillment of the orgiastic needs of your partner?
- In your sexual intercourse, how do you invite the child?
- How has your sexuality changed since your wish for a child?

Generally speaking, couples who desire a child tend to leap to the topic of sexuality. The problematic of "sex by the clock" has by now been discussed sufficiently in public that there is little shyness in speaking about it. As such, the decline of erotic passion in couples undergoing fertility treatment is no longer a stigma, but nevertheless must still be overcome as a fact. Discussing erotic passion and sexual intercourse is important in the context of fertility treatment even in cases where the couple is completely dependent on invasive medicine in its desire for a child.

At this point, we invite the couple to connect with the fire and *shen* aspect of sexuality: from fire, earth is engendered. Due to the problems with becoming pregnant, sexuality is in danger of becoming too controlled. If metal conquers fire, the pleasure, spontaneity, and passion around conception can be pushed too far into the background. Directing attention to the level of the heart and *shen* usually offers a very welcome change in the couple's love life. When man and woman (*yin* and *yang*) are able to meet with their *shen*, they share the highest pleasure and mirror the creative spontaneity of nature. To share the highest pleasure means to invite the highest. To allow the intimacy, passion, and fullness of love to return and to meet each other in sexual intercourse truly heart to heart is an invitation to the heavenly spark that could not be more powerful. In Chinese, to open the heart (*kai xin* 开心) is an expression for "to be happy." The expression "to have joy" (*you le* 有乐), on the other hand, stands for being pregnant.

Shen and *Jing*

Chapter 54 of the *Ling Shu* demonstrates that individual human corporality is unthinkable without *shen*:

"The Yellow Emperor turned to Qi Bo and said: 'I would like to know what type of qi represents the foundation of life in a person's birth, what its defense to the outside consists of, what it cannot live without, and what it depends on for its life?'
Qi Bo answered: 'The mother's qi and blood build and nourish the foundations of life [the fetus], hence the mother's qi and blood are also the defense to the outside. The shen *is something that it cannot live without, and the* shen *is also that which life is dependent on.'"*

This quotation constitutes a clear counterbalance to the one-sided emphasis on the importance of the couple's physical vitality and fertility. Without this **physical level**, without original *qi* as the expression of *jing*, conception and procreation are, of course, not possible either. In the Chinese view, *shen* and *jing* are not a pair of opposites like body and spirit in Western concepts. Their mutual connection is significant in fertility treatment as well because *shen* can change *jing*. Or in other words: working on the *shen* serves to enrich and strengthen the efficacy on the physical level. The following holds true for the *jing* level as well: always make your own diagnosis. A patient who has been examined biomedically without findings can certainly show conspicuous signs within the system of TCM. In the context of anamnesis, investigate the woman's cycle and menstruation as well as both partner's pre-existing disorders, medical history, and surgeries. Diagnosis requires the anamnesis of **both** partners. You also need to determine and discuss contradictions in everyday life, such as irresponsible physical or mental stress situations that present an obstacle for a healthy *jing* level (e.g., lack of sleep, drug-taking, competitive sports).

Clearing the physical level does not have to imply a sober crushing of hopes. On the contrary —a clear *shen* not only makes it possible to understand one's own and the partner's condition but

can also affect the condition of the *jing*, which can manifest, for example, in clearly improved lab findings, increased libido, or menstrual changes. Nevertheless, it is also possible that clearing the *shen* results in the termination of fertility treatment. It is the *shen* level that invites the heavenly spark and it is the *shen* level in which we can let go of the desire for a child.

TCM also recognizes cases of infertility in which no explanation can be found. Thus Chapter 71 of the *Ling Shu* already mentions the fact that there are people who remain childless and that this can be due to natural causes. Humans and nature resonate with each other in their appearance and creation:

"As there is grass on the earth, so the hair grows on the human body. As there are day and night in the sky, so there is sleeping and being awake in humans. As there are regions on the earth where no blade of grass will ever grow, so there are humans who will never engender children."

A distressing fixation can only be released after the impossibility of conception has been recognized on the *shen* level. This is the necessary precondition for either introducing necessary changes or peacefully accepting one's fate.

■ Discussion

Pregnancies can also occur under forced circumstances. This refers not only to sexual rape; here we can certainly also consider, for example, the view of the author Theresia Maria de Jong[6] who describes invasive methods like IVF and ICSI as "rape of the egg and sperm." We do not know yet what the results are when a child has been created in this way. The known historical Chinese texts apparently do not consider such cases; in these texts, conception does not happen without the heavenly spark. They do warn, however, against unfavorable conditions and an unlucky moment of conception because they fear negative results for the constitution of the child. We can likewise assume consequences for the constitution of those children who have been created by means of invasive fertility treatments. The practitioner should be able to recognize and name clear signs of overexertion in the couple, such as after repeated IVF or other treatments. If these invasions, from the diagnostic perspective, constitute too great a strain and limitation for physical and mental health, you should address the possibilities of treatment breaks, Godparenthood, adoption, and fosterparenting.

Concluding Remarks

Our effort to highlight the importance of *shen* in fertility treatment is rooted in the fact that the aspects of consciousness introduced here are lacking in most fertility practices. The need for help on this level surfaces in many patients in the yearning for spiritual clarification and emotional support. As in any crisis, we also find a lot of willingness to change and energy invested in fertility treatment—this area therefore offers a fertile ground for therapeutic work.

The typical emotional state of couples with an unfulfilled desire for a child, characterized by frustration, feelings of guilt, sadness, or hopelessness, demands attention. It is not uncommon for the couple to suffer from pathological traits of fixation and compulsion. For the treatment of these disorders, certain point combinations and especially points that include the term *shen* in their name are very effective. Celestial window points and dragon point combinations are suitable for treating these aspects. In dealing with the couple, however, what is most helpful for the practitioner is the presence of *shen*. Any treatment related to a conception is an individual path to the child and must involve *shen*.

> *Shen* means creativity and generative power. A change on the *shen* level also involves a change on the *jing* level as well—in this sense *shen* facilitates fertility on the physical level.

The multi-layered complexity of the concept *shen*, which we have tried to demonstrate with the quotations here, is not easy to comprehend. In our language, no term exists that can contain the extent of the many meanings of *shen*. This makes it more difficult, but also more attractive, to approach this concept. The interpretation of *shen* promoted here includes especially the search for the greatest possible clarity vis-à-vis one's own wishes, actions, and the consequences of these actions. Support on the *shen* level not always leads to the desired child. The success of the treatment manifests not in every case in the arrival and completion of a pregnancy. Nevertheless, opening to the *shen* allows the couple to engage deeply with the facts of their situation and ultimately to accept the individual reality that is grounded in inner peace and healthful clarity.

Bibliography

1. Dunas F, Goldberg P. *Chinesische Liebesgeheimnisse. Alte Weisheiten für Glück und Gesundheit.* Munich: Müller & Steinicke; 2004.
2. Fu BT (editor). *Huang Di NeiJing. Su Wen. Ling Shu. (The Inner Classic of the Yellow Emperor).* Taiwan, Daxue shuju; 1992.
3. Furth Ch. *A Flourishing Yin. Gender in China's Medical History 960 – 1665.* Berkeley: University of California Press; 1999.
4. Hua Z, Riegel AM. *Akupunktur bei Blutungsstörungen und Zyklusanomalien.* Heidelberg: Haug; 2000.
5. Huebotter F. *Die Sutra über Empfängnis und Embryologie.* Leipzig: Asia Major; 1932.
6. Jong de TM. *Babies aus dem Labor. Segen oder Fluch?* Weinheim: Beltz; 2002.
7. Jong de TM. Ein Kind auf Umwegen—künstliche Befruchtung auf dem Prüfstand. In: Doderer A (editor) *Tagungsjournal: Werde, Wachse und Gedeihe, Liebes Kind.* Idstein: Druckerei Schlosser.
8. Linck G. *Yin und Yang—Die Suche nach Ganzheit im Chinesischen Denken.* Munich: Beck; 2000.
9. Linck G. Räume der Toten—Sepulkralkultur und Ontologien im Vormodernen China. In: Schottenhammer, A (editor) *Auf den Spuren des Jenseits. Chinesische Grabkultur in den Facetten von Wirklichkeit, Geschichte und Totenkult.* Frankfurt: Peter Lang; 2003: 193 – 212.
10. Lu HC. *A Complete Translation of Yellow Emperor's Classics of Internal Medicine.* The Academy of Oriental Heritage. Vancouver: Blaine; 1990.
11. Riegel AM. *Das Streben nach dem Sohn. Fruchtbarkeit und Empfängnis in den Medizinischen Texten Chinas von der Hanzeit bis zur Mingzeit.* Munich: Herbert Utz; 1999.
12. Schmidt WGA. *Der Klassiker des Gelben Kaisers zur Inneren Medizin.* Freiburg: Herder; 1993.
13. Unschuld P. *Nan Ching—The Classic of Difficult Issues.* Berkeley: University of California Press; 1986.
14. Unschuld P. *Huang Di Nei Jing Su Wen. Nature, Knowledge, Imagery in an Ancient Chinese Medical Text.* Berkeley: University of California Press; 2003.
15. Watts A. *Der Lauf des Wassers.* Bern: Scherz; 1983.
16. West Z. *Kinderwunsch.* Starnberg: Dorling Kindersley; 2004.
17. Xing JB, Jiangong X. *Shiyue huaitai. Yueyue you taijiao. (The Ten Months of Pregnancy: Fetal Education for Every Month).* Hailaer: Inner Mongolia Culture Press; 2002.
18. Zart B. *Gelassen durch die Kinderwunschzeit.* Munich: Hugendubel; 2006.

24   Stress and Infertility

Andreas A. Noll

There is hardly another topic that is loaded with stress on as many levels as fertility. At the onset of the intention to bring a new life into this world, numerous factors manifest as "stressors": anxiety about the future, the fear of personal failure on many levels, insecurities about the couple's mutual feelings, time pressure, pressure from set norms (e. g., of fertility) and inescapable biological facts, values (e. g., laboratory or societal values) and expectations (e. g., of the rest of the family). Sooner or later, all participants complain of "being stressed," "having stress," "stressful people," and "making stress"—note the different formulations that such stressed-out participants choose.

Definitions and Mechanisms of Stress from the Western Perspective [according to *Brockhaus encyclopedia*[2]]

In 1936, the physician and stress researcher Hans Selye extended the term stress from the natural realm to the physical-psychological realm. Since then, the word has become a collective term for a variety of individual phenomena that are characterized by a state of elevated activity in the organism.

Definition

In its neutral sense, stress refers to the **non-specific adaptation of the organism to any challenge**. Most definitions understand stress as a state of the organism in which its well-being is perceived as endangered by an internal or external threat, as a result of which the organism must concentrate all its strength and apply it protectively to overcome the "danger." From an evolutionary perspective, stress is seen as the organism's reaction to stimulation and adaptation to changed environmental conditions, which is essential for its survival.

Differentiation

We differentiate between **eustress** and **distress**.

- **Eustress** is a necessary activation of the organism ("spice of life") in the form of a beneficial, health-promoting challenge that causes us to make use of our resources and thereby facilitates the further development of our own abilities.
- **Distress**, on the other hand, means a harmful excess of challenges to the organism. In recent decades, the term has been interpreted from this point of view as the result of the work- and time-related pressure in modern industrialized society, with considerable effects on individual well-being, productivity, and ability to function in society, as well as on health.

Symptoms

Stress expresses itself on all levels of the organism, for example in sweating, heart palpitations, circulatory changes in the body's periphery, behavior (e. g., aggression, excitement, or unrest), in the experience and evaluation of one's own condition. Stress can manifest in all areas of life, situations, and ages.

Causes

Triggers for stress are:
- external factors (e. g., sensory overstimulation, pain, dangerous situations)
- deficiency factors (e. g., withdrawal of food, water, sleep, or movement)
- performance factors (e. g., overload, time pressure, multiple strains at the same time, insufficient chances to recover)
- social factors (e. g., isolation)
- psychological and psychosocial factors (e. g., conflicts, uncertainty)
- times of crisis or critical life events (e. g., puberty, menopause, entry into retirement)
- changes in life circumstances (e. g., loss of a family member, divorce, unemployment, disease)

Stress wears out the nerves, exhausts, and ultimately drains our "substance." In TCM, we associate this substance with the **energy of the kidneys**—that is, kidney *jing*. This fundamental energy is, as we have read in several other contributions in this book, an absolute necessity for the creation of a child. The kidneys are the root of reproduction and development—if their energy is drained due to exertion and exhaustion, no child can receive a healthy foundation for life from its parents.

The question now is why every person responds differently to stress situations: one person gets heartburn, another headaches, the third one fits of raving madness, and the fourth one withdraws in frustration to a voracious feast. Why does one woman respond with a dwindling menstrual period while the other suffers from unbearable pain and emotional problems that turn her life into hell every month? Reduced sperm counts cause one man to despair in his sexual identity, disastrous sperm quality another.

Nevertheless, TCM definitely presents options for assigning these different reactions to stress to specific categories or patterns. With its help, we can determine where in each patient the harmonious symphony of *qi*, the up and down, inward and outward movement, is disturbed. Only the smooth flow of *qi* guarantees that blood and *qi* reach the lower burner and that the fire of the heart sinks downward to unite with the *ming men* fire to contribute mutual love and passion to the "project new life."

■ What Causes Stress?

The goal of all efforts and wishes, in both major and minor concerns, is wholeness and perfection—in the case of fertility treatment, the wholeness of the fulfilled wish and the attainment of the goal: man and woman and child.

What causes stress are the blocks on the path to that goal—be they building blocks or stumbling blocks. Some people are able to use the stumbling blocks as building blocks; others despair over a pebble. How we face obstacles depends on a variety of factors that affect the participants, such as their strength, composure (to use a detour if necessary), mindfulness, or also creativity.

Authenticity—How do we Achieve it?

Wholeness and perfection—this is the goal in minor and in major matters. Wholeness means in effect that we are content in regards to the outcome of our own expectations, satisfied and whole. It means to act the way we feel—in other words, to be authentic. A round circle—that is the feeling that we get when we are able to sit back in full contentment and satisfaction and say: "That is good, that will do." The size of the circle corresponds to the amount of self-confidence and self-contentment within the individual.

Dents and bumps, on the other hand, are deficits and excesses that move us to act or to do nothing. These are important aspects of human existence as well since they always bring us back into harmony by the desire for wholeness and roundness.

Ideas, Concepts, Feelings—Where Do They Come From?

Where does the feeling of wholeness originate? It is not anything inborn—perhaps a small part of it is, in regards to our natural destiny. But in reality it is guided by a multiplicity of societal, cultural, social, religious, and aesthetic notions—by the normative concepts determined by society:

• For whom or for what purpose do I act and live?
• What is good?
• What is right?
• What is desirable?
• What is happiness?

What is the Benchmark for our Actions and the Pursuit of Happiness?

Our personal, individual answer to these questions, this mélange of concepts, suggested from the outside as norms and assimilated by the individual as personal ethics, stems from a great variety of sources.

Until several hundred years ago, Christianity provided uncontestable answers to the questions of life, concerning the pursuit of happiness, justice, the meaning of life, and good and evil. Only Protestantism—especially Calvinism in the United States—shifted the authority of standardization piece by piece to earthly realms: the man of success shows that he is chosen, as it is said in the Bible:

• "By their fruits ye shall know them" (Matthew 7: 16)
• "Subdue the earth" (Genesis 1: 28)

From this point on, definitively from the beginning of the 19th century and the provisional end of the enlightenment period on, the highest maxim of earthly actions and striving was to be successful and rich. The wealth that was accumulated here on earth signaled that the person was chosen by God.

Benchmark: Social Accommodation

Almost four centuries after Martin Luther, people realized: God is dead! Nietzsche formulated this as follows in his book *The Gay Science (Die Fröhliche Wissenschaft)*:

"The greatest recent event—that 'God is dead,' that the belief in the Christian God has become unbelievable—is already beginning to cast its first shadows over Europe. For the few ... our old world must appear daily more like evening, more mistrustful, stranger, 'older.' ... and how much must collapse now that this faith has been undermined because it was built upon this faith, propped up by it, grown into it: for example, the whole of our European morality.[6]

Now humans were finally forced to fend for themselves. The norms originated from within themselves. It was no longer God who ruled the world but humanity—humanity is God—and so it was said: everything is possible! The human psyche, the spirit, the will as the new "inner God" was ruled by physis (nature). And now these poor humans were forced to ask themselves the question of direction. They were now left completely to their own devices, both in the minor questions as also in the very major questions of life.

The motivation, the impetus for action came to be derived from the external effect, the success in this life, the fulfillment of individual needs. The collisions that have resulted from this struggle with the external world are most of our stressors. To bring personal needs in accord with the whole, the relationship with other people, this holds the potential for conflict since the social norms—as far as they had been coined by religiously legitimized notions—are being questioned, to say the least. Nietzsche has this to say:

"The mother gives the child what she takes from herself: sleep, the best food, in some instances even her health, her wealth. – Are all these really selfless states, however? [...] Isn't it clear that, in all these cases, man is loving something of himself, a thought, a longing, an offspring, more than something else of himself; that he is thus dividing up his being and sacrificing one part for the other? [...] The inclination towards something (a wish, a drive, a longing) is present in all the above-mentioned cases; to yield to it, with all its consequences, is in any case not 'selfless.' – In morality, man treats himself not as an individuum, but as a dividuum."[7]

And thus the project "mutual child" means the collision of wishes, ideas, and needs of both partners, as well as the hypothetical needs of the future child. This situation obviously casts doubt on the conventional norm of "autonomy." Immanuel Kant writes on this topic:

"Autonomy of the will is that property of it by which it is a law to itself independently of any property of objects of volition. Hence the principle of autonomy is: Never choose except in such a way that the maxims of the choice are comprehended in the same volition as a universal law."[5]

China and the Hope for Happiness

The developments that began in the West around the 15th century were initiated in China by Confucius already 2000 years ago: the secularization of the pursuit of happiness—away from demons and gods, towards the earthly society of interconnected humanity:

"To give one's self earnestly to the duties due to men, and, while respecting spiritual beings, to keep aloof from them, may be called wisdom"[3]

And people there also asked how they could achieve wholeness and happiness in the here and now, in the earthly world of their existence. **Happiness** can be discussed and defined on different levels:
- On the **religious level**, humans strive for release from the suffering of this world, whether in the afterlife or in this life. In the latter of these, we find the interface to medicine and healing with its partly magico-religious practices.*
- The **human-social level** is concerned with the continued survival of humanity, also beyond the individual's physical existence. To bring a child into the world is an opportunity to transfer one's own ideas, and therefore also a considerable part of one's personal identity, to the next generations. Confucianism in particular

---

* Magic and healing—in this context, we may mention the "magic" of numbers (life span), values (laboratory), and doability (IVF, gene technology) —all of these have an almost "magical" effect on our patients that can be both positive and negative.

has placed great value on this aspect by establishing the mutual responsibilities of ancestors and descendants with the living as the maxim of social action (see Chapter 4).
- The third level on which to pursue happiness is the **material-realistic level**: material wealth.

In the medical model that has nowadays been accepted in part by TCM, the **concept** *ming men* helps us to answer this question.

■ The Motor—*Ming Men*

Ming is a term that is primarily used in the Confucian context, meaning "heavenly mandate." It is a potential that we carry within us and that shows us the path we have to take in the course of our lives. It is our duty to fulfill this mandate, this potential. It is the **totality of ideas** that each individual has formed about his or her very personal happiness, about wholeness on all levels (religious, social, and material) on the basis of the person's roots and socialization. *Men* means "door, gate." *Ming men* is hence the key, entryway, and motor in the pursuit of happiness.

As acupuncture point (CV-4), which lies between the two kidneys, its direction-giving fire initiates the drive to act, no matter in which direction. *Ming men* thereby unites the purpose of the essence *jing* to preserve and reproduce itself as material existence (left kidney, *yin* kidney) with the life-giving fire of the *yang* kidney, which additionally receives strong support from the "imperial fire" of the heart—connected by the *xin bao* (pericardium). The *ming men* then gives rise to the triad of lust, love, and fertility, so indispensable for the fulfillment of the wish for a child.

This urge of the *ming men* to fulfill one's personal destiny means there are **needs** to satisfy. These needs in turn result from the emptiness of certain aspects of our existence. Only this emptiness in an area of our existence, this "dent" in our round wholeness forms a need. Which in turn drives us to go outward, out into the environment, out of our isolation into social relationships. And thereby also outward into the thorny thicket of potential stress factors.

As engine for this drive, the *ming men* is indispensable for the life-sustaining and -extending functions of all viscera and bowels associated with the five phases of change. *Ming men*—in other cultural contexts called *dynamis* (Greek = "force") or *mana* (Austronesian = power)—is a governing and guiding power that is inherent in humans—explicitly directed against the notion of a specific god or of gods and spirits. *Ming men* causes us to pursue such goals as:

- happiness
- contentment
- love
- adventure
- restlessness
- progress
- leisure
- gain
- completion
- ritual
- security
- feelings
- life
- identity
- quietude
- sex
- being

■ The End of Pushing

The push to action, to the pursuit of happiness and contentment in one or another area thus serves exclusively—however selfless the goal may appear!—the satisfaction of personal needs. It ends with the satisfaction thereof and only arises out of new needs. The **pursuit of wholeness** defines itself and results from the following:

- From the **realization of deficits or excesses**, the pursuit of fullness and emptiness. Here we must note that the conventional value system both in the West and in TCM as it is received in the West generally view emptiness as synonymous with weakness; hence as "bad" and in need of treatment. Fullness (synonym: strength), on the other hand, is seen as the ideal state—regardless of the fact that fullness or strength can only exist as long as it is nour-

ished—hence per se contains emptiness within it.

- From the **juxtaposition of the self with others**. This results in sometimes awkward comparisons but also in the collision with socially or historically defined ideals of beauty, health, and wholeness.
- From **individualization, socialization, and the affirmation of self-worth**, a mutual influence of the environment on identity and vice versa, constituted from birth on.
- From the **perception of emptiness**, because this leads to fullness, and only fullness can be emptied. Or: emptiness leads to needs, fullness leads to emptying.

On the Blessings of Idleness
"In favor of the idle.— One sign that the valuation of the contemplative life has declined is that scholars now compete with men of action in a kind of precipitate pleasure, so that they seem to value this kind of pleasure more highly than that to which they are really entitled and which is in fact much more pleasurable. Scholars are ashamed of otium [leisure, idleness]. But there is something noble about leisure and idleness.— If idleness really is the beginning of all vice, then it is at any rate in the closest proximity to all virtue; the idle man is always a better man than the active.— But when I speak of leisure and idleness, you do not think I am alluding to you, do you, you sluggards?"[7]

Hence we are dealing with a system that is essentially comprised of two components:

- **The non-profit component**. This is the pursuit directed outward, into society, into the environment. It is the chase, the push for that which we are lacking. This pursuit and chase is what we normally perceive as stress. It is the restlessness, the nagging feeling of discontent, the inability to satisfy our needs and desires. **Water and wood** then—apart from the influences of other phases or viscera and bowels that we list below—are the phases that fall into disharmony and in which stress disorders like high blood pressure, burn-out syndrome, menstrual disorders or PMS, reduced sperm quality, and impotence manifest.
- **Profit component**. This is the bringing in, satiating, filling of gaps with what we need. **Earth and metal** are the phases that cause us to pause, to "do something for ourselves," and to develop a feeling for what is important in life.

317

Burn-out Syndrome

The burn-out syndrome, that is, the "burn-out" of physical and mental-emotional resources, is a gradual, creeping process. Chronic tiredness, exhaustion, lack of energy, chronic fatigue syndrome (CFS), neurasthenia, irritability, and internal restlessness are other disturbance patterns related to this syndrome.

Stages of the Burn-out Syndrome (according to Freudenberger and North[4])

- stage 1: the compulsion to prove oneself
- stage 2: increased effort
- stage 3: (subtle) neglect of own needs
- stage 4: suppression of conflicts and needs
- stage 5: reinterpretation of values
- stage 6: increased denial of occurring problems
- stage 7: permanent withdrawal
- stage 8: obvious behavioral changes
- stage 9: losing a sense of one's own personality
- stage 10: internal emptiness
- stage 11: depression
- stage 12: complete burn-out exhaustion

We have said enough here on the forces that drive us and make us push. Now let us consider the particular volatility of the stumbling blocks on our path to the goal: here we are confronted with the question why these blocks sometimes appear so gigantic to us that we immediately want to give up what we just started—but then can shrink back to ridiculous insignificance. The question of these stumbling blocks—that is the question of how we deal with potential obstacles. What is it that sometimes makes it so difficult for us to keep our sight on the truly important things, what is it that blocks us on this path and makes us stagnate?

■ Losing and Gaining Identity

First there is the basis, the starting point of *ming men*, the **identity**. What am I worth? Can I accomplish that? This means determining our self-worth by means of congruence with and demarcation from the environment. Only our environment,

the people with whom we enter into a relationship—regardless of what kind—give us feedback on our own worth. They appreciate, reject, or ignore—but each of these impulses provides a building block for our own identity.

It is the self-confidence that is fed as identity by the most diverse **social roles**. First there is the person who lives alone, defined by a comparatively broad social sphere and by the desire for twosomeness. In our context, the result is a twosomeness that is characterized by pronounced connectedness between two individuals who share a certain potential of things in common and who newly emerge together as a couple in their environment. And then the new definition as notified threesomeness.

Any departure from this position that was initially secure in every phase—secure in the environment, secure in habits and familiarity—means initially to stand on very shaky legs. The reason for this is that the change in social role and function leads to a **new definition of identity**. Two people find themselves newly in the role of potential parents, they define themselves as a couple who want a child. In this role, they find new contacts, experience new acknowledgments and frustrations. And when the child has finally arrived, yet another redefinition of roles is due—as the threesomeness of woman—man—child, with a new identity and new contacts, new acknowledgements and frustrations.

Collisions with existing structures into which we advance as we break away from everyday life are unavoidable and perhaps even trigger fear or insecurity. **Breaking away from the familiar** places high demands on our own adaptability—and can cause stress.

The need to adapt to unforeseeable conflicts results in a position of attention that allows us to be prepared for anything with due responsiveness and speed of reaction. The brief loss of familiar everyday life with all its security and clarity leads to a loss of naturalness and wholeness. Nevertheless, this gap is an emptiness that cries out to be filled. The departure into something new, the presentiment of the fulfillment of one's wishes, is a departure into uncertainty, but also into happiness. Wolfgang Bauer describes this as follows:

"[...] the feeling of a jubilant self-renunciation but also of being absorbed by a greater Self."[1]

From the daily routine, which guarantees so much security, safety, direction, and peace, the person takes off into the tingling uncertainty of a new adventure. Leaving behind rituals and familiarity, *Homo sapiens* turns into *Homo ludens*, the playful person who conjectures the perils and gains of utmost happiness beyond the security of everyday life. But nothing is safe, nothing calculable any longer. In free floating, released from the bonds of daily life and its obviousness, we find the potential for fulfilling our wishes, for happiness.

But it is just as in a game—the escape is limited, it invariably returns to the daily routine, to normality. The **return to everyday life** follows. This means farewell to curiosity, adventurousness, tingling, and longing ... And then new problems arise when we return from this excursion, from the formerly white spots of our world of experience. This is the profit stage, which usually does not receive nearly as much attention as the costly non-profit stage: New experiences, fresh impulses must be reflected on and integrated into existing values and ideas. The result of our excursion into this natural urge is a new identity, expanded by a new framework. This new element, though, does not see itself as a substitute for the old, familiar, and past, but as its extension. The old identity consumes the new one, the old is still present as strength-giving root of the flowering tree.

In fertility treatment as well, all these **three stages** of the "adventure child"—discovery of identity, departure from the familiar, and return to everyday life—include not only the potential for happiness but also for danger and various stress factors. In spite of the fact that the wood phase and the harmoniously regulating function of the liver are highly significant here by helping the couple to act in accordance with the stages and with flexibility towards any particular problems, as practitioners we can be faced with individually varying patterns.

Strategies for Harmonizing Self-awareness and Partnership

The **system of the five phases** (*wu xing*) is an elemental perspective that provides a key set of rules and regulations in the traditional Chinese worldview and its medicine. It is based on:

- a large number of fixed analogies in a chronologically horizontal synchronicity of perception (a model of thinking in which all manifestations of this world can be categorized)
- on the interplay of all five phases in the sense of a cybernetic system that self-regulates to achieve harmony.

With regard to these analogies, Confucianism in particular, which saw social existence as the highest guiding principle for individual action, ascribed specific ethics to each of the five phases. It is these ethics then that make the phase and the human emotions ascribed to it (and the correlated viscera and bowels) socially acceptable. From the moment when the person turns outwards with his or her emotions—which is, after all, the literal meaning of "e-motion"—they are no longer only an individual affair; instead, they are developed and regulated by the influences of interpersonal relationships. Every "e-motion" causes an "in-motion"—a reaction, an echo in the rest of the world. And this forms the basis for the harmonious, socially compatible conduct of the individual.

The Wood Phase and the Liver

The wood phase means for the individual that we are **developing our individuality**. *Ming men*, the kidney-based drive to develop our personality, is accepted and drives us to go outward, drives for fulfillment of personal interests and ideas. Wood means personal advancement. On this path, collisions, namely with the wood of our fellow human beings, are unavoidable and crushing; for the individual as much as for others. This struggle with oneself—one's own wants and urges—and with others—and their wants—is exhausting and a major cause of stress-related disorders like the burn-out syndrome. Social compatibility, **ethics**,

319

and hence the conduct of the individual that can take him or her out of a confrontation into togetherness, is expressed by *ren* (仁), **compassion**. The character shows a person and the number two. It means that wood only receives its social value by the fact that we can put ourselves in somebody else's place; to verify what happens with the other person, how the other person reacts when he or she is confronted with our own wishes and wants. A harmonious wood phase and hence also a healthy liver as the correlated viscus is adaptable, takes notes of obstacles and stumbling blocks in the environment, and effortlessly adjusts its conduct accordingly. In this function, the quality of the earth phase provides wood with stability.

Disharmonies
Feelings of pressure, lacking the ability to adapt to changed situations, power struggles, etc.

Acupuncture Point
LR-3, the earth point

The Fire Phase and the Heart

In the fire phase, the person and the changes in life reach the apex of *yang*. The person **connects with heaven** and hence with everything that is associated with heaven: happiness, love, the brightness of the shining sun, openness, and vastness. But these aspects in particular also harbor the risk potential of fire: in this vastness, just as in happiness and love, we can easily get lost, lose the ground under our feet, and thus completely overexert ourselves. Fire is the peak of extroversion—at this point, what should come into effect is what leads back to water, to existence and security: the metal phase. Its quality is reflected in the **ethical conduct** of fire: it is *li* (禮), **ritual**, customs and habits. Rituals and social patterns reflected the order of heaven in Confucian China. The order on earth and hence in society resembled the order of heaven. By means of a highly differentiated system of rituals, the heavenly order—represented on earth by the emperor—was reconstructed on earth; but not in the sense of mere imitation but as reality: *ji ru zai* (祭如再 "worship as if the ritual were real"[5]). Transgressions against ritual are then in fact regarded as transgressions against the heavenly order and as such inexcusable. Rituals give the heavenly fire order and structure; by providing form, they make the heart free and open, give it direction and connection to the self—to the water phase.

Disharmonies
For example, problems with entering into commitments, relationships, or social obligations.

Acupuncture Point
HT-4 *ling dao*, the metal point

The Earth Phase and the Spleen

The earth is the center of life and of the human being. This center absorbs everything that arises from change. Change means life, means constant processes and transformations in the interplay between heaven and earth, *yin* and *yang*. To juxtapose a **moment of quiet**, of pause, in opposition to these constant movements or better yet side by side with them, this is the centering and meditative power of earth. It is the aspect of pausing, of "centering," in this merry-go-round of life and the world, which sometimes turns with unbearable speed. We stop, absorb from the environment, and establish contact to the self by nurturing ourselves. The water phase is this "self-connection" for the earth, by which the earth and hence the spleen develop needs and desires. Through the earth, humans benefit from the environment, gain fullness and roundness. The social virtue, the **ethical value** associated with earth, is *xin* (信), **trust**. To nurture and be nurtured—nowadays we call this a "win-win situation" in relationships, where both partners profit from each other without feeling that they are being deceived or taken advantage of.

Disharmonies
Problems with accepting affection; insatiability, jealousy, etc.

Acupuncture Point
SP-9 *yin ling quan*, the water point

The Metal Phase and the Lung

The metal phase gives us **direction and security in life.** In addition, though, also a feeling for **boundaries**, for those that exist between inside and outside, but also for those between the self and the environment. Boundaries that are not rigid and unsurmountable, but permeable and can be extended or restricted depending on needs. Norms and regulations that are, however, observed and followed as guidelines in accordance with the sense—also a quality of metal—of one's own morality and correctness. The **ethical value** associated with the metal phase is thus *yi* (義), **righteousness and justice**. It communicates the strength and assertiveness of wood outward for metal, which by its nature tends more towards withdrawal and self-emphasis.

Disharmonies

Problems with responsibility and standards, opportunism, and doubting, for example.

Acupuncture Point

LU-11 *shao shang* ("Lesser *Shang*," i.e., young metal), the wood point

The Water Phase and the Kidney

The water phase is the source of *yin* and *yang*. In water we reach the lowest point of *yang*, but at the same time it is the powerful origin for a renewed movement towards fire in the cycle of the five phases. As such, water is **quietude and composure**, it is withdrawal and solitude, perhaps even pleasant boredom and contentment with oneself. The nature and **ethical value** of this *yin* aspect of water is *zhi* (智), **wisdom**. Wisdom does not strive, it does not push outward, towards fulfilling wishes and realizing ideas. Wisdom rests and works in stillness. Different from this, however, is the *yang* aspect of water and the kidneys: this is *ming men*, which strives for the wholeness and realization of the inborn potential for happiness as much as for adventure and the "kick." *Ming men* means **rest-**lessness, movement, dynamics, and is the root of continued growth. In it, we see the workings of *zhi* (志), the **will**, as counterpart to composed wisdom. In this respect, we find here the socially regulating authority in self-awareness, in personal identity.

Disharmonies

Problems with self-confidence, social identity, role as man or woman, power and powerlessness, etc.

Acupuncture Point

KI-3 *tai xi*, the earth point

Conclusion

In this way, the system of the five phases and, associated with it, the possibilities for influencing it by means of the correlated acupuncture points provide the practitioner with a system for intervening in the different stages of fertility treatment therapeutically. An old Confucian principle is thus put into practice: to restore harmony between the individual and his or her environment.

Bibliography

1. Bauer W. *China und die Hoffnung auf Glück. Paradiese, Utopien, Idealvorstellungen.* Munich: Hanser; 1971.
2. *Brockhaus Enzyklopädie in 30 Bänden.* Vol. 26. Leipzig: Brockhaus; 2006.
3. Confucius. The Analects. In: The Chinese Classics Vol. I. Translated by James Legge. Internet Sacred Text Archive: www.sacred-texts.com.
4. Freudenberger H, North G. *Burn-out bei Frauen: Über das Gefühl des Ausgebranntseins.* Frankfurt: Fischer; 1999.
5. Kant I. *Foundations of the Metaphysics of Morals.* Trans. Lewis White Beck. With Critical Essays ed. by Robert Paul Wolff. Indianapolis: Bobbs-Merril Educational Publishing, 1969, p. 67
6. Kaufmann W. *The Gay Science: With a Prelude in Rhymes and an Appendix of Songs* by Friedrich Nietzsche; translated, with commentary, by Walter Kaufmann. New York: Vintage Books; 1974.
7. Nietzsche F. *Human, All Too Human.* The Nietzsche Channel Website. Compiled from translations by Helen Zimmern, R. J. Hollingsdale, and Marion Faber.
8. Noll A, Kirschbaum B. *Stresskrankheiten.* Munich: Urban & Fischer; 2006.

25 Supporting the Couple in Successful and Failed Fertility Treatment

Andreas A. Noll, Gudrun Kotte, and Sabine Wilms*

The success of fertility treatment depends on a large number of factors. In addition to physiological and pathological obstacles, which are found in the physical functions of the man and the woman, we must not ignore psychological and sociocultural aspects either. The latter concern the valuation of children and of pregnancy in our society as well as norms determined by reproductive medicine. In addition, individual life and work situations, cooperation with the practitioner, and the experiences gained in the course of fertility treatment all play significant roles as well.

Ultimately, one factor that is not predictable always remains: "coincidence," "divine providence," *dao, shen,* or "fate." Neither reproductive medicine nor TCM can provide a guarantee for successful conception and pregnancy—both methods can, however, assist in creating the most "fertile soil" possible for a new life.

While reproductive medicine concentrates primarily on the removal of physiological obstacles, TCM pays additional attention to the equilibrium of all immaterial processes in their organic interplay—and thereby also to patients' psychological-emotional balance. A conversation about the potential effects of any intensive treatment with reproductive medicine on this balance is therefore one aspect of patient support that TCM can provide. At the end of any fertility treatment, we should always face healthy patients—whether there will be three, two, or even just one.

In light of the detailed contributions on supporting fertilization and conception in this book (see Chapters 19, 22, and 23), the following chapter concentrates on two aspects in the support of couples in fertility treatment:

- on supporting a pregnancy after successful conception and
- on options for additional support if the wish for a child cannot be realized

■ Supporting Pregnancy

To prepare for a pregnancy, the greatest potential and chances for success with TCM methods lie in improving the quality of egg and sperm cells. On top of that, acupuncture can have a sustained effect on resolving blockages, which has a positive impact on the psychological state of the couple. This in turn has a favorable effect on conception. After successful fertilization, TCM can prepare the supply of blood and *qi* to the uterus and thereby assist in implantation.

In principle, though, we should keep in mind that any conception that was achieved by intensive treatment can also be followed by an unstable pregnancy. This applies not only to the use of methods of reproductive medicine, such as IVF, IUI, or hormone therapy, but also after intensive treatment of the constitution and fertility with acupuncture, moxibustion, or Chinese medicinals. Below, we therefore discuss how we can support these women in the subsequent 38 weeks, to increase their chances for completing the pregnancy successfully.

Promoting the health of pregnant women and avoiding possible harm to mother and child has been a central issue in TCM for many centuries. The Chinese scholar-physician Sun Simiao (581–682 CE) was not the first, but perhaps the most famous "King of Medicine" (*yao wang*), who concerned himself with promoting the development of the fetus in the mother's womb. His book, *Bei Ji Qian Jin Yao Fang (Essential 1000-Gold Formulary for Emergencies),* became the standard classic until the 19th century and still serves as the most im-

---

* Please see *Bei Ji Qian Jin Yao Fang—Essential Prescriptions worth a Thousand in Gold for Every Emergency* (The Chinese Medicine Database, 2008) and *The Transmission of Medical Knowledge on 'Nurturing the Fetus' in Early China* (Asian Medicine: Tradition and Modernity, 2005), which were used as a source for this chapter.

portant reference text for this chapter (see also Chapter 8).

In the Chinese classics, pregnancy is commonly divided into **10 months**, counted in accordance with the lunar calendar. In each month, a different channel nourishes the child. Two months each and their respective channels are associated with one **phase**:

- wood phase: first and second month
- fire phase: third and fourth month
- earth phase: fifth and sixth month
- metal phase: seventh and eighth month
- water phase: ninth and 10th month

Each phase has its inherent quality and is introduced with dietary recommendations and behavioral instructions. The latter are related to the medical and cosmological understanding of that time and cannot always be transferred directly to the context of a contemporary Western pregnancy. The theory of fetal development that we present here in the following five sections therefore at first sight does not offer much concrete therapeutic advice for the practitioner and should not be read as such either. Its value lies primarily in the fact that it offers a new perspective on **pregnancy as a time associated with the five phases and the seasons**. A practitioner with this "Chinese" perspective can recognize, evaluate, or even treat arising symptoms preventatively in the context of the particular point in time in an innovative way.

An example: a woman with a clear weakness of the center will probably develop symptoms during the time associated with the earth phase, that is, in the fifth and sixth month. At the same time, she will respond particularly well to strengthening the center during this phase. Tuning in to the internal processes anew each month, as this theory encourages us to do, presents a valuable opportunity for both the practitioner and the pregnant woman to consciously perceive and thereby stabilize the processes inside her. While the recommendations appear to be directed strictly at the woman, the father of the developing child is invited implicitly to look inside himself as well because he also experiences all the phases of the pregnancy. In this context, a European study of the effects of paternity on men's psyche and health is interesting.[5]

Note. The quotations and the historical core of the information presented in the following sections on prenatal care in each month of pregnancy are de-

rived from the second volume of the *Bei Ji Qian Jin Yao Fang*, composed by Sun Simiao in 652 CE and translated by Sabine Wilms[6] (see als Chapter 8). Where suitable, we have modified the information from early medieval China to incorporate our modern clinical experiences. Most notably, Sun Simiao specifically warns against the application of any acupuncture or moxibustion to the channel that is associated with nurturing the fetus in each month. These prohibitions must be seen in the context of his times, when it was quite common for medical literature to contain warnings against the reckless use of acupuncture and moxibustion. Such factors as the modern clinical reality in which acupuncture and moxibustion are practiced in Western countries, the technological advances in the manufacture of much more sophisticated, safer, and less invasive needling and moxibustion equipment, as well as the special considerations in the context of fertility treatment have led us to deviate from Sun Simiao's advice in this point. Especially in the context of artificially induced pregnancies, we are frequently dealing with highly unstable processes that can respond well to supplementing treatment of the channel responsible for nurturing the fetus in each month. The strengthening effects of this strategy on the mother, which in turn then stabilizes the fetus and therefore the pregnancy, have been observed for several decades in the authors' personal practice. Unfortunately, it is, after all, relatively rare for TCM practitioners to be consulted by healthy couples turning to TCM to prepare for an ideal pregnancy. Most of our pregnant clients come with serious imbalances and symptoms that have often forced them to utilize drastic biomedical interventions in order to become pregnant. In such cases, knowing and supporting the channel associated with nurturing the fetus in each month can "make or break" the success of our therapy, especially when we see a problem in a stage of the pregnancy during which one of the parents shows a constitutional weakness. For example, if the father suffers from neurodermatitis and the mother manifests symptoms in the 7th and 8th months, this could be associated with the functions of the lung and large intestine. In such a case, we can treat certain points on the supplying channel by supplementation and thereby support the channel in its function of nurturing and protecting the fetus. Again, though, it is important to emphasize here that we should limit ourselves strictly to supplementing needling.

First and Second Month—The Wood Phase

The first 2 months are associated with the wood phase. **Wood** is the **time of great movements**, of dynamics, of change and the power of new beginnings. It is therefore not surprising that Chinese medical texts recommend much rest in this phase. The dynamic processes inside the woman's body should not be strained or aggravated by additional external movement. The pregnant woman is, however, invited to make room for her creativity and visionary power and to pay attention to her dreams. This corresponds to the wood phase and supports the power of the beginning.

According to TCM theory, the **liver channel** supplies the embryo in the **first month** of pregnancy. This channel should only be treated by stimulation with great attention in the first month.* The liver governs the activity of the muscles, sinews, and blood. In these first months, especially women with pre-existing stagnation of liver *qi* suffer from problems like mood swings, nausea, and vomiting. Tolerance to emotional strain like pressure and stress is low. It is therefore recommended that the pregnant woman not exert herself in her work. She should be able to sleep quietly and peacefully and not be afraid or worry.

Note. This and the following quotations are taken from Wilms[6]. Nevertheless, you must discuss the formulas cited here in each case with a qualified TCM practitioner in accordance with an individualized diagnosis.

"In the first month of pregnancy, yin and yang have newly combined to constitute the fetus. For cases of pain due to increased cold; sudden panic due to increased heat; lumbar pain, abdominal fullness, and tightness in the uterus from heavy lifting; and the sudden appearance of vaginal discharge, the patient

---

* The *Qian Jin Fang* prohibits the application of acupuncture and moxibustion on the specific channel.

should take Wu Ci Ji Tang *(Black Hen Decoction) to stabilize her as a precaution."*[6]

In the **second month** of pregnancy, the **gallbladder channel** supplies the fetus. You must not needle this channel for sedation at this time, in spite of the fact that the stagnation signs that already appeared in the first month seem to suggest the need for relieving the liver and gallbladder. In light of the changeable temperature sensations in this stage of the pregnancy, the lower abdomen should be warmed gently in patients with cold sensations. In addition, Sun Simiao recommends boiled, well-tasting food with a sour flavor, barley, and chicken soup. Spicy and fishy-smelling foods should be avoided. The pregnant woman should also avoid excessively hot or cold foods in these 2 months because the embryo cannot be completed if there is too much internal heat or cold. At this time, the mother should also still guard against excitement, fright, and pressure.

"For cases of decaying [fetus] and failure to complete [the pregnancy] due to increased cold, withered [fetus] due to heat, [fetal] stirring and agitation due to being struck by wind or cold, fullness in the heart, suspension and tension below the navel, rigidity and pain in the lumbus and back, suddenly appearing vaginal discharge, and abruptly alternating [aversion to] cold and heat [effusion], Ai Ye Tang *(Mugwort Decoction) is the governing prescription."*[6]

The prohibition against applying acupuncture or moxibustion on the liver channel in the first and on the gallbladder channel in the second month points to a dynamic effect that could endanger implantation and the woman's ability to hold the fetus. In principle, this classic warns against "disturbing" the channel that is responsible for supplying the child at that time. Overall, opinions differ on beneficial or harmful acupuncture points in pregnancy and on the dangerousness of acupuncture in general. In China, the use of medicinal therapy is preferred.

Because the wood phase, like the other four phases, is associated with certain colors, taste preferences, emotions, and images in the system of correlative thinking, signs that arise at this time can serve as subtle indications that the pregnant woman finds herself in the correct season—or not. Likewise, transitions to another phase can bring to light conspicuous aspects with relevance for treatment.

Third and Fourth Month—The Fire Phase

In Chinese obstetrics, the notion that the mother's inner attitude can have a formative influence on her child is found already in very early texts. Thus, the conduct of the pregnant woman in the third month was regarded as decisive for the gender of the child (see Chapter 4). This is a notion that Sun Simiao fails to elaborate on but that nevertheless plays in important role in earlier texts, such as the *Tai Chan Shu* (*Book of the Generation of the Fetus*) from the Mawangdui tombs. In China, we still find the belief that the mother's emotional state during pregnancy has a lasting effect not only on the child's health and intelligence, but also on the emotional state in his or her future life. Sun Simiao therefore recommends that pregnant women look at objects of great beauty and create internal clarity by meditating.

Both months are characterized by the quality of the **fire** phase, which corresponds to the **heart**, to **love, joy**, and a **clear spirit** (*shen*). A person's fire is harmed either by external pathogenic factors or by emotions like fright, restlessness, or excessive excitement. Behavioral recommendations therefore aim especially at a calm, cheerful emotional state. Cultivating inner harmony and joy allows the pregnant woman, the father, and the child to develop an intimate heart-connection to each other, which has a beneficial effect on their mutual well-being. Especially significant in this context is cultivating the fire of the partnership, of love and sexuality, which should be nurtured particularly consciously in this time.

The **pericardium channel**, the channel of the "messenger of the heart," nourishes the fetus in the **third month** and should therefore not be sedated. Accordingly, the pregnant woman should not be excited by grief or sorrow, nor by worries, anxiety, shock, or fright in this month; her heart and thereby her *shen* should remain calm and composed.

"For cases of cold conditions with blue-green feces, heat conditions with difficult urination of red or yellow

urine, sudden fright and fear, anxiety and worrying, flights of temper and rage, a tendency to stumble and fall, stirring in the vessels, abnormal fullness, bitter pain around the navel or in the lumbus and back, and sudden presence of vaginal discharge, Xiong Ji Tang (Rooster Decoction) [is the governing prescription]."[6]*

In the **fourth month**, the formation of all the child's viscera and bowels is completed. In addition, the mother can see the changes in her body and feels the first movements of the child. Blood and *qi* must be strengthened more and more. As a suitable diet for this month, unpeeled and nonglutinous rice as well as soups with fish and wild goose are recommended. In the fourth month of pregnancy, the **triple burner channel** supplies the fetus. It is responsible for the distribution of *qi* both in the child and in the mother. The pregnant woman should keep her body still, harmonize her emotions and ambition, and regulate her meals. This is what is called making blood and *qi* thrive, as a result of which the ears and eyes are freed. Pregnancy-related vomiting here still signals a tendency to stagnation, and restlessness and fickleness are likewise symptoms of disharmony in the triple burner.

"In the fourth month of pregnancy, for seething below the heart and desire to retch, fullness in the chest and diaphragm and lack of appetite, all of which are related to the presence of cold; for urinary difficulties, urinating very frequently like a dribble, and bitter tension below the navel, which are related to the presence of heat; and for sudden wind-cold, rigidity and pain in the nape and neck, and [aversion to] cold and heat [effusion], [fetal] stirring, perhaps from fright, with intermittent and occasional pain in the lumbus, back, and abdomen, for the fetus ascending and distressing the chest, for heart vexation and inability to get rest, and for the sudden presence of vaginal discharge, take Ju Hua Tang (Chrysanthemum Decoction)."[6]

The symptoms described in this text concern different viscera and bowels, but are all caused by a weakness in the pericardium and triple burner. For the child, a disturbance in this phase means that the development of a harmonious and joyful disposition is impeded and the completion of the viscera and bowels is disturbed.

Fifth and Sixth Month—The Earth Phase

With the **earth** phase in the fifth and sixth month, the pregnant woman has completed the first half of her pregnancy and now experiences a **stage of expansion, fortification, and stability.** Women who suffered from nausea during the first few months often experience this time as pleasant and powerful. Anything that serves to support the center is recommended; in addition to a nutritious diet especially a regular daily routine without extreme strains.

In the **fifth month** of pregnancy, the **spleen channel** supplies the fetus, and Sun Simiao warns against applying acupuncture to the spleen channel in this month. Now at the latest, the woman's middle section will clearly increase in fullness. To strengthen the spleen, the mother should focus increased attention on her eating habits: she should consume unpeeled rice and wheat as well as a harmonious mixture of beef and mutton with *zhu yu* in a thick broth, to balance the five flavors. This is what is called "cultivating *qi* to secure the five viscera." The pregnant woman should be without great hunger and should not eat to excessive satiety either, nor should she consume dry foods. She should not work to the point of fatigue and she should pay attention to dressing warmly and getting enough sleep. Avoid dryness and cold.

"In the fifth month of pregnancy, for dizziness in the head, a deranged heart, and retching and vomiting, which are related to the presence of heat; for abdominal fullness and pain, which are related to the presence of cold; and for frequent urination, sudden fear and panic, pain in the four limbs, [aversion to] cold and heat [effusion], stirring of the fetus in unusual places, abdominal pain, oppression that suddenly puts the patient on the verge of collapse, and sudden presence of vaginal discharge, E Jiao Tang (Ass Hide Glue Decoction) is the governing prescription."[6]

In the **sixth month**, the movements of the child become more and more noticeable and the strength of the muscles and sinews grows. The mother's urge to move increases, and she should certainly give in to it. Because the earth phase is responsible for the transformation and digestion of food, the text pays the greatest attention to diet in the fifth and sixth month. The recommendations are hereby very similar: All five flavors should be taken account of, especially sweet and well-tasting foods, but not in excessively large amounts. A new feature for the time associated with the stomach is the emphasis on a *yang-* and *qi*-boosting diet, which can to a large extent consist of meat. Game is especially recommended for the pregnant woman during this time. Such a diet nourishes the strength of the fetus and secures the back and spine.

For mother and child, this protein-rich diet is usually easy to digest since the **stomach channel** supplies the child in this month. At this time, do not sedate the stomach channel. Because the stomach governs the mouth and eyes, the Chinese classics assume that the mouth and eyes of the fetus are completed in the period of the sixth month. According to Sun Simiao, disorders of the earth phase manifest in very complex symptoms, with pathogenic fullness of the center (flatulence, feeling of fullness, abdominal pain) in the foreground.

"In the sixth month of pregnancy, for sudden stirring [of the fetus], alternating [aversion to] cold and heat [effusion], intestinal fullness in the abdomen, swelling of the body, fright and fear, ... sudden presence of vaginal discharge, abdominal pain as if she were going into labor; and vexation and pain in the extremities, [the patient] should take Mai Men Dong Tang (Ophiopogon Decoction)."[6]

The symptoms introduced here are, however, only a small selection among the many possible physical signs of disharmony. The mother's ability to "digest" and hold a pregnancy becomes especially apparent in this middle period. Thus, the slippery pulse that is typical in pregnancy, for example, should be detectable during this earth phase at the latest. The earth as the symbol of maternity can manifest itself during this time in increased conflicts, dreams, or encounters with one's own **mother**. The theme of the earth phase is **community**, and pregnant women should therefore particularly enjoy spending time in the circle of their family and friends during this time—it saves them from worrying and fretting.

Seventh and Eighth Month—The Metal Phase

The **metal** phase entails **clarity, structure, and processes of letting go and separating**. The general theme is **order** in all affairs, to make **space** for the newborn, and the beginning preparation for the separation of mother and child. During this time, behavioral advice focuses less on diet, but more on promoting external mobility and internal clarity.

In the **seventh month**, the **lung channel** nourishes the child. Accordingly, we must pay attention to the circulation of blood and *qi* by means of increased movement. According to the Chinese classics, the pregnant woman should challenge herself physically and keep her extremities mobile. In her movements, she should bend and stretch, to promote the circulation of *qi* and blood. In terms of her diet, several smaller meals are recommended, ordinary brown rice porridge, and non-glutinous rice, but she should avoid cold in her food and drink. With this conduct, she assists in nurturing the bones and hardening the teeth of the child; in addition, the child's skin, hair, and lungs are completed in the seventh month. The ethereal (*hun*) soul arrives as the individual aspect of the child.

You should not sedate the lung channel as the supplying channel here. Because the metal phase corresponds to the emotion **grief**, the text recommends that the pregnant woman be emotionally balanced. According to Sun Simiao, the woman should not talk too much during this time (this exhausts lung *qi*), she should not moan and complain too much, and she should not wear excessively thin clothing. In spite of the fact that the text allows and recommends movement, increased caution is advised in the care of women who had difficulties establishing a pregnancy. Too much dynamics and activity can make it difficult to hold and nourish the child. Also note that Chinese handbooks interpret movement as going for walks and ordinary activities like climbing stairs, but not as running or sports activities.

In the **eighth month**, the mother should not and cannot move as much anyway. She should prepare herself for the birth and for the child's letting go. The mother's **large intestine channel** nourishes the child, regulating letting go and

opening as the *yang* aspect of the metal phase. During the eighth month, all nine bodily openings of the child are completed. The corporeal soul *po* arrives, and the child thereby completes its facility for independent breathing and sensibility. In the eighth month, the large intestine channel should not be treated sedatingly and the woman should protect herself from cold, dryness, and wind.

"In the eighth month of pregnancy, for wind or cold strike, offenses against prohibitions, pain all over the body, abruptly alternating [aversion to] cold and heat [effusion], stirring fetus, constant problems with dizziness and headaches, coldness below and around the navel, frequent urination of a white substance like rice juice or a green or yellow substance, or accompanied by cold shivering, bitter cold and pain in the lumbus and back, or blurred vision, Shao Yao Tang (White Peony Decoction) is the governing prescription."[6]

These descriptions as well are rooted in the differentiation between external pathogenic climate factors and internal emotional triggers. The pregnant woman as well as the practitioner should therefore pay attention to both of these. Grieving or separation processes are not uncommon themes during this time, and pregnant women who are affected by such problems require especially intensive support. The metal phase corresponds to the **quality of the father**. The father of the pregnant woman, as well as the father of the child, can require increased attention. Internal and external house-cleaning and organizing can free a lot of energy for the pregnant couple during this time.

The seventh and eighth months offer a good opportunity in the care of pregnant women to **look back and evaluate** the previously experienced phases. Hereby, we can once again notice anomalies that have previously escaped the practitioner's attention. For example, if we notice that the pregnant woman is always delayed in attaining the new quality, we can carefully predict that the time of delivery is also more likely to be late than early. Every woman has her own sensitivities and individual dynamics, which reveal themselves during the pregnancy and make prognoses for the birth experience and the lying-in period possible.

Ninth and 10th Month—The Water Phase

As the phase of winter, the **water** phase is associated with **deep collection and inner stillness**, in which spring (the birth) can prepare itself. The pregnant woman should experience the quality of inner centeredness in this time because it puts her in touch with her strength and gives her a relaxed calmness for the impending delivery.

In the **ninth month**, the child is fully formed, and especially women with a difficult pregnancy are reassured by the thought that they have managed to reach this stage. A premature baby could now also survive on its own. The **kidney channel** supplies the child and should therefore not be treated with acupuncture. By contrast, anything that nourishes the kidney is beneficial: a lot of sleep, rest, good nutritious food (meat broths) and warm clothing. Pay attention particularly to warm feet, knees, and a warm back, because we can otherwise see increased pain in the area of the lumbar spinal column. The woman should not dwell in damp and cold places or overexert herself, but regular movement is considered strengthening. These recommendations, which apply to uncomplicated pregnancies, are especially fitting for women who experienced problems with their fertility and therefore bring a constitutional kidney weakness to the situation.

"In the ninth month of pregnancy, for suddenly contracted diarrhea, abdominal fullness with a sensation of suspension and tension, fetus surging up against the heart, lumbar and back pain with inability to turn or bend, and shortness of breath, Ban Xia Tang (Pinellia Decoction) [is the governing prescription].[6]

In addition to the already known signs of a disturbance, this quotation vividly describes the immediate effect of the maternal emotion—in the water phase this is **fear**—on the child. Cultivate peacefulness, confidence, and composure.

In the **10th month**, the fetus receives the *qi* of heaven and earth in the *dan tian*, as a result of which the joints close and the *shen* is fully present. The child is supplied by the **bladder channel**. Now the only thing left to do is to await the right moment for the birth, because in the Chinese perspective the child's *dao* determines the hour of birth.

You should therefore refrain from urging the woman on.

"The mother should take 'fetus-lubricating medicines,' but only after she has entered the month [of childbirth]. Dan Shen Gao (Salvia Paste) is a prescription for nourishing the fetus, to be taken in the month of delivery, lubricating the fetus and easing childbirth."[6]

The best preparation for birth is for the mother to consciously live through the water phase. In these last weeks, when the child develops only slightly but must grow all the more, it is gathering *jing*, which is extremely important for a strong state of health. From this perspective, carrying the fetus for up to 14 days past the due date can make sense and can be affirmed by the pregnant woman without any internal stress, because every day nurtures the water of the child, its kidney essence, and its primal sense of trust. When the child, the mother, and the father go into delivery strengthened in this way, the chance of delivering without obstetrical intervention is good.

Even though the successful completion of a pregnancy signifies the completion of the practitioner's task of treating a couple who wants a child, we should mention here that the **lying-in period** deserves special attention. Already valid for women in childbed without complications during conception and pregnancy, this is all the more true for women with a less robust constitution. Observing the advice of TCM regarding behavior and diet during this unique time of regeneration can lay the foundations for an unproblematic menopause later on.[1]

■ Support in Failed Fertility Treatment

The previous chapter was intended to show how Sun Simiao's "pregnancy calendar" might offer approaches for stabilizing and supporting an at-risk pregnancy. Nevertheless, the unpredictability of childbearing sometimes means that even the most outstanding knowledge of TCM and the newest methods of reproductive medicine fail to deliver the desired result. This happens, for example, when several IVF or ICSI attempts remained unsuccessful or when several miscarriages or extra-uterine pregnancies occurred. If a pregnant woman loses her child and is unable to complete the cycle of the above-mentioned "seasons," this sad situation also requires us to pay attention to the cycle of the five phases—both in the task of grieving and with regard to the question when she should attempt to conceive again.

When Can the Woman Become Pregnant Again?

Miscarriages most commonly take place during the first 3 months; up to this point, pregnancy is seen as unstable in both Western and Chinese medical theory. Forcefully promoted not only by couples but frequently also by many centers of reproductive medicine, the waiting period after a miscarriage before a new attempt is often too short. As a rule, reproductive medicine considers a period of 3 months as sufficient for recuperation and regeneration of the woman.

Nevertheless, when we consider pregnancy from the angle of TCM, we realize two things: first, the first two phases are associated with *yang* and the second two phases with *yin*. That is, the processes taking place inside the woman become increasingly profound and internal. Second, there is the division of pregnancy into **trimesters**, associated with the three treasures *shen, qi,* and *jing*:[8]

- In the first trimester, the pregnancy is governed by *shen*. The child is influenced in its creation and development more by the heavenly (*yang*) than by the earthly (*yin*) powers. The main force of growth in the child operates in the upper burner, hence the head is oversized in proportion to the rest of the body.
- The second and middle trimester of the pregnancy is associated with *qi*. The organs develop.
- The last and third trimester stands for the *jing* and thereby for the deepest and innermost layer in the human body. The child is completed and solid and gathers its constitutional strength out of the mother's *jing*.

This illustrates how significant the time of a miscarriage or premature birth is for the question of another pregnancy. With an increasing length of pregnancy, the damage and exhaustion of the mother's resources become more and more pronounced and the regeneration period becomes longer and longer.

In light of the **succession of the phases of correlative thinking**, we must moreover observe the following: a started cycle must be finished in all cases, even if the child was lost already in the first few weeks of pregnancy. We could understand this in such a way that the child's *dao* continues to affect the mother's body up to the intended time of its birth.

An example of this: a woman who became pregnant in the beginning of May loses her child in the middle of June (in her eighth week). According to doctor's orders, she waits 3 months and again becomes pregnant in the beginning of October. The due date of her first child was January 22. At this time, the woman will be in the transition period from fire to earth in her second pregnancy, that is, in her 17th or 18th week. Because the cycle of the first child is still affecting her, we should be prepared for a—albeit weakened—"birth impulse." This new knowledge allows us to understand complaints or even bleeding around this critical time in a new light and relieve them gently, in order to allow the second pregnancy to successfully run its course.

If another attempted conception does not succeed or the developing fetus is lost, we must then clarify additional realistic treatment expectations that the couple can still have of TCM in this situation. As part of this process of clarification, we reflect on the effects of the fertility treatment on the couple's relationship and sexuality whilst taking into account the particular familial and professional circumstances.

Fertility Treatment and Couple Dynamics

"Everybody knows that we want to have a child but cannot do it"—the feeling of failure on this elemental level of existence leaves deep traces in the self-confidence of both partners. The failure to meet the expectations of one's own parents, whether putative or real, to maintain the succession of generations, the expressed or implied accusation of social selfishness—all this often causes unbearable pressure and the prospect of a complete loss of perspective after the personal catastrophe of childlessness.

But the drama of this unfulfilled wish for children also has fundamental effects on the partnership or marriage. Previously hidden conflicts can come to the surface with the beginning of intensive fertility treatment and not uncommonly also lead to a fundamental break. The goal of a shared child promotes neurotic behavioral patterns that manifest, for example, in a fixation on measurements and laboratory values. Finger-pointing and mutual expedience reduce the value of the relationship to sperm and egg cells, to fulfilling the wish for motherhood or fatherhood as the sole shared goal in life. Especially after a miscarriage, not enough space or time is given to the shared grieving process. Instead, what separates the couple is projected onto the partnership itself, and the still unfulfilled wish for a child is interpreted as a relationship failure.

Love, affection, a fulfilled sexuality—when all these "soft" factors of shared life are short-changed, they can dry up sooner or later. From the perspective of TCM, however, it is precisely the mental-emotional harmony between the future parents that is one of the most important foundations for conception. To recognize and resolve such fixations, it makes sense to take an occasional treatment break or forego measuring the morning temperature. In addition, the practitioner should assist the couple in their search for other commonalities and perspectives. When we consider the medical theories and practices of TCM in such cases of forced fixation, Daoist elements in particular facilitate opening up to new ways of looking at and accepting reality. But acupuncture, dietary changes, massage, or Chinese medicinals can also determine the course for new paths and goals on the psychological level.

Alternatives—Adoption and Accepted Childlessness

Working out new perspectives together may not produce an immediate solution but can take some of the unbearable pressure off both partners. Adopting a child can be a possible alternative. But accepting childlessness can also be a chance to realize new and different perspectives on life. This does, however, require, that the role behavior and individual self-image of both partners, often colored by years of fertility treatment, receives a new direction and fulfillment.

Wherever possible, fertility treatment should be concluded with a result that is acceptable to all participants. Of primary importance is the balance in health of both treated partners. But no less important is that the partners make peace with the given situation and find an optimistic vision for the future—with or without child.

Bibliography

1. Böger H, Kotte G. Das Wochenbett in der Chinesischen Medizin. Part II. *Hebammenforum.* 2006;5:370 – 372.
2. Han J. *Mawangdui Gumaishu yanjiu (Study of the Channel Texts from Mawangdui).* Beijing: Renmin Weisheng Chubanshe; 1999.
3. Huber-Borrasch K, Kotte G, Schulze R. Die Jahreszeiten im Palast des Kindes. Die fünf Elemente der Chinesischen Medizin in der Zeit der Schwangerschaft. *Hebammenforum.* 2007.
4. Lindwedel U, Reime B. Väter: Zivilisierte Männer. *Hebammenforum.* 2007;2:104 – 109.
5. Wilms S. *Bei Ji Qian Jin Yao Fang.* Vols 2 – 4 on Gynecology. Chinese Medicine Database: 2007.
6. Lorenzen U, Noll A. *Die Wandlungsphasen der Traditionellen Chinesischen Medizin. Die Wandlungsphase Wasser.* Vol. 5. Munich: Müller & Steinicke; 2000.
7. Schulze R. Chinesische Medizin in der Geburtshilfe. Unpublished lecture notes. Berlin: 2007.
8. Zart B. *Gelassen Durch die Kinderwunschzeit.* Munich: Hugendubel; 2006.

Appendix 7

List of Photos and Illustrations

Cover: Michael Zimmermann; Photo Disc, Inc.; Dr. Beatrix Maxrath.

Fig. 6.1: Faller A, Schuenke M: *The Human Body. An Introduction to Structure and Function.* Thieme: Stuttgart–New York; 2004.

Fig. 6.2: Modified after Faller A, Schuenke M: *The Human Body. An Introduction to Structure and Function.* Thieme: Stuttgart–New York; 2004.

Fig. 6.8–6.13: Dr. Beatrice Maxrath, 2006.

Fig. 9.1–9.4, 10.1–10.4, 11.2, 11.3, and 11.5: Werner Hasselbach Design, Katharina Werner, Hamburg, Germany.

Fig. 11.1: PhotoDisc, Inc.

Fig. 11.4: Andreas A. Noll.

Fig. 19.1: © European Community, Audiovisual Library of the European Commission.

Fig. 19.2: Asklepios-Clinik Barmbek, Urology Department, Barmbek, Germany.

Further Photos: Contributing Authors.

General Index

Page numbers in *italics* refer to illustrations or tables

Prescriptions Index